A History of Modern Yoga

A History of Modern Yoga

Patañjali and Western Esotericism

Elizabeth De Michelis

continuum
LONDON • NEW YORK

Front cover photograph: by Andrea Rollefson, *Ascent* magazine, Fall 2001. The photo, shot in New York, USA, depicts a typical Modern Postural Yoga Class.

Back cover illustration: Add. Ms. 24099. Reproduced by permission of The British Library. *Khecarī-mudrā*, lit. "Space-walking seal": An advanced yogic practice in which the tongue is thrust upwards. This *mudrā* pierces the knot of Rudra (*rudra granthi*) in the central channel (*suṣumnā nāḍī*) causing the mediatator to experience union (*samādhi*) and taste the nectar of immortality. This leads to a state in which one roams in the inner spiritual sky (Grimes 1996: 166).

Continuum
The Tower Building, 11 York Road, London SE1 7NX
15 East 26th Street, New York, NY 10010

First published 2004 by Continuum

British Library Cataloguing-in-Publication Data
A catalogue record for this book is available from the British Library.

ISBN 0-8264-6512-9 (hardback)

Library of Congress Cataloging-in-Publication Data
De Michelis, Elizabeth.
A history of modern yoga : Patañjali and Western esotericism /
Elizabeth De Michelis. p. cm.
Includes bibliographical references (p.) and index.
ISBN 0-8264-6512-9
1. Yoga–History. 2. Patañjali. I. Title
B132.Y6D37 2004
181'.45–dc21 2003046285

Typeset by YHT Ltd, London
Printed and bound in Great Britain by The Cromwell Press, Trowbridge, Wiltshire

Contents

4. "God-realization" and "Self-realization" in Neo-Vedānta

PART II: MODERN YOGA THEORY AND PRACTICE

5. Vivekananda's *Rāja Yoga* (1896): Modern Yoga formulated

List of Figures and Tables

Figures

Tables

Acknowledgements

Over the years I have received much encouragement and support, both academic and otherwise, from many different quarters.

I wish first of all to thank all my family for their ongoing, manifold contributions to this project, and for unfailingly being there when I needed them. My mother, brother, sister and paternal aunts have been especially close as I was going through the period of research that led to the writing of this book: their support – material, practical, emotional, intellectual and beyond – has been truly invaluable. I am sorry that my father died years before this project was completed. As he was interested in Modern Yoga in his youth, I am sure he would have enjoyed reading this book.

I am grateful to the Modern Yoga schools and practitioners that helped me and made me feel welcome during my periods of research and fieldwork in Europe and in India. This applies particularly, though in no way exclusively, to the Iyengar School of Yoga and to the British Wheel of Yoga. I would like to extend personal thanks to Mr B. K. S. Iyengar for his life's work in the field of yoga, and to all of the staff at the Ramamani Iyengar Memorial Yoga Institute (RIMYI) in Pune for their patience and support during my period of work there. Closer to home, I would like to acknowledge Sasha Perryman for reliably guiding me through the practical intricacies and simplicities of Iyengar Yoga in Cambridge. I also wish to acknowledge the British Wheel of Yoga for providing stimulating teaching and training during earlier phases of my research. This institution's hard work and its commitment to the cultivation of yoga are widely recognized in British Modern Yoga circles and abroad. My friend and teacher Mrs Velta Wilson, herself a founding member of the British Wheel of

Yoga, deserves special mention in this context: I wish to thank her warmly for her counsel and support throughout the years.

While I thoroughly enjoyed all my studies up to BA level, I only came to academic research work relatively late in life. I was most fortunate to carry out the initial part of my post-graduate studies at the School of Oriental and African Studies, University of London, under the guidance of very gifted and generous teachers: Dr Julia Leslie, who took special care in guiding and supporting my early efforts, Dr John Marr and Professor Alexander Piatigorsky. I still remember their lectures and seminars with relish.

The University of Cambridge and especially the Faculty of Divinity and the Faculty of Oriental Studies have provided an ideal setting for my further research work. I am greatly indebted to Dr John Smith and Dr Eivind Kahrs, whose Sanskrit courses I attended in the mid-1990s. Most of all, however, I am indebted to my doctoral supervisor, Mrs Sita Narasimhan. Working with her has been both a privilege and a pleasure: her comprehensive knowledge of several relevant fields, her pedagogic skills and her unstinting support were essential points of reference as my research progressed, and remain so even now. I have especially benefited from her astounding knowledge of English, Sanskrit and more generally Indian languages and traditions of learning, and from her in-depth understanding of East–West cultural discourses and milieus. I am further very grateful to Dr Julius Lipner, who supported my early research ideas, and who has been a valued source of counsel and guidance throughout the years. I also thank him for launching the Dharam Hinduja Institute of Indic Research (DHIIR) in 1995. This Institute, established through the generosity of the Hinduja Foundation, concerns itself with carrying out research on Indic subjects in ways that may benefit both the scholarly community and society at large. As I have always been sympathetic towards the DHIIR's aims, I was delighted to be selected to take over the DHIIR's Directorship in January 2000. As DHIIR Director I would like to thank most warmly the Institute's Advisory Council, Research Groups, research projects collaborators and, last but far from least, my very capable and supportive staff for their ongoing support and manifold contributions. I would especially like to thank Mr S. P. Hinduja for making time in his very busy schedule to discuss my proposals and ideas from time to time, and Professors Ursula King and John Brockington for supporting and encouraging my work in various ways.

The DHIIR was the first research institute to be established under the auspices of the Faculty of Divinity's Centre for Advanced Religious and Theological Studies (CARTS). I wish to thank all my colleagues and collaborators at CARTS and at the Faculty for their contribution in making my years of employment here so productive, enjoyable and stimulating. Most of all I wish to thank Dr David Thompson, Director of CARTS, for his thoughtful guidance and for providing ideal conditions for the DHIIR's work to flourish.

List of abbreviations

Primary sources

CW *The Complete Works* of Swami Vivekananda; nine volumes (Arabic number after *CW* indicates volume number)
N.B. Vivekananda's *Rāja Yoga* is found in Vol. 1, pages 119–314.

YS *Yoga Sūtras* of Patañjali
Sanskrit text: Patañjali (1904)
English text: Yardi (1979)

Books by or about B. K. S. Iyengar

AY Iyengar, B. K. S. (1993 [1985]), *The Art of Yoga*. Indus, New Delhi.

GY Yogacharya B. K. S. Iyengar's 70th Birthday Celebrations (1990), *70 Glorious Years of Yogacharya B. K. S. Iyengar: Commemoration Volume*. Light on Yoga Research Trust, Bombay.

ILW B. K. S. Iyengar 60th Birthday Celebration Committee (1987), *Iyengar: His Life and Work*. Timeless Books, Porthill, Idaho.

LOP Iyengar, B. K. S. (1983 [1981]), *Light on Prāṇāyāma: Prāṇāyāma Dīpikā*. Unwin Paperbacks, London.

LOY Iyengar, B. K. S. (1984 [1966]), *Light on Yoga: Yoga Dipika*. Unwin Paperbacks, London.

LOYSP Iyengar, B. K. S. (1993), *Light on the Yoga Sūtras of*

Patañjali: Pātañjala Yoga Pradīpikā. The Aquarian Press, London.

YV Iyengar, B. K. S. (1988), *Yoga Vṛkṣa: The Tree of Yoga*. Fine Line Books, Oxford.

Modern Yoga types (cf. Table 3, page 188) and institution

MDY	Modern Denominational Yoga
MMY	Modern Meditational Yoga
MPsY	Modern Psychosomatic Yoga
MPY	Modern Postural Yoga
BWY	British Wheel of Yoga

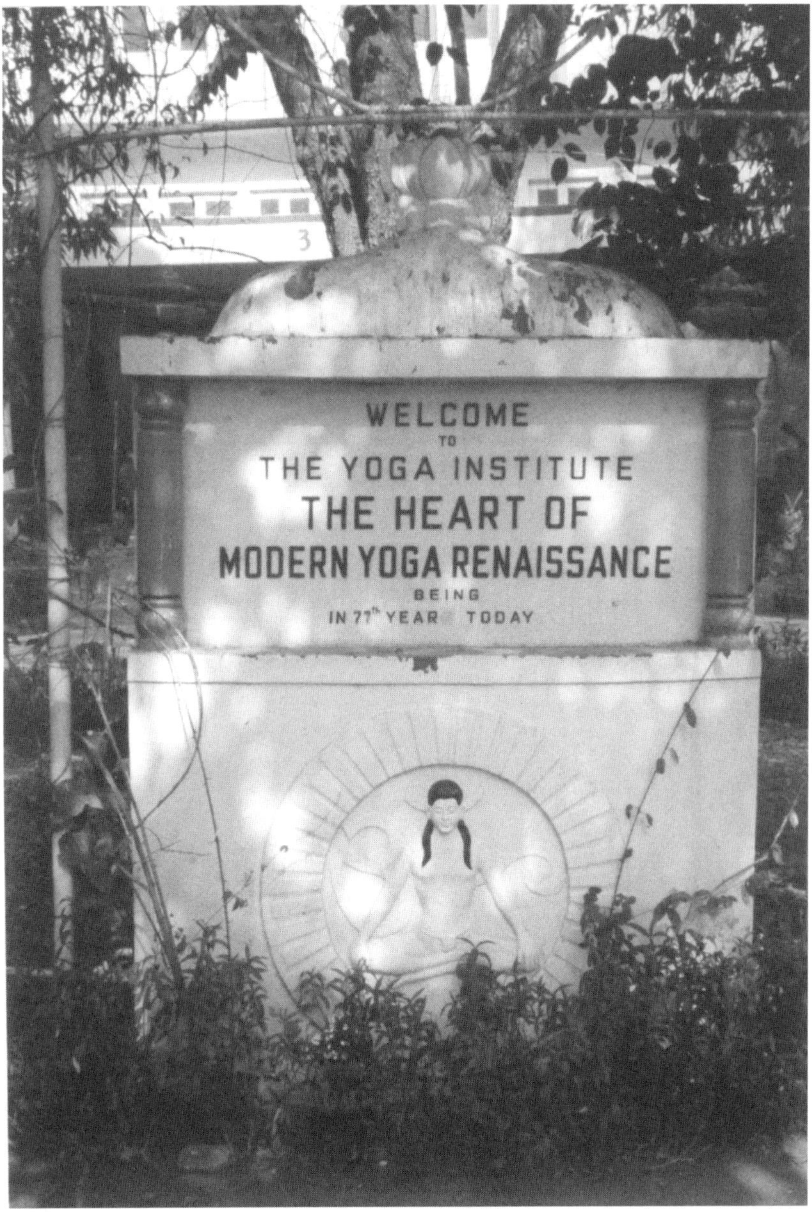

Figure 1 Plaque at the entrance of the Yoga Institute; Santa Cruz, Bombay, India. (See note 1, Chapter 6; author's photograph)

Introduction

> With no effort from us many forms of the Hindu religion are spreading far and wide, and these manifestations have taken the form of Christian science, theosophy, and Edwin Arnold's *Light of Asia*.
>
> (Swami Vivekananda *CW* 7: 287)

What is Modern Yoga?

What is this yoga? This was the question that started haunting me in the late 1980s, a decade after attending my first 'yoga classes'. I had asked myself the question before, but it had not haunted me. As anyone who has carried out a serious piece of research will know, I eventually became obsessed with it. Only, as I was progressing, my questions became more precise. And more numerous. What is classical yoga (i.e. the older forms of yoga from the Indian subcontinent, consisting of a pluri-millenarian tradition)? What is Classical Yoga[1] (i.e. yoga as outlined in Patañjali's seminal Sanskrit text, the *Yoga Sūtras* (*c.* second century CE) and in the related commentatorial tradition)? How does Modern Yoga differ from these older forms? And how did it develop its peculiar characteristics? These last two questions, eventually, became the key ones underpinning my research. My experiences of yoga as practised in Europe in fact told me (at times rationally, at times intuitively) that what I was presented with was quite different from classical forms of yoga.

Soon there were further questions that needed to be addressed in order to answer the central ones. How does 'yoga' differ from 'meditation'? And why are there so many kinds of 'yoga' even among

1. Regarding 'classical' and 'Classical' terminology see also note 10 here and Chapter 1.

the modern forms? How do they differ from each other and what do they have in common? Who contributed to create Modern Yoga as we have it today? Would it be possible to produce a typology of Modern Yoga forms showing how they relate to each other? Why are individuals across the world attracted by these modern forms of yoga? And why has such a foreign discipline taken root in so-called Western societies? *Is* it a foreign discipline? And so on and so forth. As answers emerged, of course, even more interesting questions arose. They are still coming.

Preliminary answers to these questions will be found within the covers of this book. Indeed, the present volume as a whole may be seen as a definition of Modern Yoga, especially since this corpus of disciplines and beliefs has never before been presented or discussed as a discrete historical phenomenon or as a self-standing conceptual category. For the benefit of those who need a point of reference at the very beginning, however, I will propose forthwith a brief and basic definition of Modern Yoga.

The expression 'Modern Yoga' is used as a technical term to refer to certain types of yoga that evolved mainly through the interaction of Western individuals interested in Indian religions and a number of more or less Westernized Indians over the last 150 years. It may therefore be defined as the graft of a Western branch onto the Indian tree of yoga. Most of the yoga currently practised and taught in the West, as well as some contemporary Indian yoga, falls into this category. Being only one and a half centuries old, it may well be the youngest branch of the tree of yoga, and it seems to be the only one to have stretched across the oceans to continents other than Asia. The definition 'Modern' seems precise enough to describe its age (it emerged in modern times) and geographico/cultural spread (it is pre-eminently found in developed countries and urban milieus worldwide). It also seems open-ended enough to allow for further definition and elaboration (based on De Michelis 2002: 3).

A clarification about chronology. There are two crucial dates regarding the beginnings of Modern Yoga: 1849 and 1896. The former, relating to the 150 years mentioned in the previous paragraph, refers to what seems to be the first recorded affirmation, by a Westerner, that he considered himself a yoga practitioner – after a fashion. This was the Transcendentalist Henry David Thoreau, who, in a letter to a friend, wrote: "... I would fain practice the yoga faithfully. To some extent, and at rare intervals, even I am a yogi."[2] Up to that point the West had known about (and had been interested in) yoga and *yogins*, but these were seen as altogether 'other'. Yoga, that is, was in no way perceived as an option to be taken up by Westerners; it was a phenomenon observed, studied and reported about in third person, as it were. There had, of course, been a few cases of Westerners 'going native' and becoming absorbed in Oriental (including monastic) cultures[3] – but that was another matter. In Thoreau's case yoga was taken up by a Westerner while remaining a Westerner. There is no need to examine the nature of Thoreau's yogic commitments here: what is significant is the cultural trend epitomized by his words: Westerners were starting to perceive 'yoga' as something they could engage in, not just as something 'out there'.

This religio-cultural trend became a very important and influential motif of East–West exchanges from about the last quarter of the nineteenth century onwards – possibly *the* most important religio-cultural trend, from the Indian point of view, if yoga is understood in its broadest definition. This trend took tangible form in 1896, our second important date, when the Indian reaction to Western missionary efforts took shape in the counter-missionary project of the young and influential Swami Vivekananda. The date marks the publication of his volume on *Rāja Yoga*. The great impression that the Swami made at the 1893 Chicago Parliament of Religions and the subsequent establishment of the Ramakrishna movement[4] are usually referred to as his main achievements. One of the theses of this book, however, is that his maybe less sensational but actually more long-lasting and productive achievement was the shaping of Modern Yoga, of which *Rāja Yoga* is the seminal text. In it, Vivekananda carried out a major revisitation of yoga history, structures, beliefs and practices and then proceeded to operate a translation (often semantic as well as linguistic) of this 'reformed' yoga into something quite different from classical Hindu approaches. Vivekananda's 'reshaping' of the yoga tradition – which of course he did not operate in a vacuum, but with

2. Quoted in Christy (1932: 185, 201), who refers (*ibid.*: 327, 358) to *The Writings of Henry David Thoreau*, ed. Bradford Torrey (Walden edn) Boston and New York: (Houghton Mifflin, 1906), section on *Writings*, VI: 175.
3. See, for example, the story of Csoma de Koros (Fields 1992: 283–5).
4. Following Jackson (1994: xii–xiii, 28–32), the expression 'Ramakrishna movement' will be used as a collective name to indicate all the various institutions initiated by Vivekananda in India and in the West, and continued by the monks of the Ramakrishna order.

the help, contribution, support and participation of many individuals, East and West, before and after him – is discussed at length in the present book.

After 1896 Modern Yoga flourished both in India and abroad. At the beginning of the twenty-first century it has become a global phenomenon, though its presence is in the main limited to developed urban communities.[5] The socio-historical reasons that lie behind this geographical spread are also discussed in the book, which further analyses how, from Vivekananda's time onward, Modern Yoga developed in many different ways and directions. Because of such variety, and considering the amount of in-depth analysis of theories and practices that I wished to carry out, it would have been impossible to discuss the whole of Modern Yoga in depth.

The obvious way forward was to select the type of yoga that I was most familiar with, viz. Modern Postural Yoga (or MPY, i.e. those styles of yoga practice that put a lot of emphasis on *āsanas* or yoga postures; in other words the more 'physical' or gymnastic-like type of yoga).[6] In this context Iyengar Yoga, arguably the most influential school of Postural Yoga to date, emerged as the obvious case study to concentrate on: I had a good overall knowledge of its teachings, practices and institutional structures, but I also had enough knowledge of other MPY schools to be able to draw parallels and/or comparisons.

All that was left to do after thus demarcating the field was to study Sanskrit, some yoga texts and the relevant (mainly Hindu) traditions of yoga as much as I could in the relatively limited time that I could dedicate to research. It would in fact not have been tenable, in my view, to discuss a 'new' that kept harking back to 'the old' without having at least some knowledge of the latter. How could I evaluate some Modern Yoga schools' claims that they are passing on 'the original message of the *Yoga Sūtras*' or, more generally, of yoga, if I did not know what the *Yoga Sūtras* and the yoga tradition were about?

I have been very lucky (some would say stubborn enough) to find the time and the resources to carry out this work. There are Modern Yoga practitioners throughout the world who would love to do the same but, for whatever reason, are unable to do so: I have met a number of them during periods of fieldwork and in academic circles. I

5. 'Ashrams' (see note 34, Chapter 2) and yoga centres located in isolated places are usually offshoots of the urban institutions, and tend to retain the same type of culture.
6. A typology of Modern Yoga forms, including MPY, is presented in Chapter 6 and summarized in Table 3.

do hope that my work, despite its limitations, will be of interest and of benefit to them, as well as to academics and students of Indic studies and of modern and contemporary religiosity, many of whom must have asked themselves the same questions I have tried to answer at one time or another. It goes without saying that comments, criticism, corrections and any useful piece of information that readers may be able to contribute will be gratefully received.

Before we plunge into more technical matters I would like to comment on what may be perceived as some iconoclastic aspects of the present book. The ways in which I discuss some much-loved Indian holy men or 'spiritual leaders', such as Debendranath Tagore, Keshubchandra Sen or Swami Vivekananda, may be perceived, at times, as somewhat less than respectful. This is not so, as I am convinced that all the people I discuss were sincerely committed to finding the 'right' answers to their questions, and that they were attempting to shape their lives in the light of the highest ethical principles. However, I also do perceive them as men, and therefore as fallible and in some ways limited. They were also being swept and tossed, as we all are, by the waves of history – especially so, I would argue, Swami Vivekananda. One of my strategies has actually been to attempt, as much as possible, to identify with their human predicament in order to understand their thought, motivations and actions from *their* point of view. I was also actively seeking to piece together, I will admit that much, the more 'hidden' or untold parts of their histories – though this was done not out of love of controversy, but because early in my research I found out that in order to answer my questions it was essential for me to do so.

I have also stated what I perceive to be some truths about Modern Yoga and Modern Yoga schools that may not be to everyone's liking. But there was no malice in my stating them. Quite the contrary: if I may say so without sounding patronizing, I strongly believe that if more people were to study the history, roots and beliefs of Modern Yoga more carefully (that is, among other things, by trying to exercise more intellectual discrimination), this could be of great benefit not only to practitioners of Modern Yoga, but also to academics and intellectuals in general. Modern Yoga schools would do well to encourage their students to do so, and the Modern Yoga institutions that are well off could set an example by offering grants to study the relevant disciplines at graduate and post-graduate level. Serious intellectual endeavours are often denigrated in the world of Modern

Yoga (which puts, as we shall see, great emphasis on an experiential epistemology), and if this trend is not redressed the discipline as a whole will remain lopsided.

Modern Yoga scholarship

It is true that something of a (mini) sub-field of Modern Yoga studies[7] is at last beginning to emerge, so arguably the more in-depth discussions advocated above may already have started to happen. This is a welcome development, and comes as a refreshing change from many studies on yoga published earlier, which stopped short when they came to consider (historically, conceptually or in any other way) the phenomenon of Modern Yoga.

In this emerging field of study we find publications by Joseph Alter (2000, Part II; and forthcoming), who has been working on the Indian aspects of Modern Yoga from the historical and anthropological point of view. Silvia Ceccomori's book (2001) discusses Modern Yoga in France: a look at the table of contents (accessed by Internet) shows that her coverage of the subject is quite comprehensive and, it would appear, pre-eminently historical. She does, however, place her characters within an ideological framework, and I rejoice to see that she seems to have taken due notice of esoteric and occultistic trends. Unfortunately it has not been possible to consult Ceccomori's work before submitting the present typescript and therefore I have not been able, sadly, to integrate her findings in my work. Two of my earlier articles (De Michelis 1995; 2002) reflect attempts at demarcating and describing the field of Modern Yoga, with special attention to Modern Postural Yoga schools. In them, as in the present study, I approach my subject from the point of view of the history of (religious) ideas, and my methodology consists in trying to synthetize data gathered from primary texts, historical records and fieldwork findings. Yet another contribution is Fuchs' treatment of Modern Yoga in Germany (1990), though, as in the case of Ceccomori's publication, I only found out about this work too late to be able to consult it. Hasselle-Newcombe's brief study (2002) concentrates on the contemporary picture, which is examined on the basis of sociological paradigms. Strauss' work (1997; 2000; 2002a;

7. About the use of this label for other people's work, see below.

2002b; 2003), finally, focuses on Swami Sivananda of Rishikesh, his Divine Life Society and on the career of some influential Sivananda disciples. Her historical reconstructions are discussed from an anthropological point of view.

While it is very heartening to see the beginnings of more informed, in-depth discussions of Modern Yoga, it would be good to see more humanities scholars participating in these endeavours. If this sub-field is to be built on firm foundations, the differences between modern and classical manifestations of yoga must be plotted out in detail: this requires knowledge – mainly textual and historical – of both ancient and modern/contemporary aspects of yogic disciplines and of their respective social contexts, plus the will (and patience) to compare and contrast them in systematic fashion. Without reliable landmarks of this sort it may be difficult to progress beyond relatively basic levels of exploration.

Some notes on terminology

And now a few comments about the terminology employed in the present book. I referred above to "Modern Yoga studies". It goes without saying that the 'Modern Yoga' label may not be considered useful and/or accurate by everyone. For convenience's sake, and because it has stood the test of time so far, I use it also to refer to other people's work, though they may well not employ it themselves. I would of course be open to review my thinking and terminology if more suitable labels, interpretative methodologies, or analytical tools were to be proposed.

With reference to emic[8] discussions on how to name modern and

8. Explaining the very useful methodological categories, originally appropriated by anthropologists from linguistics, and expressed by the terms 'emic' and 'etic', Hanegraaff (1996: 6–7) writes:

> Emic denotes the 'intersubjective patterns of thought and symbolic associations of the believers' or, expressed more simply, the "believer's point of view". An accurate presentation of the religion under study as expressed by the believers themselves must be the basis of research. On the part of the researcher, the reconstruction of this emic perspective requires an attitude of empathy which excludes personal biases as far as possible. Scholarly discourse about religion, on the other hand, is not emic but etic. This means that it may involve types of language, distinctions, theories and interpretive models which are considered appropriate by scholars on their own terms. Scholars may introduce their own terminology and make theoretical distinctions which are different from those of the believers themselves. The final results of scholarly research should be expressed in etic language, and formulated in such a way as to permit criticism and falsification both by reference to the emic material and as regards their coherence and consistency in the context of the general etic discourse.

contemporary forms of yoga, I can report that these have been ongoing. In itself, this is sign of a widespread intuition that 'this' (modern) yoga is not quite the same as 'that' (classical) yoga. Very often the label given to what is commonly called 'yoga' in developed societies, if further qualified, is *haṭhayoga*. This is not altogether imprecise, as it is true that Modern Postural Yoga draws heavily from *haṭhayoga* doctrines and practices. MPY is, however, also very different. As readers will find out (Chapter 7), I do take the haṭhayogic contents of Modern Yoga into due consideration (though only as one of the elements of the standard MPY make-up). But because 'this' *haṭhayoga* is different from 'that', I call it (and define it as) Neo-*Haṭhayoga*.

Another question relating to emic issues of terminology is that of 'meditation': in common English usage (i.e. in Modern Yoga),[9] 'yoga' is 'postural yoga', and 'meditation' is 'sitting meditation' – the icon of the latter being the cross-legged *padmāsana* ("lotus pose") of the *yogin* and of the Buddha. In classical Hinduism (and in Indian languages) we find much less of a gap between 'yoga' and 'meditation' – indeed the first linguistic association that speakers of Indian languages make upon hearing the word 'yoga' is with *dhyāna*, "meditation". The gap found in English is an interesting phenomenon and one that would be worth exploring in detail from a linguistic point of view. As far as my analysis was concerned, however, such a linguistic gap signalled the need to keep the 'postural' and the 'meditational' separate (at least in some cases) in order to reproduce accurately what I encountered in the field. Thus the reader will also find 'Modern Meditational Yoga' in my typology of Modern Yoga (see note 6 here); and while many Modern Yoga practitioners practise both Postural and Meditational Yoga, at some level the two may well be (and are) perceived as distinct practices.

Two important sets of terms are employed quite extensively in the present study: *esotericism* and *occultism* on the one hand and *cult* and *sect* (and the related concept of '*cultic milieu*') on the other. All are defined and discussed, with reference to the relevant secondary sources, in Chapter 1. What I would like to stress here is that they are used as purely technical terms. While they can often (especially in some quarters) be perceived as denigratory terms, this is not at all the

9. English, by the way, can be stated to be the language of Modern Yoga. This is a clear indication of its cultural roots.

way they will be used here. I simply found them to be essential analytical tools for the purposes of my work.

And, to conclude this section, a word about 'Orient', 'Orientalism' and related terms. The present book has nothing to say about the 'Orientalism' debate initiated by Edward Said (1978). When reference is made to 'Orientalism' or 'British Orientalism', the reader should bear in mind that the labels adopted are based on David Kopf's volume on British Orientalism (1969) and on the Brahmo Samaj (1979), used quite extensively to define the historical background of the events narrated in Part I.

Mention of the historical circumstances which acted as a backdrop to the emergence and development of Modern Yoga brings the discussion to more strictly scholarly concerns. As I was carrying out a preliminary review of the Modern Yoga field I found out, with some surprise, that an important cultural strand – the influence of Western esotericism – had been all but neglected in the discussions of most historians. Had this strand been of relevance only to the emergence and development of Modern Yoga, that would have been understandable: as previously pointed out, Modern Yoga studies are only in their infancy. Western esotericism, or rather the dialogue between esotericists East and West, however, has also played a key role in the shaping of modern forms of Hinduism, and this is a rather more momentous role to play. Because of this, it seemed important to bring to the attention of my colleagues what I came to call 'esoteric myopia'. The following section, discussing this topic from the point of view of Modern Yoga, also highlights some of the ways in which this limitation has affected the study of Hinduism.

Esoteric myopia

Modern Yoga draws conceptual models, themes, terminology and imagery from the classical Hindu tradition,[10] but is essentially rooted in the encounter between tradition and modernity of which the

10. For a discussion of what is meant here by 'classical Hindu tradition' see section on Classical Hinduism vs. modern Hindu elaborations in Chapter 1. The concept or category of 'Hinduism' is a notoriously controversial one. For an overview of contributions to this debate, and for his own appraisal of the problem see Sweetman (forthcoming). Sweetman's contribution is worthy of notice as it steers a well-balanced course between the Scylla of uncompromising 'Orientalist' interpretations and the Charybdis of what may be seen as ultimately self-defeating forms of radical deconstructivism.

British domination of India was the first example in history. As Halbfass notes, since Rammohan Roy's time (1774–1833)

> it has become increasingly obvious that the European, i.e., primarily British, presence in India was not just another case of foreign invasion and domination, or of cross-cultural, interreligious "encounter". Instead, it was an encounter between tradition and modernity, i.e., an exposure to new forms of organization and administration, to unprecedented claims of universality and globalization, to rationalization, technology, and a comprehensive objectification of the world. It also meant the advent of a new type of objectification of the Indian tradition itself, an unprecedented exposure to theoretical curiosity and historical "understanding," and to interests of research and intellectual mastery. (1988: 217)

As the same author further remarks, the Indian response to Europe "has many levels and facets" (*ibid.*). Numerous aspects of this East–West encounter have been explored in greater or lesser depth. One crucial interlocutor in this multifarious dialogue, however, has been consistently overlooked, namely Western esotericism. This worldview or form of thought has played an especially important role in religious matters, and its influence has been pervasive in certain modern re-elaborations of Hinduism, including Modern Yoga. This oversight has left a gap in the arguments and analyses of many otherwise valuable and accurate scholarly discussions relating to this subject.

An interesting example of this is provided by Raymond Schwab (1984: 8) who comments that 1875 marks the close of a "heroic age", covering the previous hundred years, during which the Orient was 'rediscovered' by the West. He then mentions that the end of this era was marked by two opposite events. The first was the foundation of the Parisian Ecole des Hautes Etudes in 1868, which included Indic studies as part of its curriculum: Schwab comments that the new "integral humanism" born of the Oriental Renaissance had gained official recognition (*ibid.*). The second event, "*on which it is not necessary to dwell*" (*ibid.*, emphasis added) was the appearance, in 1875, of the Theosophical Society. It is obvious that Schwab has little time for esoteric movements and for their modern manifestations. As he is more interested in the cultured aspects of Western literature and philosophy than in forms of belief and religiosity, however, the fact that he disregards these phenomena does not detract from his overall arguments.

More problematic, at least in principle, is the position of Mircea

Eliade, who in his classic work on yoga (1973) does discuss, centrally, how key religio-philosophical topics have been shaped by centuries of yoga history. As he introduces his subject and comments on the modern situation, however, he mentions the "detestable 'spiritual' hybridism inaugurated by the Theosophical Society and continued, in aggravated forms, by the countless pseudomorphs of our time" (*ibid.*: xix). Because he refuses to take into account such esoterico-occultistic groups, however, he fails to explain or even comment upon how and why these phenomena affected the yogic tradition, when it could be argued that many of his readers would have wanted (or maybe needed) to find out more about this very matter.

It is not Schwab's and Eliade's value judgements that are at stake here, but the reasons that led them to these omissions. The fact that they obviously disliked these phenomena and refused to talk about them or to acknowledge their formative influence is not going to make them go away. And neither are the alarmist cries and partisan campaigns conducted by "anti-cult" movements engaged in fighting certain (admittedly at times extreme and controversial) manifestations of modern esotericism. As aspects of esotericism and occultism become pervasive in contemporary developed societies, however, maybe the time has come to look them straight in the face instead of attacking them indiscriminately or, at the opposite end of the spectrum of reaction, pretending that they are not there at all.

Such 'intellectual myopia' towards esotericism has been especially pervasive in the study of modern and contemporary Hinduism. A relatively recent example shows the type of misunderstanding (largely caused by unawareness of esoteric trends) that the present work is trying at least in part to redress. In an interesting contribution discussing the making of modern Hinduism Ninian Smart describes, very poignantly, the "new ideology" (1982: 140) that was at the forefront of this process. His usually penetrating analysis, however, becomes imprecise when he describes Ramakrishna and Vivekananda as "pioneers of the new Hinduism" (*ibid.*: 144). While Vivekananda was indeed such a "pioneer", Ramakrishna was not – even though the official version of facts propagated by the Ramakrishna movement does represent him as such.[11] As the present work argues, the

11. Jackson (1994: xi), in his otherwise excellent study, makes an even more imprecise assertion when he writes that the movement was "launched by the two men", i.e. Ramakrishna and Vivekananda. Miller's rendition of events (1996: x–xi) is similarly slanted in the direction of uncritical emic reports.

teachings made so popular by Vivekananda (including Modern Yoga) draw only superficially from Ramakrishna's own. If we look at historical and textual evidence, rather than at conventional narratives and hagiographies, we will see that, notwithstanding his reliance on Ramakrishna as ultimate spiritual exemplar, Vivekananda was inheritor to the intellectual tradition of the Brahmo Samaj.

The type of construct proposed by Smart, in which Ramakrishna is said to be a "pioneer" along with Vivekananda, highlights a confusion that is very widespread at both etic and emic levels of discourse East and West, i.e. the confusion between 'traditional' (or 'classical', see Chapter 1) and 'modern' forms of Hinduism. Modern understandings of Hinduism, and more specifically Neo-Vedānta, have been made to represent the whole of the Hindu tradition *vis-à-vis* audiences (both East and West) that had little chance to know otherwise. Modern Western esotericism, and especially the occultistic branch of it referred to as 'New Age religion' in the present work (see Chapter 1), has been especially receptive to Neo-Vedāntic teachings, which it has eagerly absorbed and nurtured in its quest to find alternatives to Western mainstream culture.

It is in the interweaving and intersecting of these cultural trajectories that we find an interesting proliferation of Modern Yoga forms. Mapping them out and retracing their history can help us to understand the role played by esoteric currents in the shaping of modern Hinduism, and how Neo-Vedānta and New Age religion have influenced and supported each other in providing forms of religiosity suited to today's cultural temper. By exposing this so far Sarasvati-like invisible intellectual stream, certain differences between modern and more traditional forms of Hinduism, so far only sporadically acknowledged, should become more apparent. It is hoped that the contents of this book may contribute to a more mature understanding not only of Modern Yoga, but also of certain forms of Neo-Hinduism (including Neo-Vedānta), and of those forms of modern and contemporary religiosity in which 'Oriental' and more specifically Indian influences play a part.

Description of contents

Chapter 1 defines the historical and sociological frameworks used as analytical grids in the present work. Drawing mainly from

Hanegraaff (1996) and, to a lesser extent, from sociological material (Troeltsch 1931; Campbell 1972), a relatively in-depth definition of Western esotericism and of the historical developments that this form of thought has undergone from the Renaissance onward is looked into. The emergence of New Age religion at the turn of the nineteenth century (as opposed to the New Age *movement*, which only emerged in the 1970s), important because of its close connections with Neo-Vedānta, is briefly discussed in this context.

Moving next to an examination of modern Bengali intellectual circles (mid-eighteenth century onwards), a case is made for a strong (if so far largely unacknowledged) presence of Western esoteric currents in these milieus. The institutional and ideological growth of the Brahmo Samaj throughout the nineteenth century is examined from this specific angle, arguing that this modern religious movement should be seen as the structural correlative of the Western ones that contributed to the elaboration of New Age religion. Indeed, New Age religion and the Neo-Vedānta of the Brahmo Samaj, it is argued, have been in dialogue and in close creative contact from the last quarter of the nineteenth century onwards. One of the main and best-known actors in this context was Swami Vivekananda, presented in Chapter 2 as the chief ideological inheritor of a specific line of Brahmo leaders (Rammohan Roy, Debendranath Tagore, Keshubchandra Sen). Here special attention is paid to the emergence of proto Modern Yoga[12] ideas and practices: it is in fact on the basis of his predecessors' elaborations that Vivekananda would start to experiment with yogic ideas, eventually producing the earliest formulation of Modern Yoga in his *Rāja Yoga* (1896).

How Vivekananda came to compose this seminal text, powerfully bringing together Eastern and Western esoteric teachings, is narrated in Chapter 3. This chapter reconstructs the untold esoteric story of the famous Bengali 'patriot-prophet', highlighting various phases of his often tormented religious quest, his partaking of Brahmo life and ideals and, eventually, his 'turn West'. It is at this point that the Swami proceeded to assimilate cutting-edge Western esotericism and occultism, to then introduce them into Neo-Vedāntic discourses.

12. The expression 'proto Modern Yoga' is used to signify those early strands of modernistic yoga-related speculation which were eventually brought together in fully-fledged Modern Yoga.

Modern Yoga was formulated in this context and, arguably, became Vivekananda's most influential and productive contribution to modern forms of religiosity.

Chapter 4 analyses in some depth the two key Neo-Vedāntic concepts of "God-realization" and "Self-realization". Originally inspired by the central Upaniṣadic terms *brahmajñāna* and *ātmajñāna*, these English words progressively took on a semantic life of their own, and were eventually adopted (along with other Neo-Vedāntic ideas and models) by New Age religion. As they were elaborated in the same Brahmo milieus described in the preceding chapters, this chapter looks at the same historical period and place (nineteenth-century Bengal), but from the more abstract point of view of the development of religio-philosophical ideas. Side connections with related speculative currents, such as those cultivated by the Theosophical Society and by sections of the medical profession interested in hypnosis and mesmerism, are also referred to.

With Chapter 5 we move to an in-depth analysis of Modern Yoga proper. Because of the foundational role played by Vivekananda's *Rāja Yoga*, this text is examined in detail. Vivekananda's work is based on the *Yoga Sūtras* of Patañjali, the central text of the Yoga *darśana* (religio-philosophical or speculative "viewpoint"), and more specifically on Patañjali's *aṣṭāṅgayoga* ("eight limbs of yoga", *YS* II. 28 to III. 8). Mirroring the utilitarian and positivistic spirit of the time, Vivekananda attempts to modernize these teachings and to make them relevant, meaningful and useful to himself and to his contemporaries. Because he starts from largely 'disenchanted' premises, he first of all attempts to rationalize yoga's cosmology in order to make it more 'scientific'. This results in a *quasi*-materialistic *Naturphilosophie*, which will influence the rest of his elaborations. *Rāja Yoga* also introduces what we may call the two pillars of Modern Yoga theory and practice: the *Prāṇa* Model and the *Samādhi* Model. Based to some extent on Patañjali's teachings, these two models consist mainly of Neo-Vedāntic ideas mixed with Western mesmeric, Harmonial (see Chapter 3) and psychological speculations. Often adopted by New Age groups or individuals sympathetic to Oriental teachings, they will become a point of ongoing contact and interchange, and at times of complete overlap, between Neo-Vedānta and New Age religion.

Chapter 6 provides an overview of the ways in which Modern Yoga developed throughout the twentieth century, with special reference to the West and more specifically to Britain.[13] Soon after the publication of *Rāja Yoga*, 'specialist' styles of yoga started to emerge, emphasizing a variety of physical and mental practices, or specific combinations of the two. A typology of forms of Modern Yoga is provided in this context. The second part of the century witnessed the relatively fast expansion and, eventually, globalization of Modern Yoga through the three phases of Popularization (1950s to mid-1970s), Consolidation (mid-1970s to late 1980s) and Acculturation (late 1980s to date). As Modern Yoga became progressively more attuned to the secular, pragmatic and rationalistic temper of the West, it was accommodated in a twofold manner: at the margins of 'health and fitness' concerns on the one hand, and within the conceptual and institutional sphere of alternative medicine on the other.

At this point in the chapter we turn our attention to a case study of the Iyengar School of Yoga, arguably the most influential school of Modern Postural Yoga to date. The last part of the chapter sets forth the history of the school and of its founder, B. K. S. Iyengar, through the three periods of Popularization, Consolidation and Acculturation.

Following that, Chapter 7 examines the history of Iyengar Yoga from the more specifically religio-philosophical point of view. This is done by analysing the most significant textual output of the school (Iyengar 1984 [1966]; 1983 [1981]; 1993), and by combining this information with extensive data gathered over more than two decades of fieldwork in Modern Yoga circles. The modes and content of oral and written transmission of Iyengar Yoga theory and practice are discussed on this basis, and contextualized within the wider framework of Neo-Vedānta, New Age religion and, more generally, modern and contemporary forms of religiosity.

The concluding Chapter 8 refers more directly to fieldwork data and to grassroots perceptions, uses and conceptualization of Modern Postural Yoga. These data are tentatively discussed within the framework of anthropological theories of ritual. The Modern Postural Yoga session, in fact, whether engaged in under the guidance of a teacher or by oneself, emerges as an excellent contemporary example of secularized healing ritual. The standard threefold subdivision of ritual events (separation, transition, and incorporation

13. It should be noted that while the proposed overview of Modern Yoga history is based on a preponderance of British data, the developments discussed actually apply to the whole of the English-speaking world, notwithstanding smaller variations at the level of individual teachers, schools and locality.

phases; van Gennep 1965 [1908]: 11) is obvious in its structure. The polyvalence of its theories and practices, however, allows each practitioner to adopt more or less secularized interpretations of the discipline, thus making it especially suited to largely secularized and developed multicultural, multifaith societies.

PART I

The Prehistory of Modern Yoga

We Hindus are specially endowed with, and distinguished for, the yoga faculty, which is nothing but this power of spiritual communion and absorption. This faculty, which we have inherited from our forefathers, enables us to annihilate space ... Waving the magic wand of yoga ... we command Europe to enter into the heart of Asia, and Asia to enter into the mind of Europe, and they obey us, and we instantly realize within ourselves a European Asia and an Asiatic Europe, a commingling of oriental and occidental ideas and principles ... We summon ancient India to come into modern India with all her rishis and saints, her asceticism and communion and simplicity of character, and behold a transfiguration! The educated modern Hindu cast in Vedic mould!

(Keshubchandra Sen 1901: 484–5; lecture delivered in 1881)

1. Roots of Modern Yoga

> What is common to both [of Rammohan Roy's] English and . . . Bengali works is the fact that they (in contrast to Śaṇkara) relate the contents and the study of the Upaniṣads to practical and earthly matters, in particular to social goals, and not just to the goal of liberation. Here, soteriology and utilitarianism are linked together; for *all* human goals (*puruṣārtha*), and not just *mokṣa*, may be advanced through the study of the Upaniṣads and the Vedānta. Again and again, Rammohan emphasizes that being a householder, living a practical life, having worldly, temporal goals is *not* incompatible with knowing the supreme *brahman*.
>
> (Halbfass 1988: 209, original emphasis)

In order to understand how Modern Yoga developed and the role it plays in modern and contemporary forms of religion, we must first explain the intellectual and historical contexts from which it developed. As stated in the Introduction, esotericism and modernized forms of Hinduism played a key role in these developments: what is meant by these terms will now be explained at some length.

"Esotericism" as academic field of research

We owe a debt of gratitude to continental scholars for establishing modern esotericism and occultism as well-defined areas of academic study. Maybe it is because this happened only relatively recently (1990s) that 'esoteric myopia' could thrive. The French scholar Antoine Faivre pioneered the mapping of esotericism as a proper field of study and produced seminal material in this context.[1] His

1. Faivre (1992; 1994). For a summary of his work on esotericism see Faivre (1997).

Sorbonne chair, dedicated to the study of esotericism,[2] was unique until September 1999, when Faivre's younger collaborator Wouter Hanegraaff was appointed to a similar position at the University of Amsterdam.[3] My interpretation of esotericism (see below) is largely based on the work of these scholars.

As Hanegraaff points out, the "beginnings of modern esotericism are generally located in the Florentine Platonic Academy founded by Cosimo de' Medici in the second half of the 15th century and entrusted to the care of the young scholar Marsilio Ficino" (1996: 388–9). But, as discussed by Faivre (1992), the historical and cultural roots of esotericism extend as far back as Greek and Roman antiquity. In his seminal works, Faivre has defined the characteristics of Western esotericism, focusing especially on its Renaissance flourishing (fifteenth and sixteenth centuries). Building on Faivre's work, Hanegraaff (1996) has analysed the remaining four centuries of esotericism from the point of view of their relevance to New Age religion.

The publication of Hanegraaff's 1996 work on New Age religion has been especially felicitous for the purposes of the present research because many of the esoteric currents that contributed to the emergence of this type of religiosity are the same as those that contributed to the formation of Neo-Vedāntic esotericism, and thus of Modern Yoga. Indeed, it is precisely in Modern Yoga that we find a substantial overlap of New Age and Neo-Vedāntic beliefs and practices. As such, Modern Yoga became a live link between East and West: a bridge through which personal, cultural, institutional and other exchanges could take place.

The data and models drawn from the Faivre/Hanegraaff material and from other secondary sources are used in the context of my own data, based on protracted periods of fieldwork and on the study of primary sources, both classical and modern. Without Hanegraaff's timely 1996 update, however, any analysis of the role played by esotericism over the last couple of centuries would have had to stand

2. More specifically to the History of Esoteric and Mystical Currents in Modern and Contemporary Europe.
3. Where he is Professor in the History of Hermetic Philosophy and Related Currents at the Department of Theology and Religious Studies. He is also supported by two colleagues: J.-P. Brach (specializing in older aspects of esotericism) and O. Hammer (specializing in more modern forms).

on its own feet, a feat admirably managed by Godwin (1994), who, while providing us with an "intellectual history of occult and esoteric currents in the English-speaking world ... from the early Romantic period to the early twentieth century", lamented that "[t]he subject of esotericism is so new to humanistic scholarship that no conventions yet exist for its treatment" (*ibid.*: xi). Thanks to the Faivre/Hanegraaff school this is no longer the case as we are acquiring viable theoretical models to analyse esoteric contexts.[4] A summary of the characteristics of the esoteric worldview as exposed by Hanegraaff (1996: 396–401) is presented below.

The worldview of Western esotericism

First of all our author points out that a concern with synthesizing religion and science was already present in one of the main components of esotericism, Renaissance Hermeticism, and that it "has remained characteristic of esotericism right up to the present day, and is the foundation of an ever-present ambiguity" (*ibid.*: 396–7). This ongoing attempt at synthesis mirrors a deep-seated human unease *vis-à-vis* the deep epistemological split brought about by the rise of modernity within Western (and nowadays global) societies.

Hanegraaff then relates how Faivre defines esotericism: as a distinct "form of thought" encompassing six characteristics, the first four, listed as 1 to 4 below, being intrinsic (they must be present, and are separated for analytical purposes, but are more or less inseparable); the last two, listed as 5 and 6 below, being relative or non-intrinsic (they are frequently present, but need not be; *ibid.*: 397–8).

(1 to 6): Basic characteristics of esotericism

(1) Correspondences

"These correspondences, considered more or less veiled at first sight, are ... intended to be read and deciphered. The entire universe is a

4. This does not mean, of course, that the phenomena studied by Faivre and Hanegraaff were not being studied before – these authors do employ earlier sources such as Corbin and Yates, just to mention two of the best-known scholars in the field (for more details on their use of these and other sources see Hanegraaff (1996), Chapter 14). Faivre and Hanegraaff, however, systematically define and analyse esotericism and occultism in the way summarized in the present chapter, and their analytical model proved very suitable and productive when applied to my research topic.

huge theater of mirrors, an ensemble of hieroglyphs to be decoded. Everything is a sign; everything conceals and exudes mystery; every object hides a secret."[5] These correspondences are elaborated along the lines of visible-invisible, macrocosmic-microcosmic, etc. phenomena; and also along the lines of correspondences between nature (the cosmos), history and revealed texts: "the 'Book of Nature' contains the same truths as revealed in the Bible, and this correspondence may be brought to light by a visionary hermeneutics" (Hanegraaff 1996: 398).

(2) Living nature

"The vision of a complex, plural, hierarchical cosmos permeated by spiritual forces ... In combination with (1), this furnishes the theoretical foundations for concrete implementation: various kinds of magical practice, 'occult medicine', theosophical soteriologies based on the framework of alchemy, and so on, are based on it ... [t]he concept is most properly described as a form of panentheism" (*ibid.*: 398).

(3) Imagination and mediations

"The idea of correspondences implies the possibility of mediation between the higher and the lower world(s), by way of rituals, symbols, angels, intermediate spirits, etcetera. *Imaginatio*, far from being mere fantasy, is regarded as an 'organ of the soul ...' [and] is the main instrument for attaining *gnosis*" (*ibid.*: 398–9). According to Faivre this is possibly the most useful element for demarcating esotericism from mysticism; the latter aspires to "the more or less complete suppression of images and intermediaries because for [the mystic] they become obstacles to the union with God". The esotericist, on the other hand, "seems to take more interest in the intermediaries revealed to his inner eye through the power of his creative imagination".[6] But this distinction must clearly be understood as ideal-typical, as in practice there is a great admixture of the two attitudes (Hanegraaff 1996: 399).

5. Faivre (1994: 10) as quoted in Hanegraaff (1996: 398).
6. Last two quotations: Faivre (1994: 12) as quoted in Hanegraaff (1996: 399).

(4) Experience of transmutation

If it did not have implications in praxis, the concept of esotericism "would hardly exceed the limits of a form of speculative spirituality".[7] And further, "the experience of transmutation is most properly regarded as pertaining to the salvific quest for a perfect *gnosis*. . . . the principal tool to this end is the *imaginatio*, which gives access to the intermediate realms between spirit and matter" (Hanegraaff 1996: 399–400).

(5) The praxis of concordance

This is the tendency to establish commonalities between two or more traditions. Prominent examples of this element are beliefs in a *prisca theologia* or *philosophia perennis*, or the concern for a primordial "secret doctrine" as key to all "exoteric" religious traditions, as in the Theosophical Movement of the nineteenth century (*ibid.*: 400).

(6) Transmission

This component refers to the transmission of knowledge from master to disciple by way of initiation. It includes the concept of a historical genealogy of "authentic" spiritual teachers (*ibid.*).

It is also important, as Hanegraaff notes, to define what esotericism *sensu* Faivre *is not*. Esotericism, he affirms, should be explicitly distinguished

> from two other commonly encountered meanings. To define "esotericism" with direct reference to "secrecy" or a "discipline of the arcane" is overly restrictive: many manifestations of alchemy or Christian Theosophy, for instance, have never been secret but were widely disseminated. To define esoteri(ci)sm as the "spiritual center" or transcendent unity common to all particular religious traditions (as done in the so-called "perennialist" school of Comparative Religion) implies that one subscribes to a religious doctrine which is more properly regarded as an object of study. (*Ibid.*: 385)

7. Faivre (1994: 13) as quoted in Hanegraaff (1996: 399).

In fact, as Hanegraaff further points out elsewhere,

> [p]erennialists usually speak of "esoterism" rather than "esotericism". It seems useful to take advantage of this in order to distinguish between the perennialist view on the one hand, and the strongly different empirical view defended here.[8] Unfortunately, however, the distinction is difficult to maintain in translation. (Hanegraaff 1995: 110, note 24)

(7) Reformation "Spiritualism"

As previously mentioned, Hanegraaff (1996) also extends and refines Faivre's definition of esotericism. As he explains (*ibid.*: 401–3), Faivre fails to take into account post sixteenth-century developments. The latter have provided at least one new 'intrinsic' element to the esoteric tradition, namely the factor of Reformation "Spiritualism", in the sense of the term used by Church historians since the end of the nineteenth century to refer to a tradition of thought that became especially prominent in the seventeenth and eighteenth centuries (*ibid.*: 402). As he warns, this tradition should not be confused with "19th century spiritism", for which the same term is often used "as a near synonym" (*ibid.*: 403). In order to distinguish the two, i.e. the Church historical usage from the nineteenth-century spiritism one, he marks the former by the use of inverted commas (*ibid.*: 403–4), a convention that will be followed in the present work. Basing himself on earlier research on the subject, Hanegraaff lists the key characteristics of "Spiritualism" as follows:

> With reference to the classic studies of Hegler and Troeltsch, Christoph Bochinger analyzes the "spiritualist" perspective in terms of twelve closely interrelated aspects: 1. Interiorization of the expectation of a New Era and the return of Christ; 2. Spiritual hermeneutics and reliance on the "Inner Word"; 3. Opposition between religious experience and "external" knowledge; 4. Certainty about spiritual things; 5. Interconnection of God-knowledge and self-knowledge; 6. Systematic criticism or reconceptualization of traditional Church dogma; 7. Criticism of the doctrine of justification and its practical/ethical results; 8. Religious freedom and personal responsibility; 9. Religious tolerance

8. "The empirical study of religions can be distinguished from theological, positivist-reductionist or religionist approaches by its practice of permanent *epochè* (suspension of normative judgement), also known as methodological agnosticism" (Hanegraaff 1996: 4). For further details see the same source and Hanegraaff (1995).

> and criticism of Church intolerance: complete rejection of violence in matters of religion; 10. Criticism of the mediation of salvation by the Church and by external cultic ceremonies; 11. Affinity with rationalism; 12. Cosmological foundation of hermeneutics and doctrine of salvation. (*Ibid.*: 404)

Our author goes on to remark that the "spiritualist" element is "especially important because of its general relevance to the emergence of characteristically modern types of religious sensitivity" (*ibid.*: 405). We may add that it is also crucial to the present discussion as currents of Christian "spiritualism" played a central role in the shaping of Neo-Vedānta.

(8) Enlightenment and post-Enlightenment thought

Moving closer to the modern and contemporary periods, Hanegraaff details other important developments within esotericism, brought about by the impact of Enlightenment and post-Enlightenment thought. Essentially consisting of processes of secularization (including elements of rationalization and disenchantment in the Weberian sense; *ibid.*: 408, 409),[9] these represent, according to our author, "*the* decisive watershed in the history of Western esotericism", when "[t]he survival of esotericism under the condition of post-Enlightenment processes of secularization produced new and unprecedented phenomena" (Hanegraaff 1996: 406). These phenomena,

> ...in spite of their diversity, ... have emerged essentially from two broad movements, both of which are rooted in the late 18th century and have flourished in the 19th. The first of these is *Romanticism*: a movement with deep roots in the esoteric tradition, but shaped decisively by the Enlightenment and, especially, the Counter-Enlightenment. The second is most properly referred to as *occultism* .... Both movements ... can be defined as the products of a clash of worldviews. Romanticism emerged from a momentous event: the reinterpretation of esoteric cosmology under the impact of the new evolutionism. This changed the nature of esotericism forever, but left the internal consistency of its worldview essentially intact. Occultism, in contrast,

9. Concerning the complexities inherent in the concept of "secularization" see Chadwick (1990: 1–18). For a fine, concise discussion of secularization from a sociological point of view see Wilson (1988).

> came into existence when the esoteric cosmology (based on universal correspondences) increasingly came to be understood in terms of the new scientific cosmologies (based on instrumental causality). As a result, the internally consistent worldview of traditional esotericism gave way to an unstable mixture of logically incompatible elements. In both streams (and in the various hybrid combinations that emerged) traditional esoteric ideas and concepts continued to be used under new conditions but, since meaning and function depend on context, they inevitably underwent subtle but important changes. (*Ibid.*: 406–7)

Such transformations brought about what Hanegraaff (*ibid.*: 407) broadly describes as "the secularization of esotericism", of which occultism is the most characteristic expression. We follow Hanegraaff in describing occultism as

> an etic category in the study of religions, which comprises *all attempts by esotericists to come to terms with a disenchanted world or, alternatively, by people in general to make sense of esotericism from the perspective of a disenchanted secular world.* (*Ibid.*: 422, original emphasis)

> ... occultism ... is the product of a syncretism between [esotericism] and science, correspondences and causality. (*Ibid.*: 423)

Through the elaboration of a secularized esotericism various attempts were made "to update traditional tenets and present them as relevant to the secular world", resulting in the development of "religious theories, speculations and practices of a new, in-between type" (*ibid.*: 408). Aware of the complexity and elusiveness of the concept of secularization, however, Hanegraaff pinpoints four of its aspects which have played a key role in giving a specific character of "secularized esotericism" to Romanticism and in transforming "esotericism into occultism". They are:

i) the post-Enlightenment worldview that sets out to interpret the cosmos as being based on "laws of causality", as opposed to older interpretations based on "correspondences",[10]
ii) the modern study of religions (including the so-called "Oriental Renaissance" and the rise of Comparative Religion),

10. The universe, in other words, is no longer construed as an 'enchanted' or mysterious place encompassing phenomena, events and forces which are beyond human understanding, but is seen as a huge piece of machinery, the workings of which are explainable (or will at some point be) on the basis of natural laws.

iii) the rise of popular evolutionism,[11] and
iv) the popular impact of religious types of psychology. (*Ibid.*: 409)

To sum up, esotericism may be seen, for the purposes of the present study, as consisting of the following elements:

(1 to 6) original characteristics (from Faivre)
(7) Reformation "Spiritualism" (from Hanegraaff drawing on existing scholarship)
(8) Enlightenment and post-Enlightenment thought, as found in and propagated through Romanticism and occultism, by way of the secularizing effects of:
- a worldview based on causality (in the case of occultism)
- the modern study of religions
- the popular impact of evolutionism
- a rapprochement between psychology and religion.

Esotericism in classical and modern Hinduism

With a view to discussing the dialogue and cross-fertilization that took place between Hinduism and Western esotericism, let us examine any parallelism of esoteric themes between them. We shall do this with reference to elements (1) to (8) above.

(**1 to 6**): Finding parallels for Faivre's characteristics of esotericism in classical Hinduism is not difficult. Hinduism has abundant theories of correspondence, as, for example, in Sāṃkhya or Tantric

11. About which Hanegraaff (1996: 462–3) writes:

> To discuss popular evolutionism separately from the emergence of the new scientific worldview and the study of religions [i.e. the two aspects of secularization listed as i) and ii) above] ... is admittedly somewhat artificial. At least since the end of the 18th century, both developments were strongly informed by a belief in evolution and its close cognate, progress. These two terms, by the way, should not be seen as strictly synonymous: most theories of evolution have nothing to say of values, and one does not have to believe in progress in order to accept evolutionary theory ... However, ... to most people in the 19th century the suggestion of a movement from worse to better was the heart of the theory; and it is as such that popular evolutionism is important to our subject. Evolutionism understood as historical process is found neither in traditional esotericism, nor in the Oriental religions which were assimilated by Romanticism and occultism; but before the century was over, this occidental innovation had been assimilated so profoundly that it could seem as though it had never been absent.

It should be further noted that the last sentence is particularly relevant to the present study, especially as we shall come to see in our analysis of Brahmo religious ideas that Romantic reinterpretations of Hinduism were elaborated not only by Westerners, but also – a fact that is often overlooked due to esoteric myopia – by Hindus themselves.

cosmologies, or in astrology. *Brahman* or *prāṇa* could easily be postulated to correspond to the "spiritual force" permeating the universe in a general framework of living nature. Practices assimilable to imagination and mediations were often used in meditative and ritualistic fashion as amply documented from Vedic times onwards; and, of course, the experience of transmutation could be said to be the central concern of all classical forms of yoga.

As for the last two characteristics (5 and 6), the tendency to seek to establish commonalities between two or more different traditions has been quite marked within Hinduism from the times of the *Upaniṣads* and the *Gītā* through to Purāṇic and sectarian literature. The usual procedure was to affirm that all traditions had some validity, with the one under discussion being superior to all the others. Or again that Śiva was indeed a high God, but that he himself was a devotee and follower of Viṣṇu – or vice versa. The catholic nature of Hinduism is also demonstrated by its peaceful and dialectic cohabitation with Buddhism, Jainism and, to a lesser extent, Islam.[12] These syncretic tendencies would, however, have been much more apparent at the 'esoteric margins' of religion than in the mainstream. Concerning 'Transmission' there are many Hindu spiritual lineages involving direct initiation and transmission of various types of teaching from master to pupil, and these lineages have played a key role in this religion (both as theoretical structures and in practice) from at least historical times – say, 1500 to 1000 BCE – onwards.

We may also point out that several scholars use the expression "Hindu esotericism" as a matter of course.[13] The haṭhayogic and alchemical aspects of "the vast current of Indian mysticism known as tantra" discussed by White (1996: ix) show the parallelism with the early categories of esotericism (1 to 6) in plentiful ways, even though the author does not refer to his subject as "esotericism". Many of the semantic values converging in the term 'esotericism' are nevertheless found in the (Western) term 'alchemy', which he constantly employs.

Despite the above parallelism, it could be argued that there are substantial structural differences between the ways in which classical Hinduism and Western esotericism employ such categories. It could be noted, for example, that they are much more widely accepted, and

12. With notable exceptions; some current events being especially worrying and controversial.
13. For example, Hardy (1990: 117–26), while Brooks (1992: 405) and Bharati (1992: 18) explicitly connect 'Hindu esotericism' and Tantra.

indeed employed as key elements of the mainstream tradition in classical Hinduism, whereas Western esotericism is by definition somewhat marginal with regard to religious orthodoxy. In this sense it would be right to affirm, along with Hanegraaff, that to apply the concept of esotericism "beyond the sphere of the monotheistic traditions[14] is ... questionable" (1995: 109, note 20).

While this is an important problem, it need not concern us here because the intellectual trends under consideration are *modern* elaborations of Hinduism. The thinkers who cultivated these trends assimilated the 'esoteric' elements of classical Hinduism (as defined above) mainly by reinterpreting them, as we shall see, through the lenses of Western esotericism and occultism. How this happened is more immediately obvious when we examine the general conditions of assimilation of elements 7 and 8.

(**7 and** 8): These are elements much more peculiarly Judaeo-Christian and Western in form and content. Reformation "Spiritualism", Enlightenment and post-Enlightenment thought were all exported more or less wholesale from the West into Bengal during the period of British Orientalism (1773 to 1837),[15] and substantially influenced the historical processes that led to the shaping of modern forms of Hinduism including those, central to the present discussion, elaborated by the Brahmo Samaj. We should bear in mind that the cultural and technological legacies that Bengal absorbed from the West necessarily included the same stratification of discourses, however compacted by time and transmission, that one would find in the original Western setting. Once gathered into the fold of Western history the Brahmo intelligentsia, with characteristic intellectual briskness and flair, was quick to adapt both foreign and indigenous ideas to its own purposes and mental forms. The more classical elements of Hinduism – elements adaptable to "spiritualist" and occultistic treatment being among the favourite – were also revised

14. That is, Judaism, Christianity and Islam.

15. These dates are taken from Kopf's work on the subject (1969). This author explains that, as a consequence of the 1773 Regulating Acts, "Calcutta became the capital of British India" and eventually "evolved into an appropriate urban setting for expanding the channels of constructive influences from the West and for establishing new organizations offering greater opportunities for intellectual exchange between the two cultures" (*ibid.*: 16–17). The year 1837, on the other hand, is when British Orientalists attained their last great achievement, i.e. the rediscovery of Buddhist India: "The later discoveries would be made by continental Europeans or by Indians themselves" (*ibid.*: 266).

through the lenses of these later influences before being integrated in Brahmo speculations and, eventually, in Vivekananda's Neo-Vedānta. And while this group was always a tiny minority among India's millions,[16] it was this same group that eventually led India into the republican era (Kopf 1979).

At this point the modernization process became part of the national agenda, while in the meantime modernized forms of Hinduism had become the creed of most of the urbanized middle and upper classes in India as well as in the Hindu diaspora. These high-profile communities were the ones most actively involved in national and international decision-making processes, culture formation, civil representation, industrialization, commerce and finance. Certainly Neo-Hinduism did and still does carry on a dialogue with classical forms of Hinduism. From its inception, however, it was strongly informed by the values of Enlightenment liberalism, more or less orthodox Christianity and, last but not least, Western esoteric "spiritualism". In turn, it was to contribute much to Western esotericism and to certain Christian denominations (such as Unitarianism and Quakerism) over the last two centuries. Hence the developmental outlines of this phenomenon are as relevant to modernized Hinduism as they are to Western esotericism. They need, however, to be studied with reference to the specific chronological and contextual conditions found in India throughout this period.

We should further bear in mind that the Indian situation was vastly different from the Western one. While Western culture had nurtured its developing esotericism (along with many other intellectual universes) through a progression of slow and gradual historical stages, India was all of a sudden faced with an intense barrage of imported new ideas. Britain imposed this dialogue on the Orient by taking up residence in the East. As Halbfass succinctly put it: "For modern Indians, dealing with the West is not a matter of choice or predilection: it is a historical necessity and predicament" (1988: 218). The West, on the other hand, selectively steered the dialogue with the East according to its (intellectual and material) needs and wishes (Schwab 1984; Kopf 1969), except of course for causing responses in which it ended up being at the receiving end, such as various revolts, the Indian nationalist struggle and, especially relevant in the present

16. See Jackson's comment (1994: 4) that "it was always too intellectual in approach and in the end too foreign to win the acceptance of India's millions".

context of discussion, the modern Hindu missionary thrust. In other words, whereas Europe had slowly brought about its own modernist paradigm shifts from the Renaissance onwards, the ones elaborated during the Hindu period of modernization were originally introduced into India from the outside and only successively absorbed (to a point) into indigenous forms.

The British colonial enterprise in India was furthermore the first exercise of the kind actively committed to propagating Enlightenment rationalism as "the Truth". The cultural imperialism that followed forced the Indian mind to measure itself against all sorts of foreign constructs: economic, political, scientific, technological, philosophical, religious – and esoteric. These complex intellectual influences blended in with local traditions and speculations, and took strong root in India's intellectual soil.

We shall provide an analytical outline of these developments, with special reference to events that will lead to the formation of Modern Yoga, in the last part of this chapter. Further details and evidence will then be supplied in the rest of Part I. Before we proceed in this direction, however, we need to expand a little on the sociological concepts of sect, cult and cultic milieu, and finally return to Hanegraaff's definitions of New Age religion and related chronology. These constructs will in fact play an important part in our analysis of the esotericization of modern Hinduism and of the nature of Modern Yoga.

Mysticism, cult and sect

In his well-known typology, Troeltsch (1931: 993 and *passim*) defines three types of religiosity,[17] namely the church type, the sect type, and mysticism. As Troeltsch (1931: 734) explains, when the third type of religiosity emancipates itself from the more "concrete" modes of religion, such as the institutionally structured church and sect types,

> mysticism realizes that it is an independent religious principle; it sees itself as the real universal heart of all religion ... It regards itself as the means of restoring an immediate union with God; it feels independent

17. And "not simply of organisational structures", as is too often assumed in sociological literature (Campbell 1978: 147).

> of all institutional religion, ... which makes it indifferent towards every kind of religious fellowship.

It is at this point that mysticism turns into that "spiritualism" or "spiritual religion" which we described under (7) above with regards to post-Reformation developments of esotericism. This type of religiosity becomes eminently individualistic insofar as it subscribes to "the great doctrine of the Divine Seed, of the Divine Spark which lies hidden in every mind and soul, stifled by sin and by the finite, yet capable of being quickened into vitality by the touch of the Divine Spirit working on and in our souls" (*ibid.*: 738), and as such supports "a theology of the subjective consciousness of salvation" (*ibid.*: 739). Because of its stress on individual religious experience, "spiritual" religiosity exhibited "a spirit of religious toleration which granted to each individual the actual right to his own convictions". This resulted in a relativistic outlook, "since in all that is relative the Absolute is present" (*ibid.*: 750), and in a propensity towards polymorphism (*ibid.*: 745).

While church and sect types of spirituality tend to form very concrete, hierarchically ordered and clearly regulated social structures, "spiritual" religion only recognizes

> the Invisible Church ... the purely spiritual fellowship, known to God alone, about which man does not need to concern himself at all, but which invisibly rules all believers ... [T]he individual is therefore relieved of all obligation to organize and evangelize, and from all connection with ecclesiastical and sectarian organization. (*Ibid.*)

But as mystics are also human, they feel "the need for the give-and-take of intimate fellowship with other souls". The groups that they form, of a peculiarly fluid and distinctive type, are technically called 'cults' in sociological literature (*ibid.*). Hanegraaff (1996: 15), relying on Troeltsch (1931) and Campbell (1972), summarizes their characteristics by comparing them to those of the sect:

Cult	*Sect*
Individualistic	Collectivist
Loosely structured	Tightly structured
Few demands on members	Many demands on members
Tolerant	Intolerant

Inclusivist	Exclusivist
Transient	Stable
Undefined boundaries	Clearly circumscribed
Fluctuating belief systems	Stable belief systems
Rudimentary organization	Stable organization
Highly ephemeral	Persisting over time

As all these authors agree, however, these are ideal-typical models. In actual fact all three types (church, sect, and mysticism/cult) do interact and combine in many ways: significantly different formations and tendencies may also be found within the same group when observed over time; or one type may be transformed into another as the result of shifting membership and changing circumstances. This is also evident in the post-Vivekananda history of Modern Yoga: definitely cultic to start with, it will later start to develop sectarian tendencies, some of which will eventually become embodied in institutions. In the West the post-Second World War diffusion and popularization patterns of Modern Yoga, quickly followed by institutional consolidation and acculturation, have even brought about a number of attempted rapprochements with the church type.[18]

But, ultimately, cult and sect are the two types that most naturally overlap and interact. The social dynamics that Troeltsch describes with regard to sects and "spiritual religion" during the Reformation are still found in today's groups:

> In actual fact both of these religious types were constantly merging into each other. The sect aspired to the inwardness of mysticism; mysticism strove to realize the sacred fellowship of the sect. "Enthusiasm" – the result of great excitement and of the oppressive hostility of the churches – also played its part in drawing both these groups closer together. But inconsistencies and tensions, due to this partial fusion of the two types, still remained. (1931: 753)

18. There are various Christian attempts at assimilation of (Modern) Yoga forms; cf., for example, the Benedictine monks Dechanet (1993) and Abhishiktananda (1984), the Jesuit De Mello (1984), and the Anglican Father Slade (1973). A different type of assimilation, this time in the Hindu direction, is found in the International Society for Krishna Consciousness (ISKCON)'s recent (and often successful) attempts at establishing themselves as part of the Hindu mainstream.

From mysticism to cultic milieu

We have already pointed out that the associative patterns of mystic religion or "spiritualism" are fluid and flexible to the extreme, reflecting strong inward and therefore potentially individualistic tendencies. From Renaissance times in Europe, and over the last couple of centuries in India, these "spiritualist" tendencies have been reinforced by the rise of secularization on the one hand, and by the fast technological developments of communications networks on the other.[19] This has given rise to what Campbell (1972) has appropriately defined as the "cultic milieu". Introducing this concept, he observes:

> Cults ... tend to succeed very quickly and take over the characteristics of sects or else fade away in the face of societal opposition or the absence of a charismatic leader...
>
> Given that cultic groups have a tendency to be ephemeral and highly unstable, it is a fact that new ones are being born just as fast as the old ones die. There is a continual process of cult formation and collapse which parallels the high turnover of membership at the individual level. Clearly, therefore, cults must exist within a milieu which, if not conducive to the maintenance of individual cults, is clearly highly conducive to the spawning of cults in general. Such a generally supportive cultic milieu is continually giving birth to new cults, absorbing the debris of the dead ones and creating new generations of cult-prone individuals to maintain the high levels of membership turnover. Thus, whereas cults are by definition a largely transitory phenomenon, the cultic milieu is, by contrast, a constant feature of society. (*Ibid.*: 121–2)

This milieu is unified by several common characteristics:

1. The various individuals and groups composing it "share a common position as heterodox or deviant items in relation to the dominant cultural orthodoxies". This gives rise to "a common consciousness of deviance [and their] spokesmen ... thus have a common cause in attacking orthodoxy and in defending individual liberty of belief and practice. Arising from this there is a prevailing orientation of mutual sympathy and support ... [and]

19. For an in-depth analysis and discussion of the latter topic see Bayly (1996).

marked tolerance and receptivity towards each other's beliefs" (*ibid.*: 122). The latter element also receives a great stimulus from the emphasis given to the "spiritual" and mystical elements of religion which are very conducive to the acceptance of syncretic formulas (*ibid.*: 122–3).

2. There is a prevalence of "over-lapping communication structures" and of overlapping beliefs and practices (from different groups) in most cultic-milieu individuals. This further reinforces syncretization. The milieu is kept alive by "magazines, periodicals, books, pamphlets, lectures, demonstrations and informal meetings" (*ibid.*: 123). Groups are open to each other's suggestions, or mutually supportive, and they also publicize each other's ideas and events. Individuals 'sampling' groups within the cultic milieu "constitute yet another unifying force within the milieu" (*ibid.*).
3. Individuals operating within the cultic milieu share a "common ideology of seekership which both arises from and in turn reinforces the consciousness of deviant status, the receptive and syncretistic orientation and the interpenetrative communication structure" (*ibid.*). Campbell follows Lofland and Stark in applying the concept of seekership "to persons who have adopted a problem-solving perspective while defining conventional religious institutions and beliefs as inadequate" (*ibid.*) This concept prevails throughout the cultic milieu, and is applied beyond the religious field: "truth (or enlightenment)" are understood to exist "outside the purely mystical religious tradition" and to "apply equally well to the search for interpretations and explanations of non-religious phenomena ... and even in the context of the pursuit of worldly success, health or consolation" (*ibid.*: 123–4).

New Age religion vs. New Age movement

In the analysis summarized above, Campbell discusses the characteristics of the cultic milieu mainly with reference to the Western situation at the time of his writing (early 1970s). Hanegraaff, on the other hand, convincingly argues that the phenomena described by Campbell were only one aspect of a longer process, namely the nineteenth-century formation of New Age *religion*, which eventually became a self-aware New Age *movement* in the mid-1970s. Towards the end of his book, Hanegraaff (1996: 515) reiterates his definition of New Age religion as *a set of beliefs sharing patterns of common criticism directed against dominant cultural trends and formulated on the basis of a specific tradition, i.e. Western esotericism*. After this he goes on to state:

> My findings leave no other option than to conclude that the perspective which we have referred to as "New Age religion" was born in the 19th century[20] and had reached maturity not later than the beginnings of the 20th. The "cultic milieu" described by Colin Campbell continued this same perspective ... I have argued that it was only in the second half of the 1970s that this cultic milieu "became conscious of itself as constituting a more or less unified movement", and I proposed to take this phenomenon as the beginning of the New Age movement in a precise sense. If this is to be combined with the definition given above, we have no other option than making a distinction between *New Age religion* (i.e., the general type of culture criticism based on a foundation of secularized esotericism) and the *New Age movement* specifically. Although the "substance" of New Age religion has long been present, those who adhered to it clearly began to perceive themselves as being part of a "movement" approximately in the second half of the 1970s. (*Ibid.*: 522)

The above points and chronological framework, applicable with some adaptation to the development of modern forms of Hinduism, should be borne in mind as we proceed to analyse the Indian situation.

Classical Hinduism vs. modern Hindu elaborations

The chronological framework discussed below analyses the main ideological currents at work between India and the West with regard to the esotericization of Hinduism and the formation of Modern Yoga. It has been evolved by adapting the work of Friedhelm Hardy (1984), Wilhelm Halbfass (1988), David Kopf (1969) and J. N. Farquhar (1977 [1914]) in the light of my own findings. The resulting scheme is presented in Table 1.

20. See Hanegraaff (1996: 517): "The foundations of New Age religion were created during the late 18th and the 19th century, in the course of a process which I have referred to as the secularization of esotericism."

Table 1 Developments in modern Hinduism

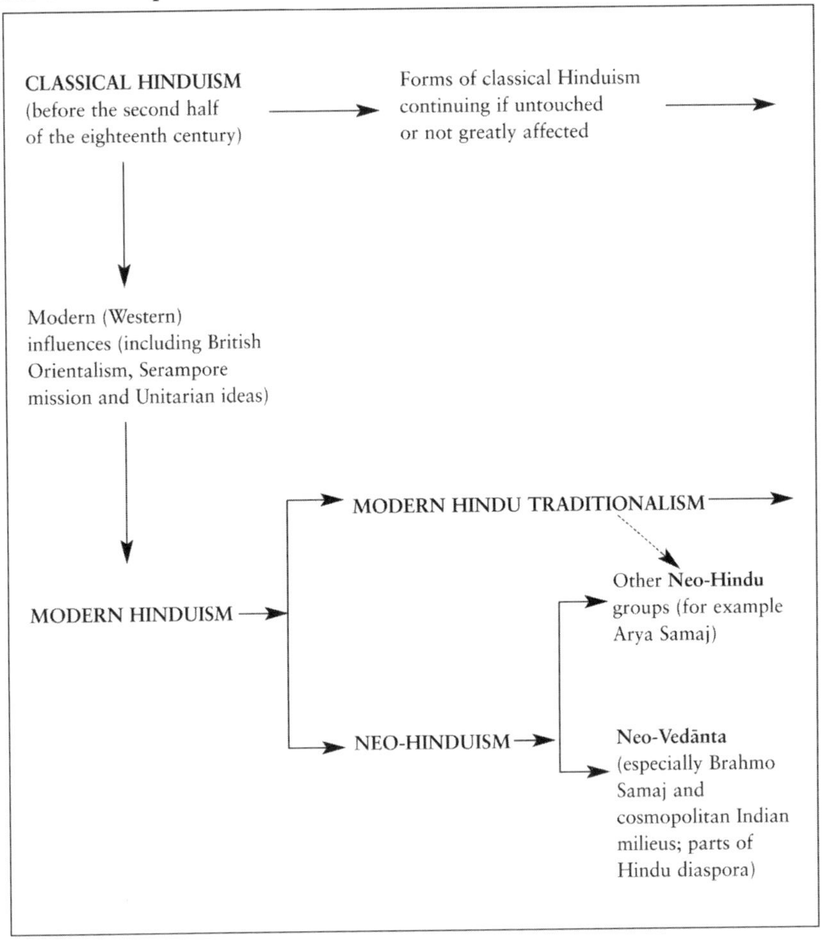

The concept of 'classical' Hinduism is used following Hardy (1984), for whom classical Hinduism is a phenomenon occurring "in a pre-18th century context", that is before the "major discontinuity … which arises through the advent of British colonial power in India … and through the process of 'Westernisation' initiated thereby" (*ibid.*: 15). It is worth noting that, in this sense, Hardy's definition encompasses what is called 'Classical' and 'Medieval' periods in some textbooks.[21] In the more specific context of yoga, the use of 'classical'

21. For example, Smart (1992, Part I, Chapter 2).

(not capitalized) will alert the reader that what is being discussed is not the 'Classical Yoga' (capitalized) of Patañjali, but all types of yoga current before the second half of the eighteenth century, including Patañjali's *Yoga Sūtras* and related commentaries.

There are other possible, more precise chronological markers for the beginning of Western influences on Hinduism. One is the 1757 Battle of Plassey (Palasī), when the British penetration of India started in earnest. As we saw (note 15 here) Kopf uses 1773 for the beginning of British Orientalism. What is beyond doubt is that by 1775 the imported culture was starting to affect traditional ways of life to a noticeable degree. This created responses and reactions in the indigenous cultures, and the Hindu ones are grouped under the general heading of 'Modern Hinduism' in Table 1 as they did not crystallize into coherent ideological movements up to 1815.[22] The term 'Hindu Renaissance' has been deliberately avoided because what has been called Hindu Renaissance over the years (whether in apologetic or analytical terms) covers too many of the phenomena found in Modern Hinduism.[23] In order to highlight the trends that led and contributed to the formation of Modern Yoga it was felt that more specific categories were needed.

The beginnings of Neo-Hinduism

One of them is the subdivision between Neo-Hinduism and Modern Hindu Traditionalism. This part of the table is taken from Halbfass, who in turn takes his framework from Hacker.[24] As Halbfass himself points out (1988: 221), "Hacker's scheme is a simplification, although a useful and convenient one". We should therefore bear in mind complexities and overlaps which blur the boundaries between these two categories when dealing with any particular piece of research.

The "Other Neo-Hindu groups" shown in Table 1 stand for such complexities, and most of all for Neo-Hindu groups which are not Neo-Vedāntic (such as the Arya Samaj), and are as such, arguably,

22. Date of publication of Rammohan Roy's *Vedāntasāra* (see below).
23. For a thorough discussion of the term 'Renaissance' as applied to the Modern Hindu context see Kopf (1969: 280ff.).
24. For a general discussion see Halbfass (1988: 210–12, 219–22). For a good discussion of the same two groups from a somewhat different point of view cf. Kopf (1969, Chapter 12 and especially pp. 192–213).

less (or differently) affected by Western esoteric trends. These parallel Neo-Hindu groups are, however, of no direct concern to the present discussion and will not be explored further.

This subdivision apart, it is clearly possible to recognize that two different overall strands develop within Hinduism as a result of its meeting with modernity: a Neo-Hindu one much more receptive to Western influences and models, and a Modern Hindu Traditionalist one not unsympathetic to modernity, but far less inclined to compromise with its dictates. As Halbfass comments:

> Traditionalism ... has also taken in and assimilated new elements, and is by no means a mere continuation of that which existed before the encounter with the West. Similarly, it is *not* possible to describe Neo-Hinduism as a rigorous break with the past and its transmission. What distinguishes Neo-Hinduism and Traditionalism are the different ways in which they appeal to the tradition, the structures which they employ to interrelate the indigenous and the foreign, and the degree of their receptivity vis-à-vis the West. Modern traditional Hinduism has preserved an essentially unbroken continuity with the tradition, and it builds upon this foundation, carries on what is already present in the tradition, even though additions are made and extrapolations occur.
>
> To be sure, Neo-Hinduism also invokes the tradition, tries to return to it, and hopes to find in it the power and context for its response to the West. Yet as Hacker emphasizes, this return is the result of a rupture and discontinuity. More important than the fact that foreign elements have been added to the tradition is that basic concepts and principles of this tradition have been reinterpreted and provided with new meanings as a result of the encounter with the West: "Neo-Hinduism ... always implies reinterpretation." The link which the "Neo-Hindus" find to their tradition is, one may say, an afterthought; for they first adopt Western values and means of orientation and then attempt to find the foreign in the indigenous... (1988: 219–20)

Neo-Vedānta started to emerge as a clearly defined ideological movement under the intellectual leadership of Rammohan Roy (Figure 2). The division from Modern Hindu Traditionalism[25] became blatantly obvious in the controversy that followed the

25. And possibly from other Neo-Hindu groups, or this differentiation may have taken place later.

publication of his *Vedāntasāra* in 1815.[26] Roy's Traditionalist opponents retorted by publishing the *Vedāntacandrikā* in 1817,[27] in which they criticized Roy (without, however, explicitly mentioning him) as *ādhunika* ("innovator") and *idānīntana* ("modernizer") (Halbfass 1988: 221, 210). Roy can thus be seen as the first influential Neo-Vedāntic author and his opponents as early theorizers of Modern Hindu Traditionalism.

Halbfass (*ibid.*: 219) points out that Neo-Hinduism has been more successful outside India than Modern Hindu Traditionalism, which "has retained a much greater vitality within India itself". This observation also applies to Neo-Vedānta, which, as we shall see through our analysis of Modern Yoga, is still expanding and growing among cosmopolitan Indians, the worldwide Hindu diaspora and across committed communities of Neo-Vedānta converts, many of whom originate from Western cultural moulds. This is only logical after we realize that Neo-Vedānta is much closer in form and contents to Western/modern culture than Modern Hindu Traditionalism. As it is within Neo-Vedānta that Modern Yoga emerged, this is the ideological current that we shall follow more closely throughout the first part of the present study.

Esoteric East–West cross-influences in historical perspective

As Neo-Hinduism was taking shape, the inner coherency of Classical Hinduism was shaken by the radical 'otherness' of many of the new ideas – the challenges of various types of Christianity and of Enlightenment and post-Enlightenment thought, as we saw, chief among them.

Some of these influences were progressively absorbed during the era of British Orientalism (1773–1837; see note 15 here). Kopf's excellent study on the subject (1969) shows how an elite of traditional Bengali literati was gradually transformed into a modernized

26. Date of the Bengali publication; an English translation of this work was published in 1816 under the title *Abridgement of the Vedānt* (see Halbfass 1988: 202, which lists Roy's publications).
27. With an attached English translation called *An Apology for the Present System of Hindoo Worship* (*ibid.*: 210).

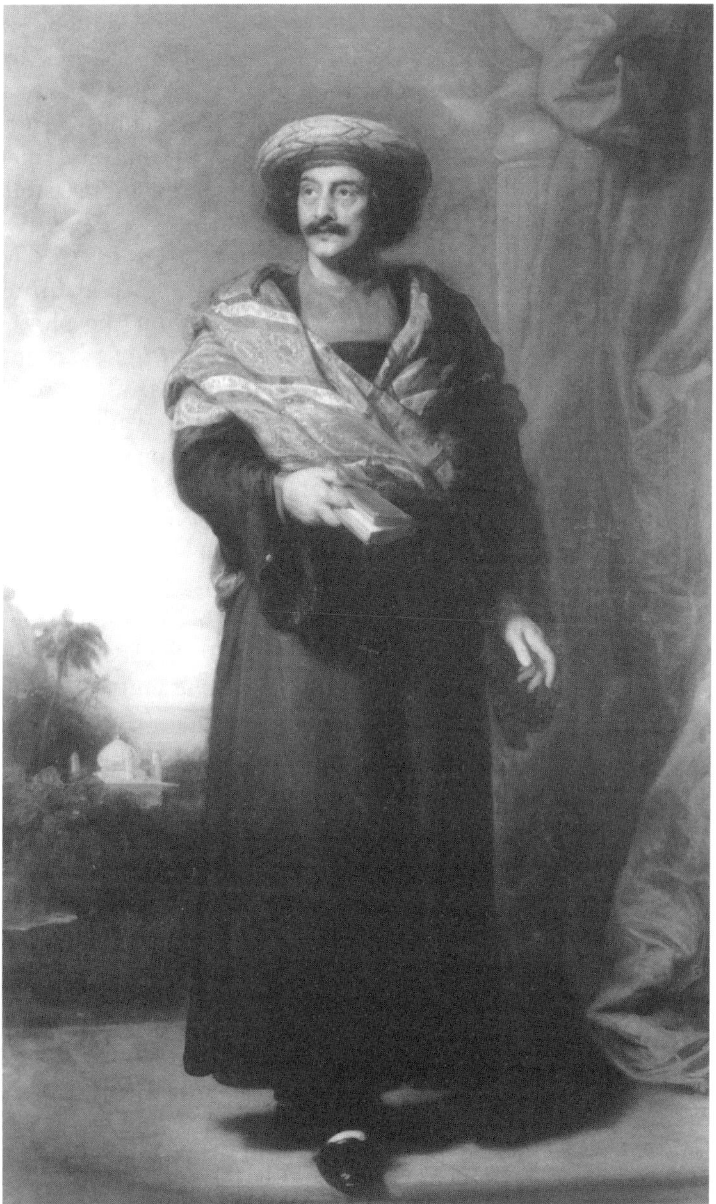

Figure 2 Rammohan Roy, *c*. 1832. Portrait by H.P. Briggs (1791–1844). (By permission of the Bristol Museum and Art Gallery)

Hindu intelligentsia[28] by means of professionalization and daily interaction and co-operation with Europeans. Both parties found common ground for discussion and common interests in areas of social, intellectual and practical co-operation. The main actors of this period were either inspired by or receptive to the egalitarian, tolerant and universalistic spirit of the Enlightenment, and modern Hindu thought was substantially shaped by such influences.

Early British Orientalists were exemplary in this sense as they were, in the main, deeply sympathetic to South Asian cultural forms. If William Jones played a key role in the recovery of the glories of Hindu culture, he was certainly not alone. Kopf (*ibid.*) has shown that the Orientalist milieu defined many of the discourses that the Bengali Renaissance would later develop, and these would be directly absorbed into modern forms of Hinduism. The Sanskritist Thomas Colebrooke, for example, "concentrated his research upon Vedic India, and by the end of his career, he had devised a new composite image of the Indo-Aryan period as an age of gold" which "was dramatically and metaphorically contrasted with the peculiarities of contemporary Hindu society" (*ibid.*: 40). In his seminal (from an Orientalist point of view) essay "On the Vedas or the Sacred Writings of the Hindus", he retraced "his discovery of 'the unity of the God-head,' or a monotheistic tradition, in ancient India" (Kopf 1969: 41). His classicist research focused on the period of Indian antiquity up to and including the world of the early *Upaniṣads*, whereas his successor H. H. Wilson extended Orientalist scholarship into 'medieval' times[29] and regionally based traditions (*ibid.*: 167–75). Thus the Orientalists left an important legacy: a reconstruction of Indian culture (including philosophical and religious beliefs, history, and so forth) based on eighteenth-century Enlightenment principles and methodology, with work done on the Vedic and 'medieval' periods proving especially influential. It was only natural that members of the Bengali intelligentsia, by definition striving to integrate foreign influences, would turn to these constructs in their attempts to adapt their culture to modern times, at the same time inevitably distancing themselves from a more conservative Hindu orthodoxy.

28. As Kopf (1969: 1–2) explains, "The term is derived from a Russian word denoting a European-educated class of professional intellectuals who found themselves increasingly alienated from Russian society and government in the nineteenth century."

29. I.e. "the history of India between the Vedas and the rise of the Muslims" (*ibid.*: 170).

There is also interesting evidence that British Orientalists themselves held rather unorthodox religious beliefs, and this is especially telling in the context of the present discussion and in view of the seminal intellectual influence exercised by this group of scholars. William Jones, for example, stated about the Vedānta that "nothing can be farther removed from impiety than a system wholly built on the purest devotion" (quoted in Mukherjee 1968: 118). In his private correspondence he admitted even more explicitly to his Hindu sympathies: "I am no Hindu but I hold the doctrine of the Hindus concerning a future state to be incomparably more rational, pious and more likely to deter men from vice than the horrid opinions inculcated by the Christians on punishment without end" (quoted in *ibid.*: 119). His biographer concludes that "Jones had faith in God and Christ as pictured in the Bible but his views were very similar to those of Dissenters such as Price or Priestley" (*ibid.*: 118). We shall hear more about Unitarianism soon.

We find similar evidence with regard to other Orientalists: Marshall (1970: 26) describes John Zephaniah Holwell as "a Christian ... of a very eccentric kind", and Alexander Dow as a nominal one. And finally we should say a few words about Warren Hastings, who, as Governor-General of India (1774–85), encouraged and actively supported the progress of Orientalist studies.[30] His patronage included commissioning the earliest translation of the *Bhagavad Gītā* from Sanskrit directly into English (1785). In its final published form, the latter work included, by way of foreword, a letter that Hastings wrote to the then Chairman of the East India Company, Nathaniel Smith (Hastings 1785). As Godwin (1994: 309) remarks, this letter may well be the first modern instance in which a European "had given credit, in print, to the fruits of yoga".

Hastings' comments were carefully worded, but they do contain a clear summary of his views on the subject. Most crucially, they reveal what the Enlightenment found fascinating about yogic and meditative practices: that effective, well-tested *techniques* of abstraction had seemingly been systematized thanks to the accumulated knowledge of generations of practitioners who had explored "new tracks and combinations of sentiment" (Hastings 1785: 9). Such experimentation led these adepts to work out doctrines "totally different from

30. "Hastings's policy was designed to encourage Orientalists and Bengalis to work together for common goals" (Kopf 1969: 178).

[those] with which the learned of other nations are acquainted" (*ibid.*). These doctrines, Hastings proposed, were "equally founded in truth with the most simple of our own" having been "derived from a source so free from every adventitious mixture" (*ibid.*). While the author's measured language betrays his awareness of treading over potentially controversial religious issues, the message is clear: Hastings is saying that Hindu contemplation and the insights it bestows are just as valid as the Christian ones, and that the Hindus' proficiency in these endeavours may even be superior to the Christians', as "even the most studious men of our hemisphere" may "have never been accustomed to this separation of the mind from the notices of the senses" (*ibid.*). Many Christians, especially in the following 'evangelical' century, would not have taken kindly to such statements. Their esotericist contemporaries, on the other hand, would agree wholeheartedly with Hastings.

The political and ideological changes that started in Britain in the second decade of the nineteenth century turned the tables on both acculturated Orientalists and Indian intellectuals. A crucial parliamentary debate took place in 1813, and the resulting India Act ended the East India Company's monopoly of trade, and opened its territories both to British commerce and to Christian preaching (Sykes 1997: 21), while in the meantime the rise of Evangelical Christianity represented by the Clapham Sect opened the doors to often questionable forms of missionary intervention. Later on, the new views of Eurocentric colonial policies resulting in Thomas Babington Macaulay's heavy-handed programme of Anglicization prevented further amicable co-operation between Indian intellectuals and the ruling British elites. Unable to return to completely traditional ways of life and prevented from elaborating a common cultural programme with the British, the Indian intelligentsia was now forced to find a different orientation:

> The Calcutta cultural mediator who for decades had responded favorably to the culture of the European (who was himself favorably impressed with Indian culture) now faced the different view that all patterns of reform were an integral part of Western civilization and that all Asian civilizations were almost by definition static and decadent. The intelligentsia in Calcutta were compelled to confront a crisis in identity. . . . Most . . . responded to the crisis by identifying with the

> Orientalist-reconstructed view of Hinduism, which they romanticized as apologists. (Kopf 1969: 272)

For different reasons, the same Orientalist constructs of Hinduism were also being adopted (and further transformed) by many in the West. There was a chronological progression in this. During the second part of the eighteenth century, we find a number of Enlightenment sceptics who, like Voltaire, were looking for intellectual weapons to attack Christian dogmas and institutions. They were soon joined by a number of committed esotericists who were earnestly seeking new and possibly more valid sources of wisdom than those the West could offer (Godwin 1994). An altogether more popular following, however, started to grow as a result of the spread of literacy in the 1830s.[31] From this time onward, Orientalist knowledge – and literary or esoteric elaborations of it – became progressively more accessible to a much greater number of people than ever before. And much of this knowledge was appropriated by esotericists East and West, who used it and reinterpreted it according to their own lights.

The contacts between these two popular esotericisms – Eastern and Western – were limited to relatively circumscribed intellectual and personal exchanges during the first half of the nineteenth century, Roy and his friends being pioneers of this trend. But a more substantial rapprochement started to take place around the middle of the century, and by 1875 the two parties were actively interacting at social and institutional levels. By this time Neo-Vedāntic esotericism was flourishing in Keshubchandra Sen, the enthusiastic and charismatic leader who followed Roy and Debendranath Tagore at the head of the Brahmo Samaj. Following the history of these Brahmo leaders will allow us to retrace the progressive occultization of Neo-Vedānta and the genesis of Modern Yoga. A basic overview of this topic is presented below, and schematized in Table 2. Further evidence and secondary details will be given in the rest of Part I.

The Brahmo Samaj and the occultization of Neo-Vedānta

Neo-Vedāntic Hinduism, eventually institutionalized in the Brahmo

31. Godwin (1994: 67) points out that in England "there was already by 1800 an artisan class eager for self-improvement and education". About the more general British context see Thomas (1988).

Table 2 Ideological developments of Neo-Vedānta in the Brahmo Samaj

Rammohan Roy (*c*. 1774–1833)
NEO-VEDĀNTIC →
ENLIGHTENMENT
(*Vedāntasāra* 1815)

Debendranath Tagore (1817–1905)
NEO-VEDĀNTIC →
ROMANTICISM

Keshubchandra Sen (1838–84)
NEO-VEDĀNTIC →
"SPIRITUALISM"

Swami Vivekananda (1863–1902)
(Narendranath Datta) →
NEO-VEDĀNTIC
OCCULTISM
(*Rāja Yoga* 1896)

Samaj, developed on the ideological foundations established by Rammohan Roy. These consisted of a universalistic interpretation of Hinduism. Inspired by Indianized versions of the Enlightenment project and influenced by Unitarian Christianity, Roy relied on a streamlined, rationalized, monotheistic theology strongly coloured by a selective and modernistic reading of the *Upaniṣads* and of the Vedānta. This Neo-Vedānta was humanistic in its concern to improve the lot of the Indian population through the implementation of social reforms and the propagation of ethical ideals. It also paved the way, albeit unwittingly, for the progressive secularization of certain strata of the Bengali population by supporting this-worldly and naturalistic interpretations of many aspects of religion.

Debendranath Tagore (Figure 3), while at first accepting the "purificationist or puritanical view of the Vedic golden age" (Kopf 1969: 202) which he had inherited in Roy's Neo-Vedānta, eventually altered the Brahmo doctrines considerably. Not only did he distance himself, like Roy before him, from central Hindu beliefs such as reincarnation and *karma*, but he also rejected the authority of the *Vedas* in 1851,[32] declaring instead that "Nature and intuition are sources for the knowledge of God. No book is."[33] In this sense Tagore brought the Brahmo Samaj more in line with Western forms of esoteric religiosity. His Romantic approach to Neo-Hindu doctrines also contributed towards shifting the Samaj closer to Westernized thought forms and further away from classical orthodoxy, a process that will then be taken up and continued by Keshubchandra Sen.

By the time Sen (see Figures 4, 5 and 6) joined the Brahmo Samaj in 1857, the rapprochement between esotericists East and West had become a reality. The thwarting of Orientalist plans of Anglo-Indian co-operation had deprived the Bengali intelligentsia of their academic interlocutors. Militant Christian missions, on the other hand, were gathering momentum and power. The only body of Western interlocutors that was now eager to communicate and co-operate with Indians *qua* Indians was that of esotericists, whether Christian or otherwise. Bengalis reciprocated, while Orient-inspired Romantic, Transcendentalist, occultistic and in due course Theosophical ideas were being propagated through a steadily growing body of literature or through lecture tours[34] and personal contacts.[35]

The cultivated Indian middle classes were expanding, especially so in Bengal: they quickly absorbed what they found congenial in esotericism, and these ideas were added to their Orientalist-reconstructed Hinduism. Just like many Western cities, Calcutta, Bombay and Madras had by now their own 'cultic milieus' and it was here that the new styles of religious associationism thrived. Farquhar (1977 [1914]) presents us with a very lively picture of such milieus, and testifies to "the rise in India about 1870 of a new spirit, which generated many religious movements" (*ibid.*: 186). The Theosophical Society and the Arya Samaj – just to mention two of the more influential associations – were both established in 1875 and in 1878 the Theosophical Society moved its headquarters from New York to India. The Brahmo Samaj was the more official and representative

32. Farquhar (1977 [1914]: 38 and 45 respectively); regarding the *Vedas* see also Kopf (1979: xxi) and Chapter 2 here.
33. From the Brahmo Samaj covenant composed by Debendranath Tagore in 1842 (as quoted in Lavan 1984: 74 and 1995: 9).
34. The lecture tour undertaken by the Theosophist W. Q. Judge in summer 1884 is typical in this respect (Judge 1980: vii).
35. Theosophy became very popular across South Asia as well as in the West.

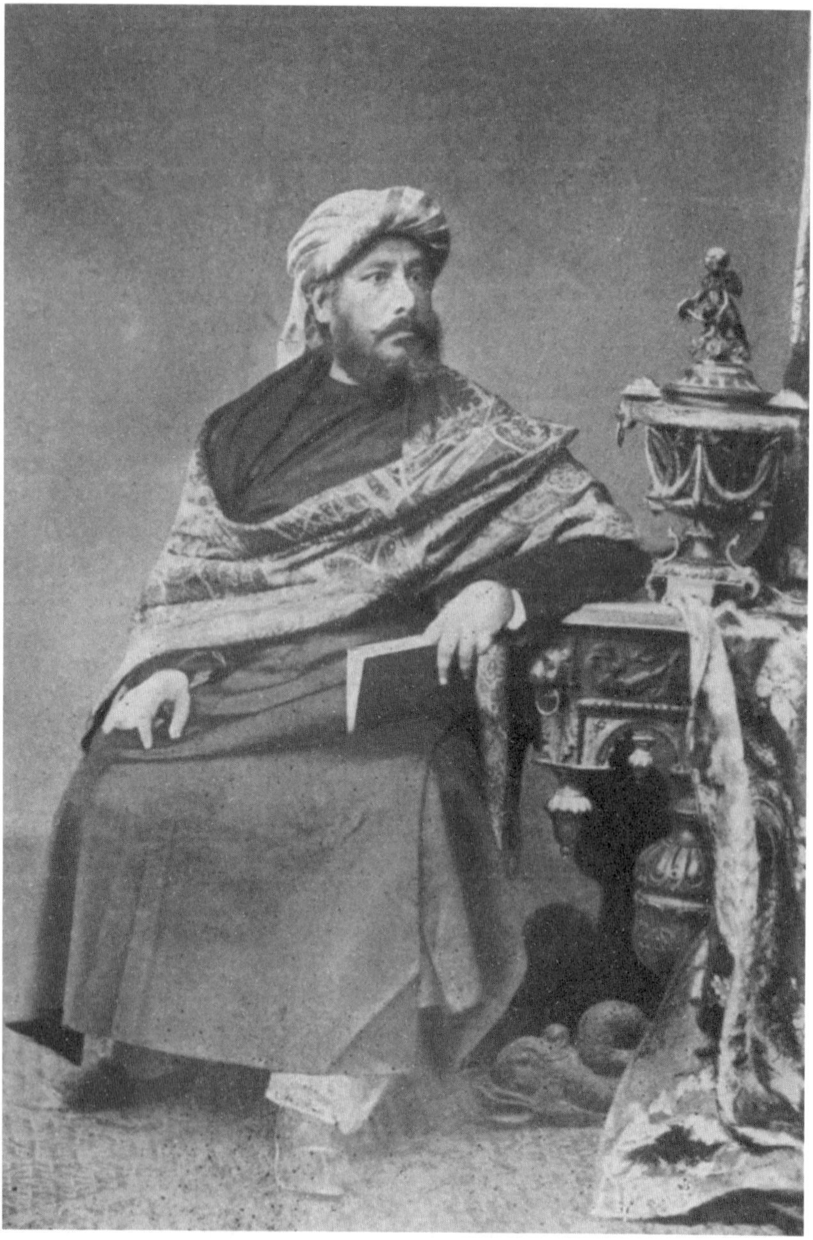

Figure 3 Debendranath Tagore at age 45. From Tagore, D. (1909) *The Autobiography of Maharshi Devendranath Tagore*. S.K. Lahiri & Co., Calcutta. (By permission of the Syndics of Cambridge University Library)

arm of this overall intellectual movement, the locus in which Neo-Vedāntic Hinduism continued to be elaborated after British Orientalism had come to an end.

Sen inaugurated Neo-Vedāntic "spiritualism" proper. His theory of "enthusiasm" as the living heart of the religious life was programmatic in this sense,[36] and may be seen as the Indian version of that radical brand of subjective Reformation "spiritualism" called *Schwärmerei* ("enthusiasm") by more moderate reformers. Early steps towards the formulation of an accessible, non-renunciatory, everyman type of Neo-Vedāntic "spiritualism" had been taken by Roy through his theorization of the *gṛhastha brahmavādin* ethos.[37] Debendranath Tagore followed with Neo-Vedāntic adaptations of the Puritan ethic, and Sen completed the process. Crucially, he also translated these ideas into lay systems of spiritual practice and into new institutional forms. As far as we have been able to ascertain, some of the practices and tenets he elaborated represent the earliest documented forms of proto Modern Yoga. His experiments in spiritually based communal living, furthermore, led to the creation of that typically modern institution, the Neo-Hindu 'ashram' (see note 34, Chapter 2), now ubiquitous throughout India and in other Neo-Hindu enclaves worldwide. For all these reasons, Sen plays a key role in the present study: his importance in the modern esoteric sphere has not been sufficiently acknowledged – for example the very direct links he had with Vivekananda. An esotericist reading of this history clearly shows that Sen was the most influential role model for Vivekananda.

Indeed, Vivekananda's debt to the Brahmo Samaj cannot be overstated. Mentioned in specialist scholarly work,[38] it hardly plays a part in less specialized etic literature, let alone in more popular perceptions. A careful study of the evidence shows that, the inspirational role played by Ramakrishna notwithstanding, Vivekananda was moulded by the formative influence of Neo-Vedānta rather than by Ramakrishna's Hinduism.

36. See his praise of "enthusiasm", written two years before his death (quoted in Hay 1988: 46–7).
37. In Neo-Hindu terminology, this may be translated as "householding spiritual seeker", meaning someone living in the world, but having some form of 'spiritual realization' as his or her main aim in life (regarding 'realization' discourses see Chapter 4).
38. Cf. Sil (1997: 52), Williams (1995a: 60; 1995b: 378), Rambachan (1994: 88), Kopf (1979: 205) and Halbfass (1988: 233), the last two being less aware of esoteric currents.

Sen opened the way to Vivekananda's full immersion into (and absorption of) Western esoteric and occultistic culture. Steeped in secularist, empiricist and Romantic ideas by way of his studies, the young Datta accessed a congenial form of (Neo-Vedāntic) Hinduism when he joined the Brahmo Samaj,[39] and it is in this context that he met Ramakrishna. His relationship with the Bengali holy man was, however, never as straightforward as popularly assumed, a fact revealed both by historical events[40] and by Vivekananda's own teachings which, just like those of the Ramakrishna movement (albeit in different ways), diverge substantially from what Ramakrishna preached (see Neevel 1976; Sil 1997; and below).

Once we become aware of the pervasive presence of esotericism in these milieus, it becomes obvious that Vivekananda's life and work manifested many of the potentialities and ideals cultivated by the more esoteric section of the Brahmo Samaj. At the 1893 Chicago Parliament of Religions the Swami produced a remarkably influential synthesis of Neo-Vedāntic esotericism. A few years later, having assimilated the highly congenial atmosphere of cutting-edge American occultism, he went on to propagate the first fully-fledged formulation of Modern Yoga with the publication of his *Rāja Yoga* (1896). He thus established what is arguably the most successful and productive branch of Neo-Vedāntic occultism to date. As we shall see in due course, his Modern Yoga teachings will also be enthusiastically adopted by Neo-Vedānta's Western partner, i.e. New Age religion.

39. He was an active member of both Sen's Brahmo Samaj of India and of the more moderate Sadharan Brahmo Samaj (see Chapter 3).
40. See studies by Neevel (1976), Sil (1993; 1997) and Kripal (1995). From certain (Neo-) Hindu points of view, works by the last two authors may be seen as provocative and iconoclastic. In a scholarly context, however, they should be judged dispassionately on the basis of accuracy, coherence and cogency of argument.

2. The religious foundations of Modern Yoga

> The higher spiritual concepts of India still appeal with a compelling force to men who have given up the observances of orthodox Hinduism and they strike a response which is not deadened by rationalism. There is a *nostalgie spirituelle* which is hard to describe.
>
> (O'Malley 1968: 788)

This chapter examines the 'esoteric history' of the Brahmo Samaj with special reference to the development of Modern Yoga. We shall discuss aspects of this modern religious movement's history that are often bypassed in the relevant literature. Apart from these aspects, the history of the Samaj is well known[1] and will not be repeated, except for the following dates, set out for the reader's convenience.

The earliest Brahmo Samaj was established in 1843, when Rammohan Roy's Brahmo Sabha (established in 1828 as a universalist theistic society) merged with Debendranath Tagore's Tattvabodhini Sabha (established in 1839 to counter trinitarian Christian conversions in Bengal). The first Brahmo schism took place in 1866, when the younger and more liberal Keshubchandra Sen seceded from the more conservative Debendranath Tagore. This gave rise to the Brahmo Samaj of India (under Sen), while Tagore's group came to be called Adi ("original") Brahmo Samaj. A second schism took place in 1878, when a more secular and socially minded Sadharan Brahmo Samaj seceded from Sen's Samaj, by then strongly

1. See especially Kopf (1969; 1979). For helpful overviews see Brockington (1989: 173–8) and Lavan (1995).

inclined towards a mystical and universalistic "spiritualism". In 1879 Sen and his followers inaugurated the Nava Vidhan or Church of the New Dispensation, headed by Sen as prophet of a new religion wishing "to convince the world that the unity of all religions was essential" (Kopf 1979: 316).

The turning point between classical Hinduism and Neo-Vedānta: Rammohan Roy's Neo-Vedāntic Enlightenment

Halbfass' statement that Neo-Hinduism involved a "rupture" or "discontinuity" with the classical Hindu tradition has been referred to in the previous chapter. One of the key players in this context was Rammohan Roy. Sparked by influences from the European Enlightenment, Roy became the cultural hero of the Bengal Renaissance[2] and is nowadays widely recognized as "the father of modern India" (Hay 1988: 15). The controversies that he initiated – most notably with the publication of his *Vedāntasāra* in 1815 and of *The Precepts of Jesus: The Guide to Peace and Happiness* in 1820 – forced others within and without the Bengal Renaissance to follow or oppose his theses, thus defining their own ideological position. He himself was the Hindu heir of a doubly cosmopolitan world: the fading one of the Indian Moguls, and the rising one of the Western Enlightenment.

His ideas and multiculturalism were, however, not altogether novel or unique: his contemporary Ramram Basu, for example, was also "receptive to Christianity", fascinated by Persian and Arabic cultures and antagonistic towards certain aspects of Hinduism, especially "the hated Brahmans" (Kopf 1969: 121). Like Roy, Basu thought very highly of the Gospel, but resisted actual conversion: "Both [men] preferred to reinterpret their own religious tradition rather than to accept an alien faith" (*ibid.*: 125–6).[3] The characteristics shared by these two Bengali intellectuals – cosmopolitan culture, historical consciousness, spiritual crisis, criticism of Hindu orthodoxy and of the 'priestly caste', a sympathetic attitude towards important aspects of the Christian message – define the Oriental version of the Enlightenment man. And it is indeed in an Enlightenment spirit,

2. Regarding the Bengal Renaissance (1800–23) see Kopf (1969, Part III).
3. For more details on Basu, who is credited by Kopf (1969: 123) with being one of the early pioneers of historical consciousness in Bengal, see *ibid.* (pp. 121–6).

reliant on eighteenth-century European intellectual strivings, that Roy started his reformation of Hinduism.

We already heard something about his interpretation of Vedānta in Chapter 1, and we will hear more in Chapter 4. Here we shall look in some detail at his position *vis-à-vis* the Christian faith. Roy's *Precepts of Jesus* stressed Christianity's ethical teachings and the role of Christ as a sublime example of their application. However, he also held that "[Jesus'] disciples misunderstood Him, and that the whole edifice of Christology [was] a huge mistake" (Farquhar 1977 [1914]: 33). This book dispelled missionary hopes that the Bengali intellectual may be on the brink of conversion and, not surprisingly, caused controversy with Christian leaders. The Serampore Baptist missionary Joshua Marshman (d. 1837) led the Christian defence, to which Rammohan replied with three *Appeals to the Christian Public* (Robertson 1995: 40). According to Robertson (*ibid.*: 41), "the *Precepts*, *Appeals* and Marshman's replies together did as much to disseminate Christian teachings [in India] as had been accomplished almost since William Carey's (d. 1834) arrival in Bengal in 1793". As far as Neo-Vedānta is concerned, however, Roy's position undoubtedly emerged as the winning and more long-lasting one.

When the controversy started, Roy was attempting to clarify his position with regard to Christian dogma by translating the New Testament into Bengali in collaboration with the Serampore missionaries. The further developments of this venture are highly significant:

> In the course of the work serious discussions arose and collaboration ceased; but one of the missionaries, the Rev. W. Adam, sided with Rammohan, and became a Unitarian in May, 1821. This led to the formation in September, 1821, of a Unitarian Mission in Calcutta under a committee of Europeans and Indians. (Farquhar 1977 [1914]: 34)

Even though this specific mission did not last, the future pattern of collaboration set to replace the fading Orientalist dialogue was established: what Neo-Vedānta was to adopt from Christianity were its more "spiritual" and esoteric teachings, as modernized, summarized, represented and propagated by Unitarians.[4]

4. For further information on the interaction between Unitarians and Brahmos see Lavan (1984).

This is where the common ground between Hinduism and Christianity could be found, and also a close overlap between Neo-Vedāntic esotericism and Western esotericism. Thus it is not surprising to hear that Marshman "charged Roy with repeating the old Arian heresy which reduced Christ to a mere man" (Roberston 1995: 40) and, we may add from the classical Hindu point of view, with reducing Hinduism to a Neo-Vedāntic-Christian *darśana*. This is how Roy "called down [on himself] the fiery condemnation of the Calcutta pandits" as well as of the Christian missionaries (*ibid.*: 41). At root, however, his was arguably the only possible irenic position, capable of retaining elements of both cultures, but in the process necessarily playing down dogma and disregarding orthodoxy and orthopraxis on both sides.

How did these developments affect the proto Neo-Hindu context? Orientalism had already been strongly influenced by Enlightenment Humanism; later Unitarian influences introduced that integrated blend of "Spiritualist" religion and Humanism which still lies at the roots of Neo-Vedāntic ideology. When Unitarianism started to influence the Bengali intelligentsia it had already assimilated humanistic values into its worldview, while at the same time retaining its theistic outlook.

Here it may be useful to review those central ideas of Unitarianism which, adopted virtually unanimously by sympathizers in India, Britain and the United States, created strong ideological and personal bonds among the individuals and institutions concerned:

> The Unitarianism that ... linked Rammohun to his British counterparts represented a new and radical approach to religion, society and ethics ... Three simple though radical ideas for the time (1815 to 1835) provided the link between the enlightened few in Calcutta and the enlightened few in England and the United States.
>
> The first was liberal religion, or the substitution of a rational faith for the prevailing popular religions of the world, which, they thought, increasingly curtailed the freedom of human beings by enslaving them to mechanical rituals, irrational myths, meaningless superstitions, and other-worldly beliefs and values. The second was the idea of social reform or emancipation in which all known penalized classes and groupings such as workers, peasants, and women were to be elevated through education and the extension of civil rights to participate fully in the benefits of modern civilization. Finally, there was the idea of universal theistic progress, or the notion that the perfectibility of

> mankind could be achieved by joining social reform to rational religion. (Kopf 1979: 3)

These cross-influences had a profound effect not only on the progressive formulation of Neo-Vedānta from Roy onwards, but also on the ongoing definition of Unitarian doctrines and sympathies. If Roy's Brahmo Samaj was strongly influenced by Unitarianism, so was Emerson's Transcendentalism strongly influenced by Roy's Neo-Vedānta. Such exchanges centred around Unitarian/Brahmo contacts, and these had been made possible by the co-operative mentality and commonality of language and values established by earlier Orientalist influences. Early Neo-Vedānta moved closer to Western-style esoteric liberalism by absorbing the values and worldview of Unitarian Christianity. This started a process of dialogue and cross-fertilization that is still active to this day.

A further important development of Neo-Vedānta took place in Bengal in the few decades before and after the beginning of the nineteenth century. This was the growth of publishing and literacy, which in turn led to the formation of a 'public opinion'.[5] The Serampore Mission, as Kopf (1969: 189–90) points out, was especially important in stimulating the promotion of local cultural consciousness. As early as 1818 the Mission established three separate journals and newspapers, after which "Bengalis followed Serampore's lead and started their own journalistic ventures, thereby greatly adding to the existing media for communication" (*ibid.*: 189). By 1822 the three main 'progressive' religious positions[6] present in the region had been given regular journalistic voices (quite apart from other *ad hoc* controversies), while foreign influences, including liberal theism and "spiritualism", were also being actively integrated into local culture.

Conditions were perfect for the emergence of a lively cultic milieu. On the one hand we find, among other things, the sudden influx of foreign (and at times contradictory)[7] ideas, with the cultural turmoil that this almost unfailingly engenders. On the other we see the fast development of communication networks facilitating the emergence

5. See Kopf (1969: 20, 72, 114, 115) and Bayly (1996: 284, 302–8).
6. These were the Serampore missionaries, the Neo-Hindus and Modern Hindu Traditionalists. For details of the three newspapers and a brief analysis of their positions see Kopf (1969: 189–92).
7. For example, the missionaries' own controversies, and their discrepancies with the British powers.

of social representation, individual expression and, last but not least, charismatic leaders. The Bengali intelligentsia was getting ready to lead India forward on the road of 'native improvement' and, eventually, of 'nation building'. It would soon be followed by the other two presidencies, Bombay and Madras, where important cultic milieus were also to develop.

Neo-Vedāntic Enlightenment to Neo-Vedāntic Romanticism

The Brahmo Samaj remained dormant for about a decade between the death of Rammohan Roy (1833) and the time at which Debendranath Tagore assumed its leadership (1843). This did not mean, however, that new ideologies and intellectual speculations did not reach Bengal during this period. If anything, the decline of Orientalism which went hand in hand with the establishment of Anglicist policies over the period 1828 to 1835 (Kopf 1969, Part V) opened India even more to Western ideas, so that modern science and humanities became part of the standard intellectual background of educated Bengalis. As the century progressed, Anglicist policies, mirroring the growth of British imperialism and of its political, financial and technological might, became more and more ethnocentric. Mill's *History of British India* (1997 [1817]), with its harsh attacks on Indian culture and *mores*, is an early example of this ideological stance. Missionary policies also became aggressive throughout what Kopf (1969: 159) calls "the Age of Alexander Duff" (1830 to 1857).[8]

The Neo-Vedāntic reaction to such challenges was taken up by Debendranath Tagore, who actively sought to neutralize missionary efforts at conversion of the younger generation, and who revived the Brahmo Samaj both institutionally and in terms of doctrinal content. His strategy worked: "Under Debendranath's devoted leadership, the Brahmo Samaj attracted numbers of Bengal's ablest young men" (Hay 1988: 38). These facts are well known. What is less well known are the esoteric, cultic and sectarian aspects of Tagore's life and work. We discuss them below, and the same procedure will subsequently be followed for Keshubchandra Sen.

8. Duff was an influential Scottish missionary. See also note 7, Chapter 3.

Tagore's intellectual background

Tagore's Hinduism, we should bear in mind, was built on the interpretative foundations established by Roy, and these were thoroughly intermixed with Western cultural models and values.[9] Tagore himself was a cosmopolitan member of the Bengali intelligentsia who was well aware of intellectual developments in the West. Oldest son of the wealthy Dwarkanath Tagore (and father of the poet Rabindranath), he was well acquainted with Western thought from early on by way of his education and through personal reading. Debendranath's son Satyendranath reports that his father received his early education at the school founded by Roy – guaranteed to have a liberal approach to knowledge – and that he subsequently attended Hindu College (Tagore, S. 1909: i). Here "useful knowledge from the West", including "European literature and European science", was "transmitted without ethnocentric bias" (Kopf 1969: 181). In his autobiography, the elderly Debendranath stated that he "had read numerous English works on philosophy" in his youth, but that they did not provide the answers he was seeking (Tagore, D. 1909: 9). There is nevertheless ample evidence that such studies helped substantially to shape his thinking, and therefore his interpretations of Hinduism.

O'Malley (1968: 67) gives us a thumbnail sketch of Tagore's eclectic predilections: he "spent three years in solitary contemplation in the Himalayas, chanted the poetry of Persian Sufis, and shared in their mysticism; but he also studied the works of Hume, Fichte and Victor Cousin, and was familiar with the principles of rationalistic philosophy". But most interesting from our point of view is how the evangelical missionary T. E. Slater – a contemporary of Tagore, who, sympathetic and sensitive to the concerns of the Brahmo Samaj, is likely to have had access to primary informants[10] – qualifies Tagore's view of Cousin. Slater (1884: 33) states that Tagore "studied Hume, Brown, Fichte, Kant, and Cousin, the last of whom he counted his greatest *guru*". A brief reminder about Cousin's (1792–1867) views

9. "Devendranath's entire religious career was based upon, and had its sustenance from, the teachings of Rammohan, his real though informal guru" (Chaudhuri 1973: 20).
10. Like Vivekananda, Slater was a delegate at the 1893 Chicago Parliament of Religions (Chowdhury-Sengupta 1998: 23).

helps us to start redressing our esoteric myopia by evidencing the less known aspects of Tagore's religiosity. This French philosopher was

> [a] spokesman for the *Juste Milieu*, which in fact stood for philosophical eclecticism. He was influenced, in turn by Locke and Condillac, the Scottish Commonsense Philosophy of Thomas Reid and Ferguson, Maine De Biran, Schelling and Hegel. Out of these elements he was able to create a fusion of ideas turning philosophy in the direction of "spiritualism". (Reese 1996: 145)

Cousin's appreciation of India as "the cradle of the human race [and] the native land of the highest philosophy" (O'Malley 1968: 801) would also have contributed to attract Tagore's sympathies. So much for Tagore's intellectual *guru*.

Hindu by birth and mystically inclined by nature, Debendranath, while taking them on board, cannot fully accept Western scientism and rationalism as his ideological bases. And neither can he, as Roy's spiritual heir, turn to classical forms of Hinduism. Cousin's eclectic synthesis provides him with a framework combining the philosophical Romanticism of German Idealism with modern empiricism. This framework is then used to further develop Brahmo Neo-Vedānta along more modern lines. But beneath the modern eclecticism and sophistication we can detect the old esoteric quandary. Tagore, like many others before and after him, is attempting to address that inescapable problem of modernity, i.e. how to harmonize 'science' and 'religion'. Like many other modern seekers, he is striving "to obtain God, not through blind faith but by the light of knowledge" (Tagore, D. 1909: 9).

Tagore's doctrinal and ritual innovations

Tagore's intellectual background is reflected in his doctrinal innovations, through which he further distanced the Samaj from classical Hinduism. We shall discuss three of his doctrinal and one of his ritual innovations, all directly relevant to the esotericization of Neo-Vedānta and to the emergence of Modern Yoga. Firstly, he rejected the authority of the *Vedas* (and all of the traditional accoutrements that this authority stood for), for which he substituted a personal epistemology of intuition based on the "pure heart". This, secondly, led Tagore to redefine the central Hindu theory of *karma* and rebirth along historicist and evolutionary lines. Thirdly, the combined influence of Tagore's novel epistemology, of the discoveries of comparative religion and of his collaborator Dutt (see below) led the Brahmo leader to theorize the establishment of a universal "natural" or "scientific" religion. And lastly, Tagore introduced a form of initiation into the Brahmo Samaj. This ritual, as will become apparent, was radically different from the forms of initiation usually found in classical Hinduism.

Intuitional epistemology

Tagore himself describes how he came to doubt the authority of the *Vedas*. He explains how, having studied the Hindu scriptures, he found that he could accept certain sections of the *Vedas* and of the *Upaniṣads*, but not others (Tagore, D. 1909, Chapter 22). Here the influence of his close collaborator Akkhoykumar Dutt (1820–86), a follower of rationalism, deism and scientism, was crucial (Kopf 1979: 49; Tagore, S. 1909: iii). More about Dutt later. As for Tagore, he eventually decided that a discriminative exegesis, capable of deciding which passages were to be accepted as normative, should be based on the understanding of "[t]he pure heart, filled with the light of intuitive knowledge", because "Brahma reigned in the pure heart alone" (Tagore, D. 1909: 75). He then concluded that "The pure, unsophisticated heart was the seat of Brāhmoism" and that Brahmos "could accept those texts only of the Upanishads which accorded with that heart. Those sayings that disagreed with the heart [they] could not accept" (*ibid.*). This obviously undermined the idea of the *Vedas* as an infallible source of revelation, a development that would be officially sanctioned by the Samaj in 1850 (Kopf 1979: 106; Farquhar 1977 [1914]: 45).

Evolutionary spirituality

In order to illustrate his difficulties with the canonical texts, Tagore quoted two passages – one cosmological, the other more didactic – relating to human life and death. The first passage (*Chāndogya Upaniṣad* 5.10.3–6) consists of what is often regarded as "the earliest systematic statement of the doctrine of karma and rebirth" (White

1996: 29).[11] This cosmological model of "photic opposition between darkness and light" (White 1996: 29) is found in several *Upaniṣads* as well as in the *Śatapatha Brāhmaṇa*.[12] Tagore could not accept this passage as containing any truth, indeed it "appeared to [him] to be unworthy vain imaginings" (Tagore, D. 1909: 76). The didactic passage, on the other hand, on how to lead a good life, he found much more convincing: one should study the *Vedas* while serving the teacher; go on to establish a pious household; support oneself by earning wealth in rightful ways; and practise self-control and *ahiṃsā* ("non-harming"). After such a life a person would, on dying, enter "Brahma-loka ... and never return ... to this world any more, no, nevermore" (*ibid.*).[13]

Tagore then proceeds to give his own exposition of human teleology. He does this by mixing some elements of these two passages with Christian concepts of heaven and hell, and with an optimistic theory of evolutive ascensional metempsychosis strongly reminiscent of Swedenborgian theories. In Tagore's vision the "Soul" (which he regards as an individuated entity as it is said never to lose its

11. The passage reads as follows in Olivelle's translation (1998):

> The people here in villages, on the other hand, who venerate thus: 'Gift-giving is offerings to gods and to priests' – they pass into the smoke, from the smoke into the night, from the night into the fortnight of the waning moon, and from the fortnight of the waning moon into the six months when the sun moves south. These do not reach the year but from these months pass into the world of the fathers, and from the world of the fathers into space, and from space into the moon. This is King Soma, the food of the gods, and the gods eat it. They remain there as long as there is a residue, and then they return by the same path they went – first to space, and from space to the wind. After the wind has formed, it turns into smoke; after the smoke has formed, it turns into a thundercloud; after the thundercloud has formed, it turns into a rain-cloud; after the rain-cloud has formed, it rains down. On earth they spring up as rice and barley, plants and trees, sesame and beans, from which it is extremely difficult to get out. When someone eats the food and deposits the semen, from him one comes into being again.

12. White (1996: 364, note 52) lists *Bṛhadāraṇyaka Upaniṣad* 6.2.13–16; *Chāndogya Upaniṣad* 5.10.1–7; *Praśna Upaniṣad* 1.9–10; *Kauṣītaki Upaniṣad* 1.2–3; and *Śatapatha Brāhmaṇa* 2.1.3.1–9.

13. The passage in question is *Chāndogya Upaniṣad* 8.15.1, which reads as follows in Olivelle's translation (1998):

> All this Brahmā told to Prajāpati; Prajāpati to Manu; and Manu to his children.
>
> From the teacher's house – where he learned the Veda in the prescribed manner during his free time after his daily tasks for the teacher – he returns, and then, in his own house, he does his daily vedic recitation in a clean place, rears virtuous children, draws in all his sense organs into himself, and refrains from killing any creature except for a worthy person – someone who lives this way all his life attains the world of brahman, and he does not return again.

"separate consciousness"; Tagore, D. 1909: 78), if sufficiently "purified",

> attains to sacred regions upon leaving this earth, and casting off his animal nature receives a body divine. In that sacred sphere he obtains a brighter vision of the glory of God, and having reached higher stages of wisdom, love and virtue he is translated to higher regions. Thus rising higher and higher ... that divine soul [is carried] onwards towards everlasting progress. (*Ibid.*: 76–7)

The heaven/hell (or rather heaven/purgatory) model comes into play when sinners have to be accounted for: "He who sins ... and repenteth not ... enters into doleful regions after death" (*ibid.*: 77). But ultimately all evolution is ascensional and progressive, as the sinner, "after having continually burnt [in the sinful regions] with the agonies of remorse for his tortuous deeds [ultimately reaches] expiation", "receives grace", and in turn starts off on the ascensional path (*ibid.*). "By the grace of God", Tagore concludes,

> the soul is infinitely progressive, – overcoming sin and sorrow this progressive soul must and will progress onwards and upwards, – it will not decline again upon earth. Sin never reigns triumphant in God's holy kingdom. The soul is first born in the human body, – after death it will assume appropriate forms and pass from sphere to sphere in order to work out the fruits of its merit and demerit, – and will not again return here. (*Ibid.*)

This important doctrinal statement of "evolutionary spirituality" should be read in the light of the comments made in Chapter 1 concerning the assimilation of Romantic thought and evolutionary theories by esotericism. It will then be clear that while Tagore definitely brings Neo-Vedānta closer to the esoterico-Romantic stream, he is still not touched by the secular and mechanistic thought forms typical of occultism. If the soul is said to be on a journey of "spiritual evolution", this is "By the grace of God": it is by an act of grace that sinners are eventually freed of their burdens. Tagore's teachings are based on strong theistic foundations and lack the more subjective and highly secularized contents typical of the later "spiritualist" (Sen) and occultistic (Vivekananda) types of Neo-Vedānta. In this sense (and in this sense only) Tagore's Brahmo Samaj has still some of the socio-religious and cultural coherence of classical Hinduism. Later in the nineteenth century this will be less and less the case, with the two younger Brahmo factions breaking loose from Tagore's aging Adi ("Original") Samaj and gravitating towards opposite poles of "enthusiastic" mysticism (Sen's Brahmo Samaj of India) and secular liberalism (Sadharan Brahmo Samaj).

"Scientific religion"

Since he started harbouring doubts about the authoritativeness of the *Vedas*, Tagore had been asking himself "what was to be the common ground for all Brahmos", finally deciding (somewhat inconsistently) that what they required was "a sacred book" (Tagore, D. 1909: 80). This led him to compose one himself, the *Brahmo Dharma* (1850), containing two sections: one 'doctrinal', the other 'ethical' (Tagore, D. 1909: 81, 83). In this he was helped by Akkhoykumar Dutt.

Proceeding to apply his new epistemological approach, Tagore "laid [his] heart fervently open to God" and the "spiritual truths that dawned on [his] heart through His grace" were taken down on dictation by Dutt (*ibid.*: 80). Thus "by the grace of God, and through the language of the Upanishads" the Brahmo leader "evolved the foundations of the *Brahmo Dharma* ... Within three hours the [doctrinal section of the] book ... was completed" (*ibid.*: 81). The second, ethical part of the book contained a code of everyday morals collated from the *Manu-* and other *smṛtis*, from the Tantras and from the *Mahābhārata*, including the *Bhagavad Gītā* (*ibid.*: 83). It is here that, according to Kopf (1979: 106), we find the official birth of the Brahmo Puritan ethic. However, as the same author points out, "the sources justifying the ethic are not from Calvin reinterpreting Moses, but from Debendranath reinterpreting Manu" (*ibid.*). From this time onward the cultivation of Puritan virtues and of "self improvement through Puritan practices" becomes prominent in the Brahmo Samaj (*ibid.*).

Dutt's rationalistic influence is evident in the second part of *Brahmo Dharma* (*ibid.*), as it is evident in his own *Dharma Nīti* (1855), in which he attempted "to apply his notion of natural law to ethics" (Kopf 1979: 51). The latter text shows how, like many post-Enlightenment thinkers, Dutt had a moving faith in the powers of science and in the predictability and trainability of humans. For him "the aim of [proper] education was the fully developed human being" who has learnt "the physical and mental rules of God" (*ibid.*: 52–3).

He recommended an educational system that would arouse "scientific curiosity" in "the wonders of the endless universe" (*ibid.*: 53), and held a positivist view of human affairs: "Human society," he wrote, "is like a machine and its pluralistic sub-units or sub-cultures are the wheels" (*ibid.*). Given such scientistic premises, Dutt also strove to define a "universal science of religion" based on natural laws of universal applicability. By 1854 he had defined the Brahmo creed in terms of a universalistic, humanist "natural religion" based on "a moral doctrine urging that good be done to others" and on the application of a this-worldly asceticism regulated by the Brahmo ethic: "The asceticism of self-inflicted torture is a perverted and crude practice ... There is no injunction of the Brahmo religion to renounce the world ... All true worshippers of God practice [*sic*] meditation, devotion, acquire knowledge and do good to others."[14] Religion, therefore, whether "natural" or "scientific", is reduced to a code of morals which must be entertained by the individual with the help of standardized, accessible spiritual practices.

If evaluated from the point of view of the formation of Neo-Vedāntic esotericism, Dutt can be seen as the opposite but also complementary pole of Tagore. This is precisely how Satyendranath Tagore describes the two men: his father was the "spiritual head" of the Samaj, while Dutt was the "intellectual leader" (Tagore, S. 1909: iii). Given that the ongoing agenda of post-Renaissance esotericism is the harmonization of 'science' and 'religion', each of the two specialists (i.e. the 'mystic' and the 'scientific humanist') could gain from interacting with the other. Co-operation would allow both to expand the range of their discourses, and to stimulate and validate each other's thinking.[15]

Their thought was exemplarily synthesized by the important (Adi) Brahmo theorist Rajnarayan Bose, possibly Tagore's closest friend and co-operator over the years. In a work published in 1863,[16] he defined Brahmoism as "the prototype for the next stage of religious

14. Dutt, *Who is a Brahmo?*, as quoted in Kopf (1979: 51).
15. *Contra* Kopf (1979: 49) who states that "It is a credit to Debendranath's broad sympathies as a leader of the reformation movement that he could recognize and support a young intellectual whose [convictions] were so alien to his own highly mystical and intimate theistic faith." Kopf, not aware of esoteric trends, overlooks the fact that post-Enlightenment "spiritualism" established a close, if necessarily ambiguous, relationship with rationalism (Troeltsch 1931: 749). Kopf's evaluation might have been applicable if Tagore had been a 'pure' mystic, rather than a "spiritualist" one.
16. *A Defense of Brahmoism and the Brahmo Samaj* (Kopf 1979: 67).

evolution in the world" and as possessing the key to the "science of religion" (Kopf 1979: 67). This key, Sen and to an even greater extent Vivekananda will argue, is pre-eminently found in the Indian traditions of yoga.

Thanks to such elaborations the idea of a "science of religion" had become common currency in Brahmo circles by the second half of the nineteenth century. What Brahmos meant by this was "the discovery of natural laws about religion [based on] the comparative study of religions carried on without sectarian bias, and leading to a unified concept of the religion of man" (*ibid.*). By this stage Tagore's Neo-Hindu Romanticism was starting to open itself up to a process of secularization. This trajectory would be continued by Sen, notwithstanding his ardent devotionalism, and completed by Vivekananda. As pointed out in the previous chapter and as apparent from the above discussion, the modern study of religions and evolutionary ideas played an important part in this secularization process.

Initiation

A striking aspect of recent and contemporary Neo-Vedāntic religiosity (including a number of Modern Yoga groups), especially in the latter half of the twentieth century, is the plentifulness and easy availability of 'initiations'. This phenomenon is linked to radical changes in the understanding and administration of these rites. Debendranath Tagore's life is once again revealing in this context, and also shows interesting parallels with Vivekananda's, as we shall see in due course. We know from Tagore himself (Tagore, D. 1909: 27–9) how he decided to establish a Brahmo initiation and how such initiation was finally administered in 1843. The Brahmo leader reports:

> ...I [reflected] that there was no religious unity among the members of the Brahma Samaj. People kept coming and going to and from the Samaj like the ebb and flow of the tide, but they were not linked together by a common religious belief. So when the numbers of the Samaj began to increase, I thought it necessary to pick and choose from among them. Some came really to worship, others came without any definite aim, – whom should we recognize as the true worshipper of Brahma? Upon these considerations I decided that those who would take a vow to renounce idolatry and resolve to worship one God, these alone would be regarded as Brahmas. (*Ibid.*: 27)

Bearing in mind the characteristics of cult and sect described in Chapter 1, it will be at once apparent from Tagore's remarks that at first the Brahmo Samaj was based on the free-flowing, loosely structured associationism typical of a cult. As membership swelled and the social profile of the group became more visible, the young leader felt the need to start making more demands on members, insisting, for example, that they should make a public declaration of their commitment by taking a "vow of initiation", i.e. by pronouncing a "declaration of faith for initiation into the Brahma Dharma" (*ibid.*). He felt the need to structure, circumscribe and organize the group by establishing a hierarchy that separated an 'inner circle' of initiates from an 'outer circle' of less committed sympathizers. All these signs clearly indicate an orientational shift from cult- to sect-type voluntaristic associationism, even though the Brahmo Samaj has always been too strongly liberal and/or "spiritualist" to become a fully-fledged, tightly structured, exclusivist sect.

We will further note that Tagore himself shaped the ritual form and doctrinal content of the initiation (*ibid.*: 27–8), which he also underwent, thus effectively initiating himself. The fact of establishing a "vow of initiation" formula is a major shift from traditional practice, as in this fashion the initiation-granting authority is appropriated by the person undergoing the ritual and withdrawn from the transmission lineage (Sanskrit *paraṃparā*). Being initiated becomes a voluntaristic, self-motivated choice as opposed to representing acceptance into a certain socio-religious structure by way of ritual assimilation granted, bestowed and administered by senior members as representatives of authority. Even though Roy's old friend and collaborator Vidyabagish actually officiated at the ceremony, there is no doubt that the Samaj's 'spiritual' authority and decisional power rested in Tagore's hands, a fact amply confirmed by events in Samaj history up to the first (1866) fission, and even up to Tagore's death, if in changing fashion. As we shall see, Vivekananda's (self-)initiation about half a century later is similarly unorthodox, only more so.

Another interesting parallel can be detected between Tagore's followers and Vivekananda's. An "enthusiastic" and emotional atmosphere pervades both groups. The same fervent "spiritualist" approach is found in the latter part of Keshubchandra Sen's career, thus marking out the transmission line from the early Tagore to the late Sen to Vivekananda as the most radically "spiritualist" strand of the Brahmo Samaj. By comparison, other strands of the Samaj will appear more conservative (Adi Brahmo Samaj of the late Tagore) or more concerned with social reform (Sadharan Brahmo Samaj). Tagore's "spiritualism" was, however, much less radical than Sen's and far less secularized than Vivekananda's.

There is much evidence showing the emotional quality of Tagore's Brahmo gatherings. Tagore himself narrates that as he and his friends sat waiting to undergo initiation "a strange enthusiasm was awakened in our breasts" (*ibid.*: 28). He then got up and pronounced his "vow of initiation" in front of Vidyabagish, who, "On hearing [Tagore's] exhortation ... and seeing [his] singleness of purpose, ... shed tears" (*ibid.*). Tagore continues: "the day of initiation into Brahma Dharma was [a] day of days ... [By] taking refuge in Brahma we had entered into the Brahma religion ... Our enthusiasm and delight knew no bounds" (*ibid.*). Two years later 500 persons had taken the vow, among all of whom there was "a wonderful brotherly feeling ... such as is rarely met with even amongst brothers" (*ibid.*: 29). When an all-night anniversary festival was organized at Tagore's gardenhouse at Goriti in the same year (1845) the group's "goodwill, affection and enthusiasm had full play" throughout the night and, when the sun rose, the group "raised a paean of praise to Brahma, and sitting in the shade of a tree adorned with fruit and flowers, [they] delighted and sanctified [themselves] by worshipping God with all [their] heart" (*ibid.*).

An incident that took place in 1848 shows how the quality and mood of congregational life had changed since Roy's time. Following Tagore's reading of a prayerful invocation at a Brahmo meeting he found that his congregation was in tears: "such feelings had never before been witnessed in the Brahma Samaj", he remarked. "Hitherto the severe and sacred flame of knowledge alone had been lighted in Brahma's shrine, now he was worshipped with the flowers of heartfelt love" (*ibid.*: 88). Indeed, as Tagore himself seemed to sense, his 'new' Samaj had shifted from the rationalistic, exoteric, liberal religiosity of Rammohan Roy to a fullness of individualistic motifs and Romantic emotional devotionalism.

About two decades later, in 1866, Keshubchandra Sen would secede from Tagore's Samaj and go on to change the nature of the association even further by establishing his own Brahmo Samaj of

India. This schism fractured the cohesion of the Samaj irreparably, and the group started on a typically culto-sectarian history of fissions and diatribes that would eventually result in a weakening of all Brahmo denominations. As for Tagore, his son Satyendranath reports that "[a]fter Keshab's separation, [he] practically retired from active work in the Samaj" (Tagore, S. 1909: xix). Debendranath Tagore's autobiography, written many years later near the end of his long life, comes to an abrupt halt with his return from the Himalayas in November 1858. Sen and Tagore met early in 1859, but Tagore refrained from reporting on the aftermath of this meeting, which was destined, again according to Satyendranath, "to work a great revolution in the Samaj" (*ibid.*: viii).

From Neo-Vedāntic Romanticism to Neo-Vedāntic "spiritualism"

This is one of the most misunderstood periods of Neo-Vedāntic Hinduism: if esoteric myopia could be compensated for when discussing earlier periods, it would really show up here. During the last quarter of the nineteenth century esoteric ideas became so widespread in educated circles both East and West that historians of religion can hardly avoid coming across one or another of their manifestations. And if they cannot recognize them, or do not have the methodological tools to analyse them, their clarity of vision in discussing the subject is bound to be affected.

A good example of this is David Kopf (1969; 1979), the otherwise outstanding scholar whose works have been used as central secondary sources in the present study. As we saw in the foregoing discussion, this author recognizes and discusses most of the key discourses of the time: Orientalist, Anglicist, Christian, rationalist, humanist, etc. He does not, however, recognize the importance of esoteric developments within Brahmo Samaj ideology. This does not affect his treatment of British Orientalism (Kopf 1969), but becomes marginally noticeable in his treatment of Debendranath Tagore and Dutt (see note 15 above) and very noticeable in his treatment of Sen (Kopf 1979, Chapter 9), in whom Neo-Vedāntic esoteric "spiritualism" finds its full flower.

Kopf's overall appraisal of the Brahmo leader's religious career is revealing in this context: "Keshub's New Dispensation", Kopf states, "was one of the great intellectual achievements of the nineteenth century" *ibid.*: 316). Sen's teachings, however, as we shall see in the remaining part of the present chapter, were not especially novel or unique if seen from the point of view of the ongoing East–West elaboration of esotericism. Also, while Kopf does point to the existence of ideological links between Sen and Vivekananda (*ibid.*: 314, 205), he does not seem to realize how crucial these links were to the formation of the most socio-politically influential form of liberal modern Hinduism, i.e. Neo-Vedānta. It could indeed be argued that if the Sadharan Brahmo Samaj represents the secular substratum of what Kopf (1979) calls the "modern Indian mind", Sen's New Dispensation represents its esoteric one – far less known but nevertheless extremely influential. These two modes of thought, in fact, while opposite, are also strongly complementary in this characteristic *forma mentis*, which casts the foundational esoteric polarity of 'religion' and/vs. 'science' in characteristic Indic mould. The unselfconscious Neo-Vedāntin, not altogether 'religious' and not altogether 'secular', is likely to hold them both at once: albeit in neatly compartmentalized fashion.[17] As we shall see more fully in Chapters 3 and 4, these were the foundations on which Neo-Vedāntic occultism would progressively be built from the last quarter of the nineteenth century onwards.

The Eastern outreaches of Western esotericism

If occultism would start to take root in Bengali cultic milieus from about the 1970s onwards, we should not forget that Western esotericism had been present in the subcontinent for much longer. Freemasonry, which was already becoming established in India by the 1760s,[18] is a good case in point, and possibly much more directly relevant to the shaping of Brahmo ideas and to the formation of Neo-Vedāntic ideology than can be shown here.[19] Freemasonic endeavours would have been highly compatible with, if not similar to, Brahmo religious universalism. Freemasons are in fact "joined

17. See Warrier (2000) for fieldwork evidence clearly pointing in this direction – though this is not the way the author interprets her findings.
18. Lodges had been established in Calcutta (1730), Madras (1752) and Bombay (1758); see Gould (1920: 317).
19. I am not aware of any published material discussing the spread and influence of Freemasonry in India over the last couple of centuries. Any such study would no doubt contain very interesting data.

together in an association based on brotherly love, faith and charity. The one essential qualification for membership is a belief in a supreme being" (Goring 1995: 182). Freemasonry is "non-political" and "open to men of any religion" (*ibid.*), and its leaders think it is "more expedient only to oblige [members] to the religion in which all men agree, leaving their particular Opinions to themselves; that is, to be *good Men and true*, or men of Honour and Honesty, by whatever Denominations or Persuasions they may be distinguished".[20]

From the seventeenth century, Freemasonry was favoured by a substantial number of European aristocrats (Goring 1995: 182), and this tradition seems to have continued in colonial India. The Earl of Moira (later Marquess of Hastings), for example, not only succeeded Lord Minto as Governor-General of India in 1813, but also acted as Grand Masonic Master for that country (Gould 1920: 318). A quarter of a century later in Bombay Dr James Burn laboured "to throw open the portals of Freemasonry to native gentlemen", and his efforts were crowned with success in 1843 with the establishment of the Rising Star of Western India Lodge. By the early 1880s "it was the fashion with the Indians to become members of the Freemasonry. Lawyers, Judges and Government officials were its members. Thus, the membership gave a chance to mix with the high dignitaries and officials."[21] By 1920 there were 183 lodges in the three presidencies (Gould 1920: 318).[22]

Such ideals of religious universalism, however, were not found exclusively among Freemasons. The rationalistic optimism of the Enlightenment had encouraged a number of visionaries and intellectuals to work out their own systems of religiosity and/or of social utopia, as amply demonstrated by Godwin (1994). Some connections can be found between British Orientalists and these innovators as these circles seem to have overlapped, at least to some degree. In 1782, for example, General Charles R. Rainsford, a Freemason,

20. Williams (1974: 15–16, quoting from "Freemasonry" entry in *Encyclopedia Britannica* (Vol. 9; Chicago, 1960: 735)).
21. Williams (1974: 15, quoting Bhupendranath Datta).
22. Presumably 1920, as the source consulted explicitly states that the text was "abridged, revised, rewritten and updated". It has so far not been possible to cross-check this information with the two previous editions (1882–87 (2 vols) and 1903).

> published a call to alchemists, Kabbalists and Freemasons to join a new "Universal Society," intended to "conciliate all doctrines, and even all interests, making constant use of all its talents and directing all its energies to the general wellbeing of the whole Earth, and the particular advantage of the country in which it is established". (*Ibid.*: 104)

One of Rainsford's esoteric associates was Peter Woulfe, who was also a follower of the apocalyptic prophet Richard Brothers (*ibid.*) – the very same visionary that the Orientalist Nathaniel Halhed believed in and championed in the second part of his life (Marshall 1970: 9, 30).[23] We have further seen how other Orientalists had esoteric leanings in Chapter 1.

Far more detailed research would be needed to reconstruct such patterns of connection and interaction and the ways in which these affected Indian religious sentiments. What is clear, however, from a relatively superficial study of the sources is that strong undercurrents of Enlightenment universalism and radical philanthropy, also key ingredients of Sen's religious synthesis, were already well established in Western esoteric discourses by the end of the eighteenth century, when British Orientalism brought its modernizing influence to bear on the Indian subcontinent.[24] The Brahmo Samaj adopted such traditions, along with the liberal and to a degree esoteric creed of Unitarianism, and attempted to give them a Hindu form. From Roy through to Sen and Vivekananda, the Brahmos would shape and defend their Enlightened, Romantic and "spiritualist" Neo-Vedānta, and attempt to defuse the perceived threat of Christianity by absorbing numerous Christian themes and forms into it. These ideological developments were in good part based on the Neo-Vedāntic appropriation of the Western esoteric motif of India's spiritual superiority. Indeed, this ideological theme became an

23. For Halhed's biography see Rocher (1983), who comments: "Halhed often subsumes in his own person the incongruities of his time. The Age of Reason was not free of mystical and aberrant beliefs ... It was troubled by the revelation of Eastern doctrines and life styles, to which it reacted with alternate gusts of enthusiasm and disdain" (*ibid.*: vi).
24. As Kopf points out (1979: 351, note 9), "The universalist aspect of Bengal renaissance ideology has generally been ignored in favor of Westernizing and nationalist aspects" – a lacuna which he tries to fill, but only with limited success as he does not realize that the universalist religious theme is predominantly connected with esoteric discourses.

important weapon in the Neo-Hindu apologetic armoury. Let us see in more detail how this came about.

India responds as 'esoteric Other'

With regards to the West, Troeltsch (1931: 749) describes the rise of "mystic and spiritual religion" (i.e. cultic esotericism) as the rise of the "secret religion of the educated classes". This description could similarly be applied (*mutatis mutandis*) to the emergence of cultic milieus and the propagation of Neo-Vedāntic ideology in India. The Bengali intelligentsia, however, did not need to keep its religion "secret". While Western "spiritualism" and Romantic esotericism were often critical of Christian orthodoxy and orthopraxis, and hence were better not flaunted except in cases of extremism, the corresponding Neo-Hindu forms could easily be presented and interpreted as a moving away from the 'superstitions' and 'idolatry' of classical Hinduism towards a more promising (from a Christian missionary and colonial point of view) 'theism'. What may have appeared as dangerous marginalism bordering on heresy in Europe could easily be read as a turning away from 'heathenism' and a rapprochement towards Christianity in the Indian context. Given enough time, Hindu theists would hopefully turn into Christian converts. From the point of view of a budding Indian nationalism, on the other hand, these discourses could be seen as themes of a renascent Hinduism, a "scientific religion" purified of its outdated traditions through eager acquisition and adaptation of modern approaches to knowledge.

These peculiar conditions produced one important consequence: the ideological space occupied by East–West religious discourses remained remarkably unstructured, as socially authoritative fora capable of monitoring the quality of intellectual production were never created. The elaboration of Neo-Vedāntic ideology, and possibly of Neo-Hindu ideology at large, remained therefore wide open not only to creative experimentation and innovation, but also to dilettantism and egocentric self-affirmation. This trend was reinforced by the gradual shift of British colonial rule from Orientalist to Anglicist policies, a change that further increased the structural divide between socio-political powers and the elaboration of modern Indian religious culture.

Furthermore, by the first half of the nineteenth century a rather Romanticized and mythologized 'India' had also become one of the two main "spiritual" interlocutors of Western esotericism, the other one being 'Egypt'.[25] This tallied with the important motif of the 'gnostic superiority' of Indians. Already adumbrated, as we saw, by Orientalists, this theme was later adopted by Neo-Vedāntins[26] and elaborated into important apologetic motifs such as the one postulating the constructive co-operation of a "spiritual East" and a "materialist West" (King 1978).

If these developments can be seen to have their source in the Western colonial enterprise and especially in the socio-political domination that was part and parcel of British Orientalism, it should not be assumed that Indians did not play an active role in them. Quite the contrary, those Indian minorities that out of interest or choice came to identify themselves with progressive, modernist and liberal ideas – Brahmos foremost among them – immediately started to play an active role in shaping such constructs. And some among them – those that are most relevant to the present discussion – gladly took on the cloak of "spiritual advisers" and "experts", with or without encouragement from Eastern and Western admirers.

It is thus that we witness the appearance of the first Neo-Vedāntic *gurus* (see below), who, with their entourage of practitioners and theorists, started to propagate more or less coherent Neo-Vedāntic teachings within India and, eventually, abroad. These individuals actively contributed to the shaping of some forms of 'alternative religiosity', many of which would in due course come under the umbrella of New Age religion. Both Campbell (1972; 1978) and Hanegraaff (1996) acknowledge as much, but do not discuss the role

25. Both Hanegraaff (1996: 442–62) and Godwin (1994, Chapters 14–17) have traced this theme back to its roots, and have pointed out how it also implied a major conceptual shift away from Christianity:

> Originally, esotericists had pointed to Hermes and Zoroaster as the fountains of a perennial wisdom which had attained to full flower in Christianity. Now, in a secularized climate and under the impact of the new knowledge about Oriental religions, the sources of wisdom were moved increasingly eastward and Christianity was believed not to have fulfilled but to have corrupted them. (Hanegraaff 1996: 448)

The same authors also show how similar ideas were widely popularized by the Theosophical Society (Hanegraaff 1996: 448–55; Godwin 1994, Chapters 14–17). In this context see also Bevir (1994) and, regarding more modern aspects of the same phenomenon, Cox (1979).

26. See, for example, Rammohan Roy who, in 1819, wrote: "by a reference to history it may be proved that the world was indebted to our ancestry for the first dawns of knowledge which sprang in the East" (quoted by Sil 1997: 50).

played by Neo-Vedānta in any detail as they look more closely at the Western rather than at the Oriental or Orient-inspired aspects of this phenomenon.

This, however, creates its own problems, as, for example, in Campbell (1972: 125) where Buddhism and Hinduism are said to be "widely disseminated throughout the cultic milieu" because they have "mysticism as their central ingredient". Here Campbell fails to realize that what he is discussing are not these religions in their totality, but Neo-Buddhist[27] and Neo-Vedāntic versions of them, i.e. the characterizations of Hinduism and Buddhism most frequently found in the cultic milieu. These are represented as overwhelmingly spiritual and mystical, while the more complex, culturally and chronologically layered religious contents that are rooted in the traditions' classical periods are usually left out or over-simplified. And while contemporary representatives of classical Hinduism are likely to consider Neo-Vedāntic spokespersons hardly authoritative in matters of religion, the liberal, modernist and revivalistic factions which propagate the ideological core of Neo-Vedānta in the contemporary world are the most vocal (and anglophone) on the global stage, and have no compunction in suggesting that their own views are representative of Hinduism as a whole. Thus many who do not have the time or inclination to examine these groups' claims end up believing that Neo-Vedānta is all Hinduism is about.

As previously mentioned, however, more critical and discriminating studies on Neo-Vedānta and related subjects are starting to appear. This will no doubt help to shed light on important aspects of modern religiosity East and West, including Modern Yoga and the flourishing of modern-style meditative practices. In this context, the following discussion on our next Brahmo leader will prove of special relevance.

27. Here I am implying that different but somewhat comparable processes of modernization have happened in Buddhist contexts. For interesting pointers in this direction see Gombrich and Obeyesekere (1988) and Sharf (1995).

Sen as charismatic Neo-Vedāntic leader

Keshubchandra Sen played an important role in the elaboration of Neo-Vedāntic constructs: generally as ideological forerunner of Vivekananda and more specifically as creator of prototypical forms of Modern Yoga.[28] Chronologically and ideologically positioned between Tagore's Neo-Vedāntic Romanticism and Vivekananda's Neo-Vedāntic occultism, Sen progressed throughout his life from the former towards the latter, despite having introduced "enthusiastic" Neo-Vaishnava devotionalism into the ritual life of the Brahmo Samaj. Indeed, such forms of devotionalism should be understood as attempts to compensate for the sense of disenchantment brought about by the rationalistic interpretations of religion which were becoming common at the time: throughout Sen's most active years (1858 to 1884), the secular spirit started to penetrate Western culture in depth[29] and, as usual, Bengal followed closely.

Born in Calcutta in 1838, Sen died at the relatively early age of 45 on 8 January 1884. By all accounts he was endowed not only with great energy and a very dynamic character, but also with an extremely charismatic personality. Kopf (1979: xvi), for example, credits him with having gathered some of the best men into Brahmoism from 1860 onwards. Debendranath Tagore stated that "Whatever [Sen] thought in his mind, he had the power to express in speech. Whatever he said, he had the power to do. Whatever he did, he had the power of making other men do" (as quoted in Sen 1938: 29). Both Tagore and Sen's closest collaborator Protapchandra Mozoomdar refer admiringly to his handsome physique and striking presence (Kopf 1979: 259; Sen 1938: 51). These impressions are confirmed by two photographs showing a handsome, well-groomed man bearing a resolute and self-assured expression and having obvious stage presence (see Figure 4 for one of them, for the other see Sen 1938: facing page 100). Just like Vivekananda, Sen was known for being a good actor (Kopf 1979: 254; Sen 1938: 18). All of these

28. Following my specific analytical bias, I will mainly endeavour to expose the generally little known cultic and esoteric aspects of Sen's life. For a somewhat hagiographic overview of his life see the well-structured work by Sen (1938); for a similar account, but from a liberal Christian missionary point of view see Slater (1884); for a sympathetic scholarly appraisal see Kopf (1979, Chapter 9 and *passim*). A very synthetic overview of Brahmo history, including Sen's ideological developments, may be found in *ibid.* (pp. xxi–xxiii).

29. See Chadwick (1990: 18), who points out that the forty years between 1859 and the end of the century were crucial in this respect.

characteristics, along with his rhetorical abilities and perfect command of English, must have much enhanced his leadership qualities and charismatic potential.

Sen's charisma was also felt in the West: the Orientalist Max Müller describes the deep impression made by Sen on the British public during his 1870 visit to Britain:[30] "I have been struck, when lecturing in different places, to find that the mere mention of Keshub Chunder Sen's name elicited applause for which I was hardly prepared" (reported in Sen 1938: 77). Sen toured and lectured extensively during this visit, and the accounts of his trip clearly show that he was lionized by both liberal Christians and, in somewhat lesser measure, by esoteric groups such as the Swedenborg Society (*ibid.*: 83). His biographer reports that "invitations poured in to preach from Unitarian and Congregationalist pulpits" (*ibid.*) but, following the tradition established with Roy, Unitarians were the most supportive of, and interested in, the Brahmo leader (*ibid.*: 87). As soon as Sen returned to India there was a new flurry of "lectures, pamphlets, propaganda, open letters to the authorities, newspaper agitation, resort to legislation" (*ibid.*: 101).

Sen was not only a born leader, but also an activist: starting in 1854 at sixteen years of age and hardly stopping throughout his life, he "establish[ed] schools, classes, societies and fraternities" (*ibid.*: 11). In youth, as in his more mature age, he "founded them, fostered them, unremittingly worked for them ... turning his associates into ardent fellow workers under his guidance" (*ibid.*: 11–12). From 1859 or 1860 onwards he regularly gave highly exhortative (and later in life emotional) *extempore* speeches and sermons (*ibid.*: 19, 28), and these were published and circulated in a Bengal where, in Sen's own words, the number of "improvement societies, friendly meetings, debating clubs, literary associations, etc. ... [was] hourly increasing" (*ibid.*: 20). By 1865 his Brahmo "mission work proceeded apace, more educational institutions sprang up, and tracts and pamphlets multiplied. There was no end of activity" (*ibid.*: 53). He seems indeed to have contributed enthusiastically to the "over-lapping communications structures" of the nineteenth-century Bengali cultic milieu.

30. Sen sailed from India on 15 February 1870, reached London on 21 March 1870 and was back in Calcutta on 20 October 1870 (Sen 1938: 74, 104). Regarding Sen's visit to Britain see also Collett (1871).

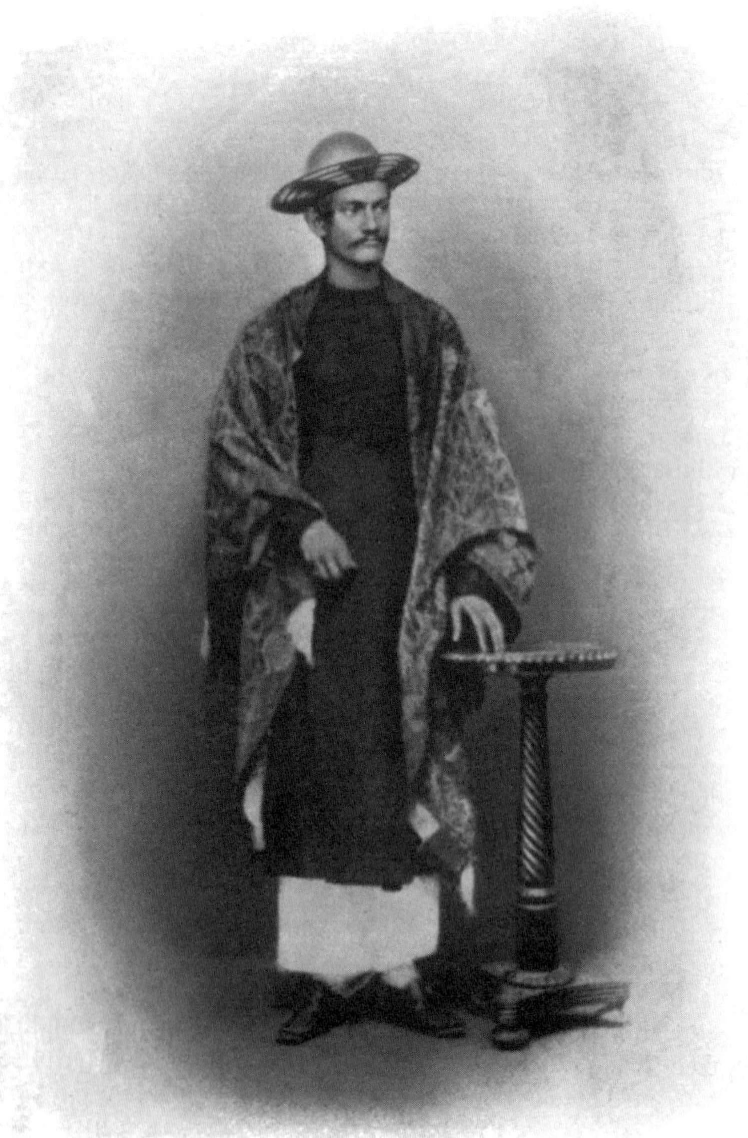

Figure 4 Keshubchandra Sen in 1859. From Sen, P.K. (1938) *Keshub Chunder Sen*. Keshub's Birth Centenary Committee, Calcutta. (By permission of the Syndics of Cambridge University Library)

Sen's religious career

Most of the religious associations established by Sen were highly cultic in nature, with a very loose structural organization effectively centering on Sen himself, always the undisputed leader. One of the earlier ones, the Sangat Sabha, was established in 1860 as a "circle for intimate spiritual fellowship" (*ibid.*: 25). Protapchandra Mozoomdar, future Brahmo leader and one of the participants, describes how the group was composed of "steadfast followers of Keshub", who

> met frequently, and with fiery zeal of self-reformation, laid bare their whole hearts, freely and frankly discussing their own faults, courted mutual aid and criticism, and under Keshub's guidance made most genuine progress in spiritual and moral life ... in them Keshub found congenial spirits; he magnetised them; they magnetised him; and together they formed a nucleus of organisation out of which the best materials of Keshub's subsequent movements were supplied. (Quoted in *ibid.*: 25–6)

As for administrative procedures, Sen (*ibid.*: 25) states that "There were no fixed hours, no formalities observed, ... no restraints, no programme ... It was soul-force that brought them together ... and determined the proceedings of the Sabha."

Sen relied on this type of unstructured, voluntary, inward-looking associationism, typical of cults, throughout his life. When he seceded from Tagore to form his own Brahmo Samaj of India in 1866, for example, "there was no constitution, no governing body, no rules. Everything was left in Keshab's hands" (Farquhar 1977 [1914]: 46). This, however, meant that his groups were only held together by his charisma, and that they would have fallen apart without him – as they in fact did: Hay (1988: 46) reports that "Of Keshub's work little remained after his death in 1884." Even more to the point, a contemporary Brahmo (Naidu 1895: 20) commented: "The present condition of the Samaj is very deplorable. Since the death of Keshub dissensions among his followers and disunion among his missionaries prevail ... Each missionary does his own work in his own way."[31]

Throughout the middle part of his career, however, Sen tried to

31. Cf. also Slater (1884: 133) and Kopf (1979: 284–5) with regard to problems between Mozoomdar and Keshubchandra Sen's family after Sen's death.

provide Brahmoism with stronger doctrinal structures. He sought, for example, to formulate a viable Brahmo theology by repeatedly attempting (1859, 1867 and 1871) to establish a Brahmo theological school.[32] These ventures failed because the interested parties could not resolve "the conflict between individual religious experience and systematic knowledge" (Kopf 1979: 79): obviously a problem rooted in the Samaj's strong cultic bias, or in what Kopf describes as "a certain prevailing resistance by Brahmos to the intellectualization of their faith and the crystallization of its main ideas into a commonly held theology" (*ibid.*: 82). This is confirmed by contemporary primary sources: aspiring theologians were accused of expecting the Samaj to give up "justification of [*sic*] faith, right of private judgement, priesthood of every believer, and all other achievements of the reformation", and of leading it towards "dry intellectualism" and "scholasticism among a few".[33] This strong anti-intellectualism and the Christian ideological bias reflected in the choice of terminology will remain prominent characteristics of esoteric and occultistic Neo-Vedānta.

In 1875, Sen met Ramakrishna (Sen 1938: 117), who was thus introduced to Brahmo circles and, through them, to the world. The two relished each other's company, and Ramakrishna's influence and example surely played a part in leading Sen to adopt even more radical "spiritualist" views and practices: by 1876 Sen "had retreated almost full circle to an antitheological position", and "was no longer interested in active social reform but had turned instead to meditation and the comparative study of major religions" (Kopf 1979: 79, 139). In the meantime a substantial number of Sen's followers started to resent their leader's complete centralization of power, and his justification of some of his actions by asserting that he was the recipient of "adesh or direct messages from God" (*ibid.*: 139). This led to a split in the Samaj, the seceding group going on to establish the more moderate and socially engaged Sadharan Brahmo Samaj in 1878.

So far we have highlighted the strong cultic and charismatic characteristics of Sen's movement. While these were definitely the more prominent, we also find that some sectarian tendencies did emerge in

32. The first attempt was carried out by Debendranath Tagore and Keshubchandra Sen together, the second and third by Sen only (Kopf 1979: 79).
33. Kopf (1979: 83) quoting K. S. Ghose, *The Rise of Scholasticism in the Brahmo Samaj* (Calcutta: Naba-bidhan Publications Committee, 1940).

the association from the beginning of the 1870s, showing most notably in the establishment of lay religious communities. These tendencies never took over the movement completely, possibly also due to Sen's early demise, but they were significant in that they provided the human and institutional context in and through which Sen could elaborate his unique doctrinal and ritual innovations.

These lay religious communities started off by drawing inspiration from Protestant liberal and "spiritual" Christianity, but eventually emerged as truly acculturated Neo-Vedāntic institutions. The two prototypical communities founded by Sen show us this developmental pattern. The first one, called *Bharat Ashram*,[34] was established in February 1872, lasted for five years and was strongly influenced by the "Unitarian gospel of social reform" that Sen was following at the time. As Mozoomdar (quoted in Sen 1938: 113) points out, this first ashram was important because from it "began the steady development of the apostolic community which almost to the last day of his life formed Keshub's great ambition".

The second community, more interesting with regard to our discussion of Modern Yoga, was established in 1876 in the village of Morepukur near Calcutta. Called *Sadhan Kanan*,[35] this institution showed substantial signs of acculturation, and may be regarded as prototypical of the Neo-*Sannyāsa*[36] ashrams that are currently found all over India and wherever else Neo-Vedāntic Hinduism has struck root. Established shortly after Sen had turned his back on the idea of "social gospel", this institution placed "[v]ery great stress ... on meditation and retirement from the world" (Sastri 1911: 270). It is in this context that Sen started to formulate more universalistic and eclectic forms of Neo-Vedāntic religiosity including, as we shall see shortly, prototypical forms of Modern Yoga.

34. "Indian hermitage". The Sanskrit term *āśrama* is the traditional name used to describe the forest dwelling of sages and anchorites.
35. "Forest abode for religious practice" or, in more emic terms, "for spiritual culture".
36. Meaning Neo-Vedāntic renunciation. Neo-*Sannyāsa* may be seen as the evolved and institutionalized monastic form of Roy's *gṛhastha brahmavādin*, to which Tagore contributed Neo-Vedāntic initiation and Vivekananda Neo-Vedāntic renunciation. Vivekananda himself will define what a Neo-*Sannyāsin* is by telling his monks: "You are not like ordinary worldly men – neither householders, nor exactly Sannyasins – but *quite a new type*" (*CW* 7: 222, emphasis added). For comments on the more secular version of Roy's original concept see note 37, Chapter 1.

The semantic range of the term may overlap with what is called *brahmacarya* (the individual being called a *brahmacārin*) in Neo-Vedāntic circles, meaning various degrees of lay renunciation. Cf. also Gombrich and Obeyesekere (1988: 205–6, 216–18) with regard to the corresponding modern Buddhist phenomenon, called *anāgarika*.

By 1880 Sen was approaching the culmination of his religious career, and in the four years preceding his death his utterances became increasingly emotional in tone, hyperbolic in style and "spiritualist" in content. He also started to elaborate peculiarly Neo-Vedāntic forms of ritual and religious symbolism. This is strikingly evident in a report of how he proclaimed his "New Dispensation" doctrine in January 1881:

> [Sen] appeared on the platform, with twelve of his missionaries around him, under a new red banner, on which were inscribed the words Naba Bidhan (Nava Vidhāna), that is, New Dispensation, and also an extraordinary symbol made up of the Hindu trident, the Christian cross and the crescent of Islam. On the table lay the Scriptures of the four greatest religions of the world, Hinduism, Buddhism, Christianity and Muḥammadanism. Four of the apostles were specially appointed that each might study the Scriptures of one of these religions. Henceforward, the phrase Brāhma Samāj falls into the background, and Keshab's body is known as *The Church of the New Dispensation*. (Farquhar 1977 [1914]: 56)

Turning more and more towards "enthusiastic" and syncretic forms of belief, Sen was soon affirming that his Nava Vidhan was the culmination of Judaism and Christianity. In 1882 he proclaimed that "[t]he Old Testament was the First Dispensation; the New Testament the Second; unto us in these days has been vouchsafed the Third Dispensation", that is, his own church (quoted in *ibid.*: 63). As Lavan (1995: 17) summarizes, "what Keshub was doing was truly radical within Hinduism – [providing] an apologetic and new dimension of eclecticism for his faith".[37]

The influence of American Transcendentalism

Sen's "eclecticism" was mainly based on a universalistic and religionist interpretation of the modern discipline of comparative religion: a theoretical approach that he inherited from Tagore's Neo-Vedānta and which was reinforced by Transcendentalist influences. As for the apologetic contents of his thought, consisting of his direct and indirect claims that Hinduism was the most advanced religion in

37. For a detailed analysis of the second half of Sen's life, including the emergence of his "New Dispensation", see Damen (1983).

'spiritual' terms, this was based on his appropriation and powerful application of the esoteric motif of India's spiritual superiority.

It is important here to acknowledge fully the influence of Transcendentalist ideas, as these were crucial in shaping Sen's thought and that of many other Brahmos during the second part of the nineteenth century. A very direct influence was exerted by the Unitarian missionary Charles Dall, who arrived in India in 1855 and became a close friend of Sen, then only a youth. It was through Dall's efforts that "thousands of copies of the complete works of Channing, Emerson and Parker were circulated among Brahmos" (Kopf 1979: 16), and we know that as early as 1858 Sen was drawing from the writings of Parker and Emerson to prepare his lectures (*ibid.*: 30).

American Transcendentalists greatly emphasized 'intuition' and 'true reason' (as opposed to analytical understanding) as sources of knowledge. They were also convinced that the new discipline of comparative religion would prove the concordance of all religious traditions, and that such findings would lead humanity to a higher religious synthesis. Of all non-Christian religions they admired Hinduism most, and it will be remembered that one of them, Thoreau, was the first recorded Westerner to claim, in 1849, to be practising yoga. Emerson's Romantic idealism and especially his concept of the Over-Soul, allowing for a diffused but personally accessible dimension of the divine, were particularly influential. Emerson believed that by cultivating self-reliance and self-development all human beings could attune themselves to the Over-Soul, and thence draw inspiration, guidance and support. This 'inward turn' of Emersonian philosophy, placing a direct point of access to the metaphysical in each individual's psyche, lies at the root of Hanegraaff's third 'mirror' of secularization, concerning the psychologization of religion. This trend is also visible in Sen's thought, as he is the first to introduce this important element in Neo-Vedānta.

Some of these innovative concepts were already part of Sen's thought early on in his religious career, and can be found in the first series of lectures that he delivered when about twenty-two years old.[38] Here we can already see his enthusiastic temper and charismatic drive, his passion for modernity, his "spiritualist" inclinations (now turning psychological), and his vision of a new type of reli-

38. Twelve lectures were delivered and published in the form of monthly tracts ("Tracts for the Times") starting June 1860 (Sen 1938: 19, 147).

giosity that would combine all these elements into one. In the lecture entitled "Signs of the Times", he affirms:

> Freedom and progress are the watch-words of the 19th century. It is likewise beginning to be felt that true faith does not consist in an intellectual assent to historical events, but in earnest and steady reliance upon the ever-living, ever-present Deity ... Many an earnest soul is strenuously protesting against the worship of the "dead letter" – antiquated symbols, and lifeless dogmas, and vindicating the living revelations of the spirit within ... A strong yearning after the living and the spiritual is thus clearly manifest. Nor, again, does the controversial and jealous spirit of sectarian dogmatism fall in with the catholic views of the age. History has portrayed in frightful colours the mischievous effects of sectarianism, and has fully proved that *opinion* cannot serve as the bond of religious confraternity – that which is local, contingent and specific cannot constitute the basis of a church. Such a church as stands upon what is above time and place – upon catholic principles of Faith and Love, such a church as shall establish the brotherhood of man, many are looking forward to with eager expectations. (Quoted in Sen 1938: 22–3)

Sen's decidedly anti-intellectual recommendations are offset in his thought by a reliance on "subjective revelation", which he opposes to "book revelation" and defines psychologically as "a state of mind, an actual fact of consciousness".[39] He affirms: "We account revelation as the only way through which we come in contact with the saving truths of the spiritual world" (*ibid.*: 23). Such revelation he also refers to as "intuition" and "inspiration" in his contemporary and later work.[40] He further assigns a "primary" and a "secondary" meaning to the term "revelation":

> ... if revelation is taken in its primary and literal signification, viz., knowledge communicated by God, it is possible only as a fact of mind, and cannot therefore be identified with books or other external objects ... If on the other hand revelation is understood in the secondary acceptation, viz., whatever teaches us precious doctrines, and elevates

39. Eleventh tract, on "Revelation" (Sen 1938: 23). We may also note that the eighth and the ninth tracts are entitled "Testimonies to the Validity of Intuitions", nos I and II (*ibid.*: 147).
40. Slater (1884: 170) points out that Sen's doctrine of "intuition" is "similar to that propounded by [the Unitarians] Mr. Theodore Parker and Mr. F. W. Newman" (*ibid.*), and also compares it to Victor Cousin's doctrine of religious intuition (*ibid.*: 171).

our moral and religious conceptions and feelings, far from being confined to the texts of any particular book as the exclusive sacred repository of divine truth, it extends over all books that inculcate truth – nay it embraces the whole universe as a living revelation. Such is our doctrine of revelation. (Quoted in Sen 1938: 23–4)

The whole programmatic "spiritual" and esoteric agenda of Keshubchandra Sen is already here in a nutshell. However, in the following years Sen would amplify it, developing Tagore's themes of evolutionary and "scientific" religiosity in their ethical and "spiritual" implications. He would also embellish his teachings with a mixture of Hindu, Christian and comparative religion motifs and, with the help of his missionaries,[41] enthusiastically propagate them throughout the Indian subcontinent. This same message would be eagerly interiorized by Vivekananda, who, as we shall see, will develop it in his own specific ways. Through Vivekananda and his Ramakrishna movement, finally, the Neo-Vedāntic message will spread widely both in India and in the West.

But Sen's most momentous, indeed paradigmatic shift must be seen to be in the epistemological domain: from Tagore's 'selective' intuition of revelation based on Hindu canonical (if no longer infallible) texts Sen progresses to a Transcendentalism-inspired concept of individual experiential revelation defined psychologically as "a state of mind". With this conceptual step the transfer of religious authority from 'outer' sources (metaphysical, but socially upheld and validated) to 'inner' ones (individually induced and validated) is completed.[42] It will be pre-eminently on the strength of this shift that Modern Yoga will be conceptualized as the experiential core of a universalistic "scientific religion" (Sen/Dutt) and as the empirical, "scientifically worked out" method to access such an experience (Vivekananda CW 1: 128).

Sen's proto Modern Yoga

Sen's re-elaboration of the esoteric motif of India's spiritual superiority took place relatively late in his life: it consisted, most importantly, of a revivalistic interpretation of yoga as best method and core

41. Sen first conceived the idea of a Brahmo missionary effort in 1861 (Kopf 1979: 258), and renewed his efforts in this sense after seceding from Tagore in 1866 (*ibid.*: 318–19).
42. This central development of Neo-Vedāntic ideas is discussed from a linguistic and semantic angle in Chapter 4.

achievement of all religious striving. This change in religious idiom may be illustrated by comparing two further photographic portraits of the Brahmo leader. In the earlier one Sen is shown in prayerful attitude, with hands joined and eyes cast heavenward, in altogether Christian iconic mode (Figure 5); in the latter, taken the year before his death, he is portrayed in the cross-legged attitude of the yogi sitting among greenery on a tiger skin and with a renouncer's pot (*kamaṇḍalu*) beside him (Figure 6). Considering that he was a progressive, highly Anglicized householder with no monastic affiliation whatsoever, this style of portraiture must have been highly unconventional indeed.

Sen's revivalistic interpretation of yoga had a more theoretical and a more practical side. With regard to the former, we saw above how Sen made a distinction between "primary" and "secondary" types of revelation in the lectures he delivered as a young man. Eventually, in 1869, Sen would systematize what he saw as different types of "revelation" into a threefold model of the ways in which "God manifests Himself to us". These were: "through external nature, through the inner spirit, and through moral greatness impersonated in man" (Sen 1901: 143), or through nature, "inspiration"[43] and history. As will be noted, manifestation through "nature" and "history" allows Sen to integrate modern knowledge[44] into his belief system. "Inspiration" through the inner spirit, however (or primary "revelation" or "intuition"), is repeatedly stated to be the most powerful, complete and valid type of religious experience, the other two being classified as secondary:

> Nothing ... can bear comparison with the almighty power of Inspiration – the direct breathing of God's spirit – which infuses an altogether new life into the soul and exalts it above all that is earthly and impure. It is the more powerful, being God's direct and immediate action on the human soul, while the revelation through physical nature and biography [i.e. history] is indirect and mediate ... The highest revelation ... is inspiration, where the spirit communes with the spirit face to face without any mediation whatsoever. (Sen 1901: 89–90)

If up to this relatively early lecture (1866) Sen was still elaborating

43. Or "communion with God in the soul" (Sen 1885: 4).
44. More specifically an idealist view of history (along the lines of Hegel and Schlegel, where history is seen as an expression of the divine) and a mixture of Romantic and positivist views of science.

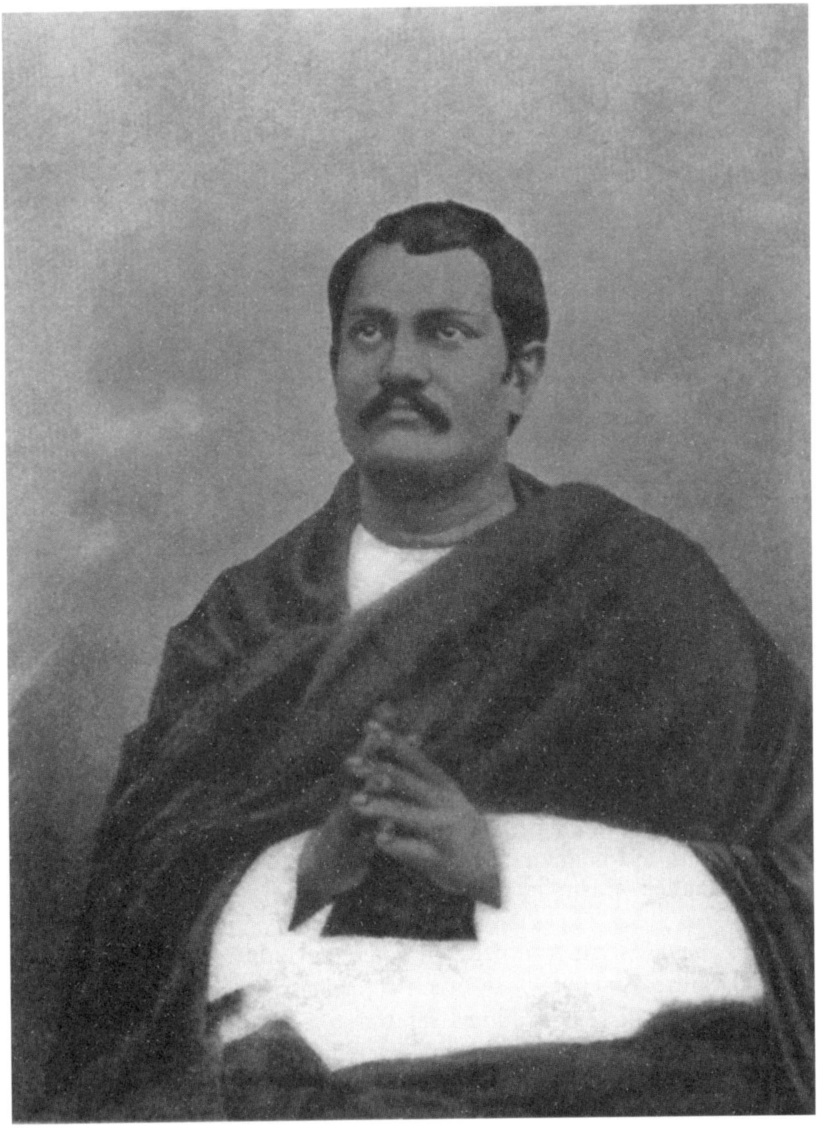

Figure 5 Keshubchandra Sen at prayer. From Sen, P.K. (1938) *Keshub Chunder Sen*. Keshub's Birth Centenary Committee, Calcutta. (By permission of the Syndics of Cambridge University Library)

what was his own variation of Transcendentalist philosophy, by 1875 the more peculiarly Neo-Vedāntic slant that his theories were taking was becoming apparent:

> The subtle Hindu mind has always been distinguished for its spirituality. It penetrates the hard surface of dogmatic theology, and evolves and deals with the deeper realities of faith. It loves communion with the Spirit, and abhors matter as an unreality ... The idea of perceiving the Indwelling Spirit, far from being foreign, is eminently native to the primitive Hindu mind. (Sen 1901: 207)

We see that Sen starts to build his Neo-Vedāntic apologetics on the more esoteric layers of Transcendentalism by representing "the Hindu mind" as pre-eminently spiritual and as peculiarly gifted in its ability to access "revelation".

The following year, 1876, Sen was to translate such theories into practice. This was also the year in which the *Sadhan Kanan* was established. Sivanath Sastri provides us with an interesting sketch of life at the *Kanan*:

> Here many of the missionaries of the Samaj spent with him [Sen] most of the days of the week in meditation and prayer, in cooking their own food, in drawing water, in cutting bamboos, in making and paving roads, in constructing their cabins, in planting and watering trees, and in cleansing their bedrooms. As marks of their asceticism they began to sit below trees on carpets made of the hides of tigers and of other animals, in imitation of Hindu mendicants and spend long hours in meditation. (Sastri 1911: 270)

This, as previously mentioned, sounds remarkably like contemporary Neo-Vedāntic ashrams, with much constructive '*karmayoga*'[45] being carried out, and regular times set out for devotional and spiritual practice. Such a set-up would, however, have been highly innovative at the time. Sastri's evident perplexity about Sen and his associates spending time "meditating *in imitation* of Hindu mendicants" must have been shared by many of his contemporaries. Sastri continues:

> It was towards the end of this year that Mr. Sen introduced a fourfold classification of devotees. He chose from amongst his missionaries four

45. I.e., ideally, 'work carried out carefully, selflessly and joyfully for the sake of the community' in contemporary Neo-Vedāntic diction.

> different sets of men to represent four types of religious life. The *Yogi*, or the adept in rapt communion, the *Bhakta*, or the adept in rapturous love of God, the *Jnani*, or the earnest seeker of true knowledge and the *Shebak*, or the active servant of humanity. These four orders were constituted and four different kinds of lessons were given to the disciples of the respective classes. (*ibid.*: 270–1)[46]

We already heard with regard to the elaboration of Dutt's Brahmo ethic that "All true worshippers of God [should] practice [sic] meditation, devotion, acquire knowledge and do good to others" (see section on "Scientific religion" earlier in this chapter). Now Sen took up this lead to provide his community with a system of practice catering for all "four types of religious life". Dutt and Sen, in other words, were striving to define new schemes of religious and ritual life, schemes that would suit the secularized mentality of the last quarter of the nineteenth century. As in the case of Vivekananda's *sannyāsins*, it was a matter of finding "a new type" (see note 36 above). In Sen's fourfold system of practice we find the prototypical form of what will later become a core teaching of Modern Yoga, i.e. Vivekananda's model of the '4 yogas' (*Rāja-, Bhakti-, Jñāna-* and *Karma-yoga*).

It is also at the *Sadhan Kanan* that we find the young Narendranath Datta, the future Swami Vivekananda, enthusiastically partaking of the Brahmo religious life. Much evidence suggests that by the time he turned twenty-one he had already assimilated not only the full range of Brahmo teachings, including Sen's own, but also the latter's flamboyant style. We further know that the future Vivekananda remained in Sen's entourage up to the time of the latter's death (see next chapter), and that he seriously entertained the idea of becoming

46. As this is a central point, and little known, Slater's version of the fourfold division will also be given:

> In 1876, this movement took a new and more definite form in the 'Classification of Devotees' ... This classification is fourfold, and comprises *yoga*, or intense contemplative communion with the Divine Spirit; *bhakti*, or love of God; *gyān*, or study, research, and thought; and *seba* or *karma*, the service of fellow men. The *yogī* (one who cultivates *yoga*) lives in the spirit world, and aims at the subjugation of his nature. The *bhakta* loses himself in intense love for God. The *sebak* delights in active deeds of benevolence. Special initiative services are held for those who wish to enter the several departments. Into the fourth class we find Brahmic ladies have been initiated. (1884: 78; Slater quotes as his sources the *Theistic Annual* for 1877 and the *Indian Mirror*, 27 February 1876)

The above report is especially interesting as it highlights the modern usage of *seva* and *karma* as synonyms. This semantic shift happened most likely through Christian influences with the Victorian concept of 'good works' acting as the conceptual link between *karma* and *seva*.

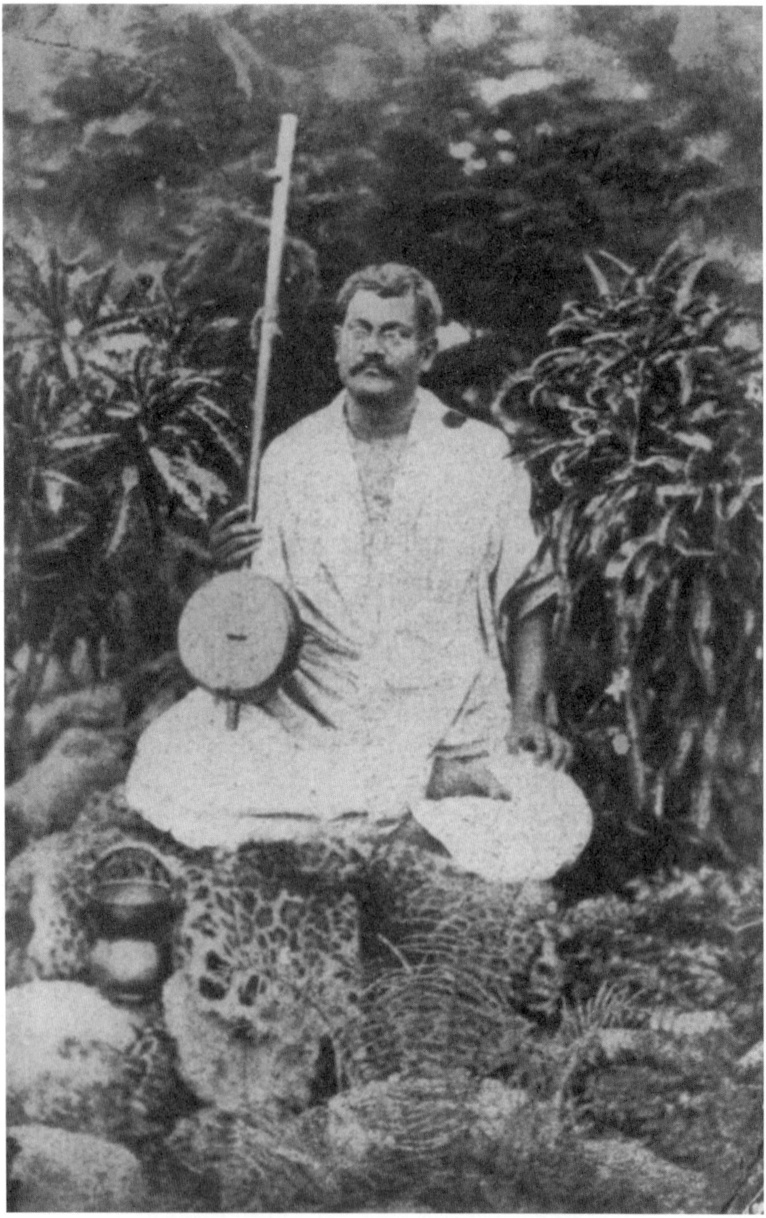

Figure 6 Keshubchandra Sen at Simla, 1883. From Sen, P.K. (1938) *Keshub Chunder Sen*. Keshub's Birth Centenary Committee, Calcutta. (By permission of the Syndics of Cambridge University Library)

one of Sen's missionaries.[47] Despite his later repudiation of Brahmoism,[48] ideologically speaking Vivekananda's Ramakrishna movement should be seen as a most successful continuation (and implementation) of Brahmo ideology drawing from both Nava Vidhan and Sadharan branches of the Samaj. All these developments, crucial to the future development of Neo-Vedāntic Hinduism (and of Modern Yoga), will be discussed in more detail in the next chapter.

As for Sen, his apologetic and revivalistic formulation of yoga grew even stronger in the period before his death. By 1881, while preaching the creed of his New Dispensation, we find that Sen characterizes "Hindus" not so much as having developed an outstanding tradition of adeptness in yoga practice, but as actually possessing an almost genetically in-built "yoga faculty":

> We Hindus are specially endowed with, and distinguished for, the yoga faculty, which is nothing but this power of spiritual communion and absorption. This faculty, which we have inherited from our forefathers, enables us to annihilate space and time... (Sen 1901: 484)

It was the cultivation of this "yoga faculty" that concerned him more and more towards the end of his life, and when he passed away he left unfinished a text on the subject (Sen 1885).

This concern tallied with his long-held theory of 'divine humanity', a well-known Swedenborgian theme that would surely have been represented among the many intellectual currents found in the Calcutta cultic milieu. Thus as early as 1866 he was applying the Christian concept of the incarnation to the whole of humanity: "True incarnation is not ... the absolute perfection of the divine nature embodied in mortal form ... It simply means God manifest in humanity; – not God made man, but God *in* man ..." (Sen 1901: 61). "For it must be admitted," he further reasoned, "that every man is, in some measure, an incarnation of the divine spirit ... If, then, incarnation means the spirit of God manifest in human flesh, certainly every man is an incarnation" (*ibid.*: 62–3). Towards the end of his life, Sen had come to see the "yoga faculty" as the means to access such 'divinity' and to make it operative in the world.

By this stage proto Modern Yoga and the "spiritual power" of the

47. See introductory quotation to next chapter.
48. Cf., for example, *CW* 6: 263; *CW* 8: 477–8; *CW* 9: 22.

"Hindu mind" had become powerful apologetic themes in a world of divided ideologies and contrasting allegiances. As such, they were to become one of the most effective rhetorical weapons of Neo-Vedāntic esotericism. This is what they continue to be up to the present day, though each interpreter puts them to a different use depending on inclination and circumstance. One of the most famous of these interpreters, and indeed the creator of fully-fledged Modern Yoga, was the Swami Vivekananda. It is to him that we now turn.

3. Vivekananda and the emergence of Neo-Vedāntic occultism

But for Ramakrishna I would have been a Brahmo missionary.
(Swami Vivekananda)[1]

The previous chapter has highlighted some of the ways in which Neo-Vedānta developed throughout the first three quarters of the nineteenth century. By 1875 this modernized tradition was being represented by apologists both East and West as an exemplary form of spirituality. An ideology of self-perfecting voluntarism and ethical activism sustained the Brahmo ethic, while more secular discourses gravitated towards definitions of religion as "scientific" and progressive, towards utilitarianism and towards the individualization and psychologization of spiritual experience. It is at this time that Narendranath Datta, the future Swami Vivekananda, comes on the scene (Figures 7, 8 and 9). Born on 12 January 1863 in Calcutta (Jackson 1994: 22), the Swami achieved fame in the West, and an almost mythical status in India, where he is still respected and revered by many as, among other things, the harbinger of a modern and dynamic form of missionary Hinduism to the West.

1. As reported by Vivekananda's brother (quoted in Williams (1974: 15 and 1995b: 378)).

Vivekananda: spiritual hero or esoteric seeker?

Swami Vivekananda did indeed play a pivotal role in the context of Neo-Vedāntic esotericism and of Modern Yoga. Not quite a Neo-Hindu philosopher, not quite a militant nationalist, he nevertheless became a cult figure and a popular ideologue in both fields. Most of all, however, he was the first Indian to succeed in acting as an effectual bridge-builder between Eastern and Western esoteric milieus, much as Unitarians and Theosophists had done the other way around. In a way, he was the proud nationalistic and indigenous counterpart of these groups. This explains why he has been adopted by popular mythology as the archetypal nationalistic religious hero, whereas an important body like the Brahmo Samaj was never included in the religio-nationalistic pantheon, despite the fact that it was politically and institutionally far more influential.[2]

A substantial amount of literature has been produced over time on Vivekananda and his work. The overwhelming majority of these studies is hagiographic in tone, while a fraction of them, based on more stringent critical and historical methods, concur on showing the Swami as a much more tormented and paradoxical individual.[3] These different readings are well exemplified by two schematic overviews of Vivekananda's life provided by Williams (1995b: 373) and reproduced below. They will allow the reader to operate an instant comparison.

2. See Kopf (1979) concerning the last affirmation.

3. Narasingha P. Sil (1997: 23–5) discusses these sources, and makes a clear case for the need and importance of further studies along these lines (*ibid.*: 11–13). Rambachan (1994), while not a biographical study, should be consulted by anyone interested in an in-depth discussion of Vivekananda's ideas and of their influence within the context of modern and contemporary forms of Hinduism.

Sil's careful (if cutting) discussion (1997) has two great advantages: firstly, its author compares and contrasts specific aspects of classical and modern Hinduism so as to highlight which is which (as does Rambachan; this is an obvious but often neglected procedure). Secondly, Sil makes extensive use of essential (and sometimes recent) Bengali sources without which it would be nearly impossible to compose a realistic picture of the subject. As Sil himself states (*ibid.*: 12): "It is absolutely essential that Vivekananda's achievements be assessed after a careful perusal of all extant sources, especially those in Bengali ... [A]ny uncritical reliance on the existing translations is bound to be precarious, because most often those authorized by the Ramakrishna Order have been doctored or censored." For further sources see below and notes 38 and 40, Chapter 1.

(1) Archetype of the spiritual hero	**(2) Historical periods of doubt and faith**
I. Wondrous Child: – visions – meditations	I. Childhood: 1863–78
II. Exceptional College Student: – master of Western thought – independent thinker	II. College: 1879–86 – Brahmo Samaj – Freemason – Sceptic
III. Carefully trained by Sri Ramakrishna	III. Ramakrishna's disciple: 1886–89
IV. Warrior Monk: – conquers West – awakens India	IV. Renewed search: 1889–90 V. Break with Ramakrishna *gurubhāis*: 1890 – re-establishing contact from America: 1894 – return and founding of Order: 1897–1902

Variations will be found across different authors as to the detail of the above two schemes, but a comparison of the general tone is what is meant here. The biographic material composed along the lines of the first scheme is well known, readily available, and need not be discussed here.[4] But some of the 'alternative' findings of the type exemplified by Williams in scheme (2) above are very suggestive in the context of the present study, and will be discussed below. Our main sources for this discussion will be Jackson (1994), Sil (1997) and Williams (1974; 1995b).

Vivekananda's esoteric biography I: India

Childhood

There is very little historical evidence for this period of the Swami's life. Datta's father, who was a lawyer (Sil 1997: 38), is described as having

4. A concise version of what could be described as a common knowledge appraisal of Vivekananda may be found in Hay (1988: 72). Most standard emic works on Vivekananda will be found in Sil's bibliography (1997: 236–45), including Bengali and English primary sources, and in Williams (1995: 396–7, notes 3 and 4). His Eastern and Western Disciples (2000 [1912]) and Rolland (1966 [1930]) may be quoted as representative.

"rational, progressive ideas" (Williams 1995b: 375). As we shall see later, he encouraged his son to join a masonic lodge: he cannot therefore have been much of a Hindu traditionalist. His general views seem also to have contrasted with his wife's "deep and traditional piety" (*ibid.*). Such lack of coherence in the religious and ideological make-up of the parental home might have given a deep psychological root to Datta's later religio-philosophical ambivalence and consequent seeking.

Schooling

In scheme (2) above, Williams refers to a period of scepticism in the young Datta's life.[5] Williams may be right in tracing the genesis of Vivekananda's scepticism to his school years. However, this is a trait that will remain with the Swami for the rest of his life, as shown by his writing and pronouncements. Obvious as it is, this aspect of the Swami's psychology has not been sufficiently stressed. Such 'scepticism', however, should be understood more as an emotional state or mood than as an intellectual, let alone philosophical, conviction. These are important facets of Vivekananda's personality, which undoubtedly contributed to make him an 'esoteric seeker' rather than a 'spiritual hero'.

His educational curriculum may go some way towards explaining these tendencies. The available evidence indicates that for substantial periods of time he attended the institutions established by two well-known educators: the Bengali intellectual Ishwarchandra Vidyasagar and the Scottish missionary Alexander Duff.[6] Both men embodied powerful intellectual positions attempting to synthezise tradition and modernity, both were convinced rationalists, but most of all both fostered a secularist spirit in their charges.[7]

In addition to this we know that as a student the young Datta was keenly interested in Western philosophy. This led him to explore,

5. See also Brajendranath Seal, a classmate of the future Swami, who "recalled the latter's bitter intellectual cynicism, his restlessness, and sardonic wit" (Kopf 1979: 204).
6. See Lipner (1998: 64–5). Williams (1974: 18) further points out that Vivekananda passed his First Arts Examinations ("a sort of half-way house to the undergraduate degree" according to Lipner (1998: 65)) at the Scottish Church College in 1881.
7. Kopf (1979: 47) describes Vidyasagar as "an ardent rationalist" who "was known to be a dedicated humanist and a professed atheist". He was also one of the main exponents of "indigenous secularism as against the Westernized variety". As for Duff, he was "one of the most intellectually gifted missionaries to serve in India" (*ibid.*: 159) and, "by stressing science and reason at his school and at his Scottish Church College, he unwittingly produced secularists" (*ibid.*: 45–6).

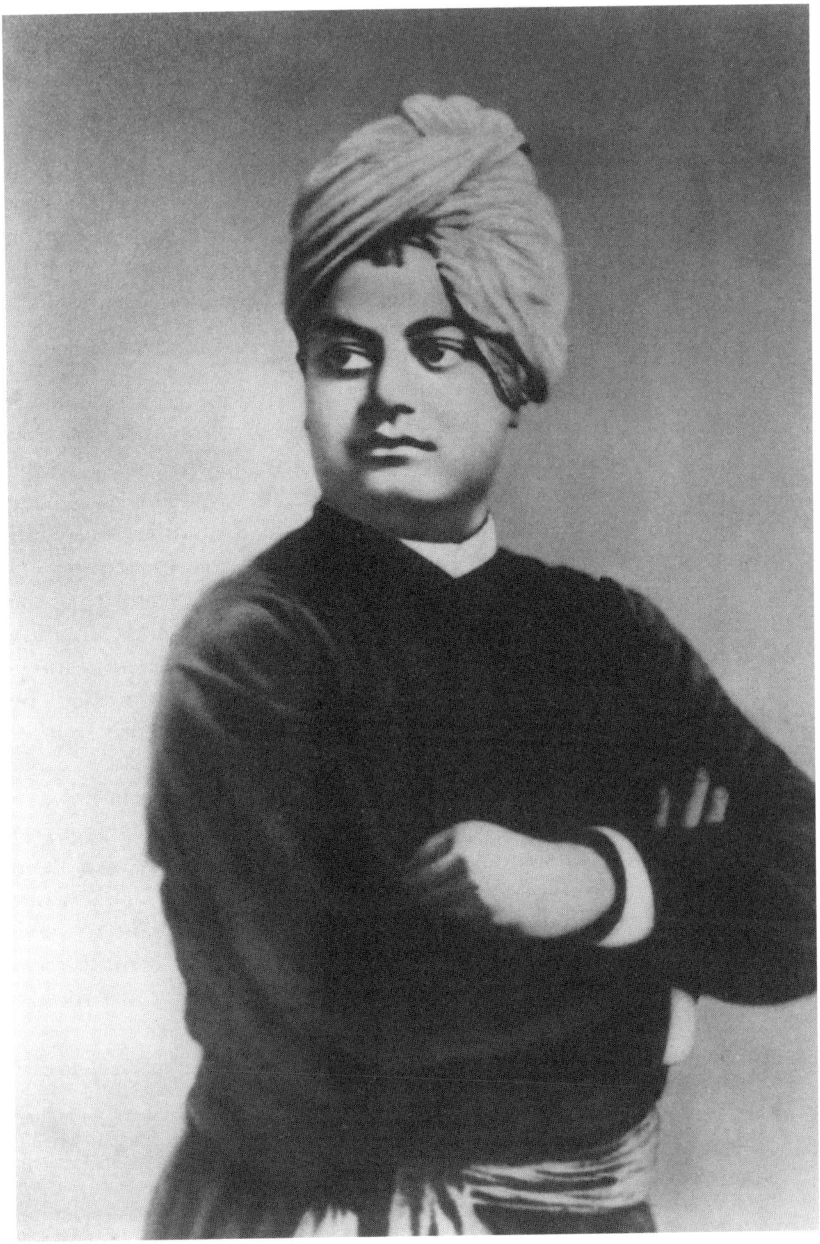

Figure 7 Swami Vivekananda at the Chicago Parliament of Religions, September 1893.

even though reportedly not in great depth,[8] the works of Hume, Kant, Fichte, Spinoza, Hegel, Schopenhauer, Comte, Spencer, J. S. Mill and Darwin (Sil 1997: 30). These intellectual influences left a deep mark in the future Vivekananda's mental make-up. We see this clearly in his recurrent attempts to use Western intellectual paradigms in his speeches.[9] From the specific point of view of the present study, however, the most important result of his education was that it provided him with a vocabulary and with conceptual frameworks that would allow him to communicate with (and impress) English-speaking audiences in the West.

In short, the young Datta seems to have been more of a charismatic "dreamer and visionary" (Sil 1997: 175) than a systematic thinker. Maybe Romantic influences, Neo-Vedāntic or otherwise, have not been sufficiently explored in the context of critical scholarship on the Swami. While subject to bouts of 'scepticism', he seems to have been very receptive to the idealistic emotionality of Romantic poets. His colleague Seal, for example, commented how, after prescribing "a course of readings in Shelley" to Datta, the latter found that the British poet's "Hymn to the spirit of a glorified millennial humanity moved him as the arguments of the philosophers had failed to move him". The budding Neo-Advaitin was especially impressed by Shelley's belief that the universe "contained a spiritual principle of unity" (Williams 1974: 19).

Later in life Vivekananda would also speak highly, especially when addressing Western audiences, about Edwin Arnold's *The Light of Asia* (1879),[10] the amazingly successful poem[11] that emerged from the Romantic milieu of American Transcendentalism. This work became an instant bestseller, and as such it can be said to have popularized a Romantic image of 'the Buddha' as prototypical 'Oriental sage'. The Swami was well aware of the effect that Arnold's

8. His fellow student Brajendranath Seal remarked that Datta "did not appear ... to have sufficient patience for humdrum reading – his faculty was to imbibe not so much from books as from living communion and personal experience. With him it was life kindling life and thought kindling thought" (quoted in Williams 1974: 19). Sil (1997: 30) concludes his survey of evidence by stating that "In spite of being an intelligent individual, Naren was neither a brilliant student nor an accomplished scholar."
9. Rambachan (1994: 30, 87–90, 107–8, 128–31) discusses specific instances of this.
10. Cf. references to the poem or to Arnold himself in *CW* 1: 86, 407; *CW* 2: 61, 155; *CW* 3: 511; *CW* 4: 319; *CW* 6: 97; *CW* 7: 287, 429; *CW* 8: 97.
11. It went through at least a hundred editions in England and America and was translated into numerous languages including, according to the 1884 *Trübner's Record*, Bengali and Sanskrit (Almond 1988: 1).

poem had on Western audiences: "Have you not seen even a most bigoted Christian, when he reads Edwin Arnold's *Light of Asia*, stand in reverence of Buddha, who preached no God, preached nothing but self-sacrifice?" (*CW* 1: 86). Thus Arnold's Romantic creation may well have functioned as a sort of role model for the young Bengali seeking to find his identity.

In his quest for the less-publicized facets of the Swami's personality, Sil (1997: 161) also highlights the youthful Datta's keen admiration for, and even enthusiastic impersonation of, the French leader Napoleon. Sil does not make this connection, but if we superimpose Arnold's Buddha onto the more martial and energetic figure of Napoleon we actually come very close to the Vivekananda cherished by popular imagination. Two of the Swami's most famous portraits, taken during the 1893 Parliament of Religions, have a definite 'Napoleonic hero' look about them (see Figure 7 for one of them).[12] Other photographs, showing him cross-legged or just seated upright, draped in flowing robes, gaze turned inward under closed eyelids, the hint of a smile on his lips, attempt to repropose the timeless icon of the meditating Buddha (Figure 8). Another portrait, taken soon after Vivekananda's return to India (February 1897; Figure 9) is also interesting for its similarity with Sen's 'yogic' portrait discussed in the previous chapter (Figure 6): the composition is almost identical, down to the surrounding foliage and the *kamaṇḍalu* (renouncer's pot).[13] With regard to the production of these icons we will remember that Keshubchandra Sen who, like Vivekananda, had a well-developed sense of the theatrical, had in his own days already experimented with the photographic medium in similar ways.

Brahmo

The point that Vivekananda repudiated his Brahmo past later in life but was nevertheless deeply influenced by it has already been made. Testimonials of people from his entourage confirm that he was

12. The other portrait similarly shows him with arms crossed in front of his chest, a self-assured and somewhat daring expression on his face, but this time as a full figure (for a reproduction see Chetananda 1995: 59). For an extensive and informative record of Vivekananda and Vivekananda-related photographs see *ibid.*
13. However, Sen's *ektār* ("one-stringed" lute) is likely to have been chosen to signify his penchant for ecstatic devotionalism, after the manner of Bengal Vaiṣṇavism, whereas Vivekananda's book clearly proposes him as more of a *jñānī*. Sen is portrayed with an *ektār* also in several other photographs (see, for example, Kopf 1979: 256 and Sen 1938: between pages 184–5).

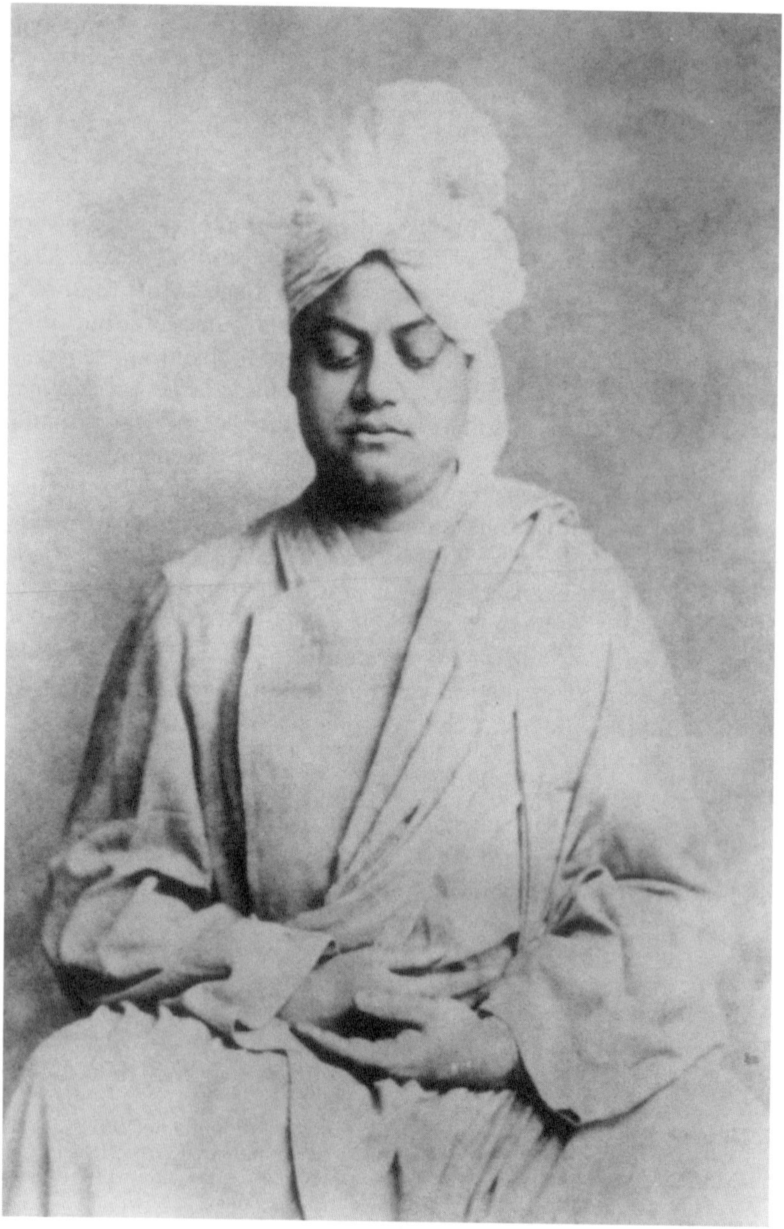

Figure 8 Swami Vivekananda in London, December 1896

thoroughly involved in Brahmo life and activities over the formative years around his twenties. Williams (1974: 11) reports that Narendranath Datta's name was on the original roll of the Sadharan Brahmo Samaj. Vivekananda's own brother, on the other hand, states that from 1881 to 1884, the year of Sen's death, the future Vivekananda was active in Sen's "Band of Hope", which sought "to wean away the young men from the path of smoking, drinking, etc." (quoted in Williams 1995b: 378). Vivekananda's biographer Isherwood further states that the Swami joined the Nava Vidhan in 1880 (Kopf 1979: 205, note 47), and according to Mallik, an older contemporary (quoted in Banerji 1931: 344), Vivekananda was more attracted by the Sadharan Brahmo Samaj at first, and later by Sen's Nava Vidhan.

In view of the cultic fluidity of late nineteenth-century Calcutta (described in the previous chapter), it should not come as a surprise that the young Datta was active in both Brahmo denominations. As Lipner points out,

> the social and, in important respects, the intellectual boundaries between the different Samajes were fluid ... those interested could move freely and exploratively between the Samajes...
>
> ... in the cultural hothouse that Calcutta was at the time, there was a great deal of overlap and criss-crossing socially, religiously and/or intellectually among the [Brahmo] circles. (1998: 65–6)

Under such circumstances there would have been no need, especially for younger members, to be totally committed to one or the other of the camps. But apart from this, the young Datta's involvement with the Brahmos, and the active role that he took in some of Sen's projects, are beyond doubt.[14] Of special interest to us is that the future Swami, accompanied by a friend, would often join "picnics and musical festivals in a suburban garden called the 'Hermitage'. Here they would have musical fiestas and animated discussions on ... things, religious and social, political and philosophical" (quoted in Lipner 1998: 65). This 'Hermitage' could only have been Sen's *Sadhan Kanan*, and here the young Datta would have been powerfully

14. "K. K. Mitra, who also knew Vivekananda in the early 1880s, has stated that the latter engaged in Brahmo activities, attended Brahmo meetings, lived among Brahmo students, and loved to sing Brahmo songs" (Kopf 1979: 205, note 48).

exposed not only to this leader's example and teachings, but to his living *oeuvre* as manifested in his Neo-Vedāntic ashram.

Freemason

Before we examine the relationship between Ramakrishna and Narendranath Datta, a few remarks should be made about the latter's membership of the Calcutta Freemasons' Lodge. The young Datta joined the lodge at some point before 1884 (Williams 1974: 15). His father encouraged him to join, as both Vivekananda and his brother were to explain later, so that he would get to know influential people who may later help him in his career (*ibid.*). Datta's father, who, as we saw, had rationalist and progressive tendencies, was obviously not concerned by the religious and ethical implications of such a move. In any case, the young Datta's involvement in Freemasonry, however superficial, must have given him an early insight into the structure, contents and social network potentialities of esoteric associationism. The freemasonic ideals of "equality, social reform, philanthropy and a 'common denominator' approach to religious unity" (*ibid.*: 15; 1995b: 379) would have further reinforced the highly compatible Brahmo beliefs he held.

Ramakrishna and Vivekananda

Ramakrishna may well have died unnoticed and unremembered, as have so many other Indian holy men before and after him, had he not entered into Sen's orbit. After Sen's death (1884) he became the focal point of attention for many young Brahmos who suddenly found themselves deprived of their charismatic leader. Within two decades of his own death (1886), he had been adopted as the spiritual head of Vivekananda's Ramakrishna movement. While Ramakrishna's Hinduism was virtually untouched by modern influences, he was eventually proclaimed worldwide as a master of Neo-Vedāntic "God-realization". This was moreover done in the context of discourses charged with Christian overtones: his translated sayings are known as *The* Gospel *of Shri Ramakrishna* (Gupta 1978 [1907]; 1984 [1942]) for which a *Concordance* has been compiled (Whitmarsh 1989); the members of his inner circle of followers were his *apostles*; Vivekananda was presented as a novel St Paul (see details of his initiation below) and his letters are classified as *epistles* in his

Collected Works, and so on. A reactive assimilation strategy is obviously at work here.

Commonplace accounts describe the relationship between Ramakrishna and Vivekananda as idyllic and reciprocally affectionate. Critical scholarship, however, once again brings up more ambiguous (and realistic) vistas: the Calcutta cultic milieu was charged with social, religious and psychological tensions, especially in the latter part of the nineteenth century. This dense atmosphere reflects on our story. Neither the young Datta nor his master were straightforward characters. While Ramakrishna was obviously a natural mystic endowed with an engaging and lively personality,[15] his spiritual struggles have nothing of the straightforward one-pointedness of the younger and equally famous modern South Indian saint Ramana Maharshi.[16] Vivekananda also emerges from recent scholarship (see note 3 above) as a forceful but rather paradoxical character. That the relationship between the two Bengalis was somewhat fraught and occasionally strained therefore comes as no surprise.

Williams (1974: 17) reports that to start with Datta was under the impression "that Rāmakṛṣṇa was an 'idolator' and that he and his devotees were intellectual inferiors". At first he also thought that the Bengali holy man was "a brain-sick baby, always seeing visions and the rest" (*CW* 8: 263). Such harsh judgements are maybe not so surprising if we think that they came from a twenty-year-old educated and Anglicized Brahmo of impulsive character.

According to Williams (1995b: 380–4), the relationship between the two Bengalis developed as follows: Ramakrishna and the future Vivekananda met in December 1881, after which Datta more or less shunned the older man, despite the latter's proclamations of affection. In 1884 the young Datta faced a series of bereavements: his father and Keshubchandra Sen both died within less than two months of each other.[17] This must have had deep personal and emotional repercussions because both men had been central to the future Swami's life: the first one as life guide and natural source of authority and support, the second as role model (however unacknowledged). What is more, these events resulted in the total collapse of his social

15. The mixture of charm, wit, sensitivity, spirituality and common sense that were all part of the man are evident from a reading of *The Gospel of Shri Ramakrishna* (Gupta 1978 [1907], 1984 [1942]), even in its English translations.
16. See Kripal (1995), Sil (1993, 1997). Regarding Ramana Maharshi see Osborne (1994).
17. 25 February (Sil 1997: 41) and 8 January (Williams 1995b: 382) respectively.

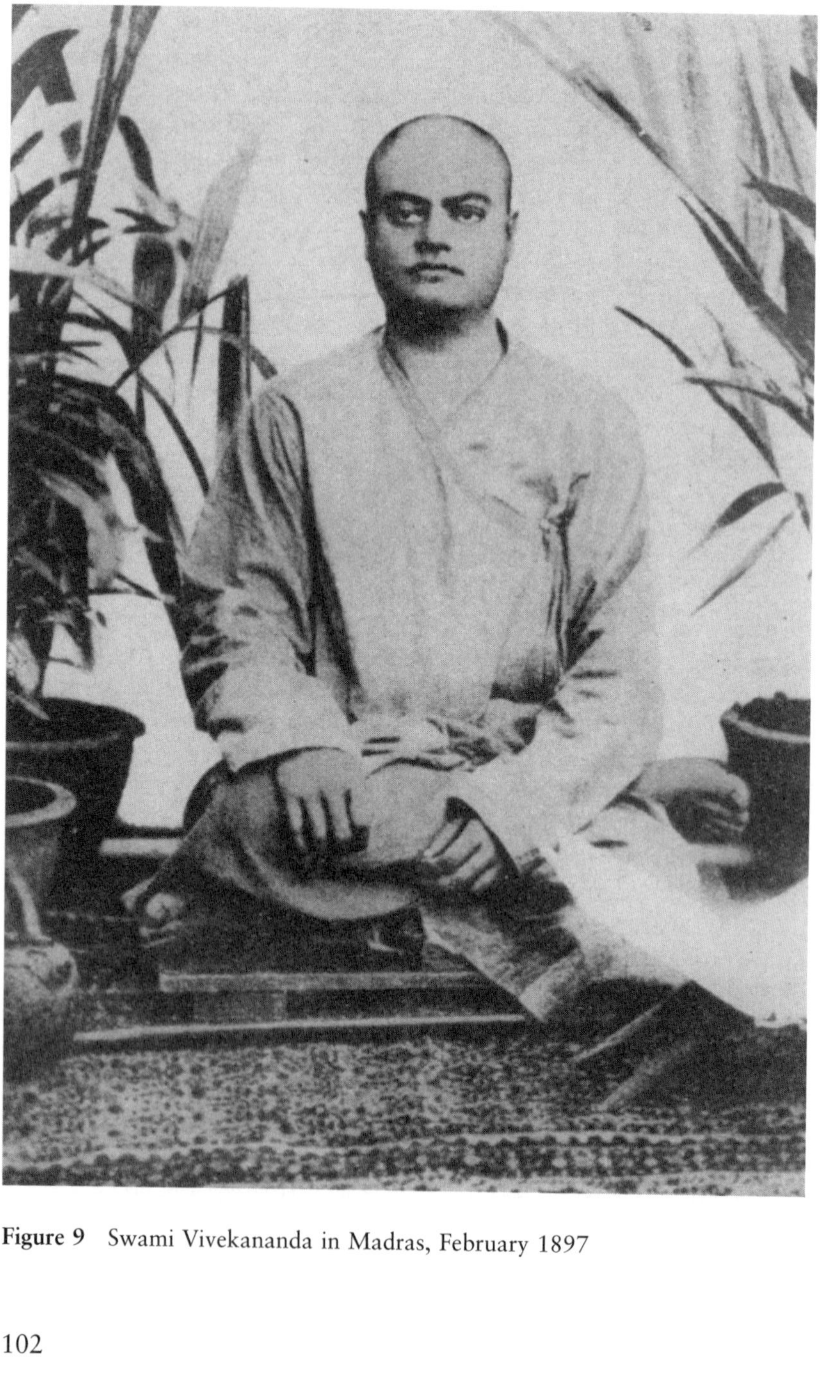

Figure 9 Swami Vivekananda in Madras, February 1897

and family networks: his father's passing away left the family financially ruined and bitterly divided, giving rise to a prolonged period of financial crisis and emotional turmoil.[18] We also saw how Sen's Samaj was left in shambles after the leader's demise, and this was the young Datta's main social circle. He does not seem to have coped well with these unexpected pressures and responsibilities:

> Sudden confrontation with the harsh realities of life was quite upsetting, almost traumatic, for the inexperienced and easygoing Narendranath. In spite of his reputation at college for his eloquence, erudition, and leadership qualities and the fact that his lawyer father had connections in influential circles, Naren never did manage to procure a suitable employment except for a short stint as a school teacher.[19] We have a graphic account of his predicament: "I had to look for a job even before the period of mourning was over. I went from office to office barefoot and hungry, carrying an application for a job ... But I was unsuccessful everywhere." Unable to cope with abject poverty, the shocked college graduate ... became a regular visitor to Dakshineshwar. (Sil 1997: 38)

As standard narrations indicate, Ramakrishna was all too happy to offer counsel, reassurance and comfort to the younger man. Speculating on the basis of available evidence and of existing scholarship, Sil (*ibid.*: 40) concludes:

> It is most certainly a fact that [Ramakrishna] provided a deep psychological support to the flamboyant but flabbergasted young man facing a crisis of career and family responsibility. Indeed as Dr. Kakar has written, Narendra was under intense mental strain, highly vulnerable and suggestible when he came close to the Master, and the "mighty mentor" stepped into the void of his would-be disciple's life which had been rendered utterly chaotic after his father's death. Thus there might have developed a "quasi-therapeutic relationship" between Ramakrishna and Narendranath.

Rather than this quasi-therapeutic relationship, hagiographic narrations of the Ramakrishna-Vivekananda relationship represent Ramakrishna carefully grooming the young Datta according to the

18. See Williams (1974: 61 and 1995b: 380).
19. He lost his job "apparently upon complaints from the upper-class boys that he did not know how to teach properly" (Sil 1997: 44). Eventually he also gave up his law studies (*ibid.*).

established method of personally passing on one's spiritual legacy through initiation within a *guru-śiṣya paraṃparā* (traditional "teacher-pupil transmission"). But even here historical evidence, as we shall soon see, does not tally with these accounts. After examining a wider range of sources, one is led to ask questions concerning the ways in which Vivekananda came to appropriate and interpret Ramakrishna's spiritual legacy.

Ramakrishna's spiritual transmission

Ramakrishna and Vivekananda were not to spend much time together after their rapprochement as the older man passed away on 16 August 1886. At this point the question of spiritual transmission becomes crucial, especially with regard to the validation of Vivekananda's subsequent work and influence. What concerns us here is not to pass judgement on the religiosity of a specific individual, but to evaluate the strengths and qualifications of a spiritual teacher, as this is how the Swami later presented himself and how the Ramakrishna movement has presented him ever since. Here the question of initiation becomes important.

There is a distinct lack of clarity in the evidence relating to the spiritual legacy passed by Ramakrishna to the young Datta and his Brahmo cohort. We shall now discuss the available evidence,[20] but before we do so it is important to clarify the following with regard to available textual sources in this context: Gupta (1978 [1907]) is a text based on Gupta's original *Śrī Rāmakṛṣṇa Kathāmṛta* ("Nectar of the Story of Ramakrishna"). Written in Bengali, the latter is widely reputed to be the most reliable and comprehensive record of Ramakrishna's life and sayings.[21] Gupta (1978 [1907]) was composed and translated by Gupta himself, and as such may be regarded as the most reliable source in English.[22] Gupta (1984 [1942]), on the other hand, while based on the original *Kathāmṛta*, is by now known, at least among scholars, to have been substantially shaped by its translator, Swami Nikhilananda. As such, it should be taken as the

20. Though regrettably we have no access to the Bengali sources.
21. This text was published in five volumes (1902, 1905, 1907, 1910 and 1932), and the author's name used for these publications was 'M', for Mahendranath Gupta (Gupta 1978 [1907]: xi).
22. Information on the history of this text and on the Bengali *Kathāmṛta* is given in the "Introduction to the 1978 edition of the Condensed Gospel" found in the 1978 and subsequent editions.

Ramakrishna movement's 'official' version of events rather than as a straightforward translation of the original.[23]

So what is the evidence we do have about Ramakrishna's spiritual transmission? Williams (1974: 36) reports that all the Master did was to ask Datta to "take care of the boys" (i.e. the other young devotees), but quotes no source for this affirmation. Nikhilananda (1984 [1942]: 70) provides a more literary version of Ramakrishna's words: "I leave these young men in your charge. See that they develop their spirituality and do not return home", but again one finds no trace of a corresponding passage in the main body of Gupta's (1984 [1942]) text. Ramakrishna's affection for and attachment to "the boys" does shine through in Gupta's accounts of the Master's life (1978 [1907]; 1984 [1942]), but the reasons why they should have remained together, in what form or for what purpose are never entered upon. One fact is certain, however: Ramakrishna never formally initiated the future Vivekananda and the other young devotees.[24] This is a stark fact that both Vivekananda and the early Ramakrishna movement have been at pains to underplay and to counterbalance with informal or 'mystical' types of initiation.[25]

The most polished example of 'official' narrative concerning how the Ramakrishna order was established, perhaps unsurprisingly, is the one written by Nikhilananda (1984 [1942]: 70). Typically, it consists more of interpretative emphases than of facts, and there is no straight reference to matters of spiritual transmission in Ramakrishna's own teachings. Nikhilananda narrates that Ramakrishna spent a week at a disciple's house in Calcutta after having been diagnosed with cancer: "During this week he dedicated himself practically without respite to the instruction of those beloved devotees who had been unable to visit him oftener at Dakshineswar. Discourses incessantly flowed from his tongue, and he often went into samādhi" (*ibid.*: 67). Whoever reads the relevant section of Gupta's reports

23. Nikhilananda's Introduction to this book (Nikhilananda 1984 [1942]) is, however, listed separately in the bibliography as it is an explicitly autonomous source.
24. He did, however, initiate into *sannyāsa*, according to Swami Nikhilananda (1984 [1942]: 33), the "great pundit" Narayan Shastri and maybe also Gauri, another scholar.
25. See, for example, Datta telling Gupta, after Ramakrishna's passing away, that while at Cossipore the Master had "transmitted his power to [him]" (Gupta 1984 [1942]: 985); or Vivekananda's later (1901) and more spectacular report of a similar transmission (reported by one of his disciples in *CW* 7: 206–7). This latter narration was then incorporated by Nikhilananda (1984 [1942]: 72) in his 'official' version of events.

(1978 [1907]; 1984 [1942]), however, is likely to be disappointed: Ramakrishna's discourses and his ecstasies are in no way different to the ones found in all other parts of the book.

Nikhilananda's story proceeds: after this week the Master was moved to Śyāmpukur (in the northern section of Calcutta), and it is at this point that

> [t]hese young men, under the watchful eye of the Master and the leadership of Narendra, became the antaranga bhaktas, the devotees of Sri Ramakrishna's inner circle. They were privileged to witness many manifestations of the Master's divine powers. Narendra received instructions regarding the propagation of his message after his death. (Nikhilananda 1984 [1942]: 67)

But here again no traces, not even oblique references to these momentous events, can be found in Ramakrishna's words.[26] Nikhilananda nevertheless continues in the same vein:

> The Master did not hide the fact that he wished to make Narendra his spiritual heir. Narendra was to continue the work after Sri Ramakrishna's passing. Sri Ramakrishna said to him: "I leave these young men in your charge. See that they develop their spirituality and do not return home." One day he asked the boys, in preparation for their monastic life, to beg their food from door to door without thought of caste. They hailed the Master's order and went out with begging-bowls. A few days later he gave the ochre cloth of the sannyāsi to each of them ... Thus the Master himself laid the foundation of the future Ramakrishna Order of monks. (Nikhilananda 1984 [1942]: 70)

As before, one finds no mention of these important happenings in the main body of Gupta's (1984 [1942]) text. As for contrasting evidence, Sil (1997: 45) reports that on 19 January 1886 Ramakrishna "worried ... over the wearing of ochre-colored (*geruā*) clothes on the part of Naren and a few others, when these were presented to them

26. All evidence we find about this training consists in Gupta's comment (1984 [1942]: 886) that "[a] band of young disciples, led by Narendra, was preparing to renounce the world and dedicate their lives to the realization of God and the service of humanity". The *Condensed Gospel* version (Gupta 1978 [1907]: 284), is equally vague: "To the younger disciples, headed by Narendra, this great and unique service for the Master [i.e. tending him in his final illness] led the way to the great renunciation of the world of which they are the most glorious examples in the present day. For was not Sri Ramakrishna their living Ideal, a unique example before their very eyes – who had given up the world and its so-called pleasures for the sake of God?"

by Huṭko Gopal".[27] Importantly, he also points out that "[t]he master did not wish [Datta] to become a *sannyāsī* during the lifetime of his mother" (*ibid.*).[28]

We do, however, find an 'official' report of the actual act of renunciation undergone by Datta and his cohort in the literature of the Ramakrishna movement. These events took place on 24 December 1886, a few months after the Master's death. It is a striking narration:

> ... subtle things were happening, knitting the brothers together. It all found expression one night before a huge Dhuni (sacred fire) in the compound ... Meditation lasted a long time. When a break was made Narendra began to tell the story of Jesus, beginning with the mystery of his birth through his death and resurrection. Through his eloquence, the brother-disciples could catch something of the apostolic fervour that had impelled Paul to spread the Christian gospel far and wide in the face of adversities. Narendra charged them to become Christs themselves, and so aid in the redemption of the world; to realize God and to deny themselves as Jesus had done. Standing there before the sacred fire, their faces lit up by the flames, the crackling of the wood the sole disturbing sound, they took the vows of renunciation before God and one another. The very air was vibrant with their ecstatic fervour. Strangely, the monks discovered afterwards that all this had happened on Christmas-eve! (His Eastern and Western Disciples 2000, Vol. I.: 196).[29]

One cannot but wonder at the total unorthodoxy of this initiation, which in its exalted fervour and strong Christian contents is much more reminiscent of Sen's "enthusiasm" and theories of "divine

27. Gupta (1984 [1942]: 975), on the other hand, states that the ochre cloth was donated by Ramakrishna to the young devotees. It would be interesting to read Gupta's Bengali version of these events, if he narrated them.
28. Vivekananda's mother, Bhuvaneshvari Devi (1841–1911) outlived her son. For her portrait and dates see His Eastern and Western Disciples (2000, Vol. I: facing page 16).
29. Williams (1974: 36–7) quotes the same passage from an earlier edition of this work. Comparing the two versions is instructive in terms of the shifting emphases found in official Ramakrishna movement literature. In the earlier version the Christian element is even stronger than in the quoted version. One also notes that in the more recent edition a further paragraph is added to the quoted one, arguably in an attempt to validate the initiation. In it one of Vivekananda's group of monks is reported to say, retrospectively, that "[Ramakrishna] had already made us sannyasis. That attitude was strengthened at Antpur", i.e. where the described event took place (His Eastern and Western Disciples 2000, Vol. I: 197). As in other instances, the language is more suggestive than affirmative, and somewhat ambiguous.

humanity" than of Ramakrishna's Hinduism. It is also, importantly, a self-administered initiation, with no links to religious authorities or structures of any sort.[30] In this more technical sense it brings to mind Debendranath Tagore's own initiation (described in Chapter 2). It is also a perfect example of how far the development of the cultic milieu and of its forms of individualistic religiosity had come in Bengal by this stage.

After Ramakrishna

After Ramakrishna's death, during the period 1886 to 1892, Vivekananda "began his peregrination of India ... and he came in contact not only with the masses throughout the length and breadth of the country but also with the feudal chiefs and petty princelings" (Sil 1997: 49–50). Throughout these years Williams (1974: 36–41, 47–59; 1995b: 384–8) traces various periods of doubt, study, seeking and wandering, summarized in phases III to V in scheme (2) at the beginning of this chapter. We do not need to follow these intellectual and geographical 'peregrinations' in detail, thus we will just look at the final outcome of these years of wandering.

In late December 1892 the future Vivekananda "reached the southern tip of India at Kanyākumāri (Cape Comorin), completing his journey to the cardinal points of India" (Williams 1974: 57). According to Vivekananda's own *post-facto* recollections, it is at this point that he "hit upon a plan". He reasoned:

> We are so many Sannyasins wandering about, and teaching the people metaphysics – it is all madness. Did not our Gurudeva [Ramakrishna] use to say, "An empty stomach is no good for religion"? ...
>
> Suppose some disinterested Sannyasins, bent on doing good to others go from village to village, disseminating education and seeking in various ways to better the condition of all ... through oral teaching, and by means of maps, cameras, globes, and such other accessories ... We have to give back to the nation its lost individuality and *raise the masses*.
>
> To effect this, the first thing we need is men, and the next is funds. Through the grace of our Guru I was sure to get from ten to fifteen men

30. Another ceremony, during which "Naren initiated all his *gurubhāis* into *sannyās* by performing *Virajā Hom*" is reported by Sil (1997: 49) as having taken place "in the third week of January 1887". But this again leaves open the question of Vivekananda's own initiation.

in every town. I next travelled in search of funds, but do you think the people of India were going to spend money! . . . Therefore I have come to America, to earn money myself, and then return to my country and devote the rest of my days to the realisation of this one aim of my life.

As our country is poor in social virtues, so this country is lacking in spirituality. I give them spirituality and they give me money. (*CW* 6: 254–6, original emphasis)

Vivekananda's straightforward characterization of East–West relations is sobering. The details of his plan for social uplift tie in perfectly with his Brahmo and Neo-Vedāntic background. Indeed, his ideas and propositions are just further developments of Sen's own. As in the case of Modern Yoga vs. Sen's proto Modern Yoga, or in the case of Neo-Vedāntic occultism vs. Neo-Vedāntic "spiritualism", what Vivekananda did was to adapt his ideas and teachings to more thoroughly secularised and materialistic conditions.

The shift from one position to the other may be seen by comparing the above passage with a corresponding one from Sen's literary corpus. In 1877, as Narendranath Datta was just a child of eleven, the Brahmo leader proclaimed:

Let England baptize us with the spirit of true philosophy. Let the sages of Aryan India baptize us with the spirit of heavenly madness. Let modern England teach hard science and fact; let ancient India teach sweet poetry and sentiment . . . Let me have only fifty young men from our Universities, trained in science and philosophy, and baptized with the spirit of madness, and let these men go forth, as missionary-soldiers of God, conquering and to conquer, and in the fullness of time the banners of truth shall be planted throughout the length and the breadth of the country . . . (Sen 1901: 326)

Sen's language may be more flowery and Romantic, his rhetoric more idealistic – but the common thread linking the two programmes is undeniable. Here we may usefully refer to the testimony of contemporaries. Mallik is one of the few primary sources stating clearly the continuities between Sen's and Vivekananda's programmes and ideologies:

[Vivekananda] owed the beginnings of [his] spiritual culture to the pattern set by Keshab Chandra . . . By whatever name Vivekananda might have been known he was a reproduction of Keshab Chandra.

> The followers of Vivekananda have signalised their activities by undertaking philanthropic work and in this they are only carrying out the *Seva Sadhan*[31] that Keshab Chandra first introduced in the Brahmo Samaj . . . (Quoted in Banerji 1931: 345–6)

Despite Datta's repudiation of Brahmoism, his nation-regenerating programme, and his very own role within it, will ultimately turn out to be cast very much in the form of Sen's missionary enterprise. As Sen had expanded Debendranath Tagore's plan out of the confines of Bengal to apply it to the whole of India, so Vivekananda would eventually expand Sen's plan out of the confines of India to the whole of 'the West', believing as he did (and as he was made to believe) that he possessed 'spirituality', that elusive entity that would heal the ailing Western soul. In order to do this he had to acculturate his message, which he did by entering into a creative dialogue with the circles that accepted and supported him, i.e. with Western cultic milieus.

Vivekananda's esoteric biography II: the West

With Vivekananda's first voyage to the West we come to the high point of his life. The young Swami reached America in July 1893 and would remain in the West up to December 1896. It is during this time that Neo-Vedāntic occultism was created: *Rāja Yoga*, its seminal text, was published in 1896. In this tract, as we shall see more specifically in Chapter 5, Vivekananda gives shape to Modern Yoga by blending Neo-Vedāntic esotericism and avant-garde American occultism. Thus Neo-Vedāntic ideology became an integral part of Western occultism and, conversely, Western occultist ideas were integrated into Neo-Vedānta. These ideas were then transmitted back to India by way of Vivekananda's thought and example and also, importantly, by way of the influential Ramakrishna movement he created.

Vivekananda at the Parliament of Religions

Vivekananda's main aim upon leaving India was to attend the Chicago Parliament of Religions, due to take place in September 1893. Travelling with very meagre funds, he ran out of money soon after his

31. "Religious practice of service"; this prefigures what is usually referred to as '*karma yoga*' in contemporary Neo-Vedāntic circles.

arrival. By a stroke of luck, however, he came to be 'adopted' by prominent members of the local cultic milieu.[32] His newfound friends, impressed by "the handsome monk in the orange robe" who spoke "perfect English",[33] took him under their wing. From then onwards he was looked after and supported by them, and eventually he also started earning money by giving talks and classes and by becoming the recipient of donations. With his hosts and companions he acted as a wise counsellor and teacher, as a friend and as "a soiree ornament ... entertaining the wealthy and the curious" (Williams 1995b: 388).

That he was accepted so promptly and so unconditionally tells us something about his charisma, his adaptive skills and about the open-mindedness of his hosts as individuals and as Americans. But it tells us just as much about the fascination exercised in cultic milieus by Oriental teachers, who would be implicitly understood by romanticizing Westerners to be providers of genuine teachings, whatever their credentials.[34] Vivekananda knew how to reinforce and make use of these sympathies:[35] he was, for example, only too eager to assert the superiority of Hinduism over other religions[36] and to reinforce assumptions that all Indians are routinely trained to be outstandingly 'spiritual' and religiously observant.[37] In this sense we could say that, if Sen was the first Neo-Vedāntic *guru* to make use of these apologetic strategies in India, Vivekananda was the first Neo-Vedāntic *guru* to successfully use them abroad. He would not be the last.

The Parliament of Religions itself was of course an avant-garde intellectual manifestation of the activities of the same cultic milieus,

32. Jackson (1994: 29) lists of some of them.
33. As described by Harriet Monroe, a major figure in early twentieth-century American poetry (quoted in *ibid.*: 26).
34. For a cutting but heartfelt insider's critique of the 'gnostic superiority of Indians' motif see Mehta (1993). Siegel's hilarious but earnest modern *guru* parody is based on the same theme (1991: 303–316).
35. See Halbfass (1988: 229): Vivekananda "adopts Western motifs of self-criticism and the search for India and transforms them into aspects of Hindu self-assertion ..." Regarding Vivekananda's work outside India see Sil's sober evaluation of his "Conquest of the West" (1997, Chapter 11), which tones down the triumphant notes of propaganda we have become accustomed to hear.
36. In his main Parliament of Religions address he states that Hinduism is the most resilient of the three "prehistoric" religions, the other two being Zoroastrianism and Judaism (*CW* 1: 6); that it encompasses Buddhism and Jainism (*ibid.*: 6, 19); and that it is superior to Christianity (*ibid.*: 11, 15).
37. See, for example, his assertion that "In India they teach children never to eat until they have practised or worshipped ... a boy will not feel hungry until he has bathed and practised" (*ibid.*: 145).

East and West. This said, it will be clear why the Brahmo Samaj and the Theosophical Society were invited as official representatives of Hinduism (Chowdhury-Sengupta 1998: 22). As Vivekananda had not been invited to contribute to the proceedings, he had to submit an application to the relevant administrators. This he did by introducing himself as a monk "of the oldest order of *sannyāsis* ... founded by Sankara" (Williams 1995b: 388).[38] He also asked both Brahmos and Theosophists to validate his application. Interestingly, the Theosophical Society refused to offer any help when he stated that he had no intention of becoming a member (See *CW* 3: 208–10). The Brahmo Samaj, on the other hand, supported him by way of their representative Protapchandra Mozoomdar, whom we already mentioned in the previous chapter. Sitting on the Parliament's selection committee, Mozoomdar "accepted Vivekananda's late application without a letter of invitation and allowed him to participate in the Parliament by classifying the Swami as a representative of the Hindu monastic order" (Sil 1997: 188).[39]

Vivekananda's assimilation of Western occultism

By the end of the Parliament of Religions in September 1893 Vivekananda had become a media celebrity. On the strength of this he started "working for a lecture bureau, drawing large crowds, earning fairly large sums of money and speaking in the major cities of the East, South and Midwest" (Williams 1974: 59). In July 1894 he quit the bureau, and between the end of July and the beginning of August 1894 he "delivered a series of lectures at the Greenacre Conferences in Elliot, Maine, sponsored by Christian Scientists. The fall of 1894 was spent in Boston, Chicago and New York, responding to the invitations of the wealthy" (*ibid.*: 60; regarding conference dates see *ibid.*: 133).

Vivekananda's involvement with Christian Scientists yet again confirms that he gravitated in cultic circles. His own teasing but

38. In the first of his Parliament addresses he similarly professed, with typical hyperbole, to belong to "the most ancient order of monks in the world" (*CW* 1: 3), though, as we saw, he had not undergone a traditional monastic initiation. For further details and sources regarding Vivekananda's claims and monastic status see Sil (1997, especially Chapters 2, 3 and 4) and Williams (1995a: 58–9, 61, 94; 1995b: 388).
39. According to Vivekananda, Mozoomdar later became somewhat resentful of his success at the Parliament (*CW* 3: 210–11; cf. also Sil 1997: 152, 159). The Swami was also supported by Harvard Professor John Henry Wright who gave Vivekananda "a strong letter of recommendation" (Sil 1997: 194).

largely sympathetic report (*CW* 6: 259–62) of the Greenacre "queer gathering" (*ibid.*: 259) shows how easily he blended in with American esotericists.[40] A couple of months later (25 September 1894; *CW* 6: 263–77), writing to his fellow monks back in India, he commented on the Theosophists and the many spiritualists and Christian Scientists found in America. Christian Scientists, he said, "are Vedantins" in the sense that "they have picked up a few doctrines of the Advaita and grafted them upon the Bible" (*ibid.*: 270). Something of the sort may well have been happening. But, as we shall see in our discussion of *Rāja Yoga*, the opposite was definitely taking place too: Vivekananda would be grafting the occultistic teachings that he came to know in America – and which he obviously found convincing – onto his own (already esotericized) interpretations of Hinduism. It was on the basis of the teachings that he was quickly absorbing from his Western cultic entourage that he was to evolve his (occultistic) understanding of (Neo-)Vedānta.

Vivekananda soon realized that the big American cities of the East were good places to spread his message. In August 1894, less than one year after the Parliament of Religions, he reported to one of his followers that he would lecture in New York and Boston, the latter being described as "a good field" (*CW* 9: 29).[41] And indeed Versluis (1993: 316) confirms that at the end of the nineteenth century Boston "was home to devotees of many exotic cults and beliefs. Asian religions were ... assimilated into the mixture of Theosophy, occultism, astrology, mind reading, psychic research, mesmerism, and other avant-garde alternatives to traditional religions." The same author quotes (*ibid.*) Kathleen Pyne to the effect that this same city "was filled with adherents to the cults of India and Egypt ... From "thinking persons" on down to the level of shopkeepers and dressmakers, most Bostonians took it for granted that "psychic force" was

40. A few extracts about this proto-Woodstock gathering (the latter also presided over by a Swami) will suffice: "[The participants] do not care much about social laws and are quite free and happy ... You will be astounded with the liberty they enjoy in the camps, but they are very good and pure people there – a little erratic and that is all ... I teach them Shivo'ham, Shivo'ham, and they all repeat it, innocent and pure as they are and brave beyond all bounds ... Here God is either a terror or a healing power, vibration, and so forth" (*CW* 6: 259–61).

41. By Christmas 1899 he is convinced that also the Pacific coast is "a great field" where, as he remarks, "[t]he Raja-Yoga book seems very well known" (*CW* 8: 486).

a reality, while the language of mind-cure could be heard in everyday conversation."[42]

Such was the milieu into which Vivekananda settled and started to propagate his teachings. It was, *mutatis mutandis*, the social group corresponding to the Bengali cultic milieu from which he himself came. Except that these American circles were far more widespread, affluent, secularized, individualistic and far more intent on engaging in "occult" endeavours (about which see below). It was therefore not surprising that, with relatively minor adaptations on both sides, he was readily accepted and accepting. This pattern of social interaction continued throughout his stay in the West: embraced by the more fluid, unchurched, affluent strands of the cultic milieu, he in turn adapted to them. Flattered by their admiration and support, he also admired them, and the reciprocation of positive feelings led to mutual assimilation.

Harmonial Religion: Metaphysical beliefs and mesmerism

At this point we must take a step back in time to find out what had been going on in Western cultic milieus over the last few decades that would be of relevance to the future development of Modern Yoga, i.e. what Vivekananda came in contact with as he settled into the Western cultic lifestyle.

An element of great relevance is the strong presence of 'Harmonial Religion' or 'American Harmonial Piety'. As Fuller (1989: 49–53) explains, this type of religiosity was not a direct development of Swedenborgian teachings, but was based on these teachings' form and vision: "That is, they lent an ideological matrix to a wide array of activities and gave them a certain plausibility they might otherwise have lacked" (*ibid*.: 49). Fuller further elaborates:

> Swedenborg's doctrines gave the nineteenth century its most vivid articulation of a form of piety in which "harmony", rather than contrition or repentance, is the sine qua non of the regenerated life . . . The deity – here conceived as an indwelling cosmic force – is approached not via petitionary prayer or acts of worship, but through a series of inner adjustments. As the barriers separating the finite personality from

42. The 'cultic' tradition was long-established in Boston: Fuller (1989: 42) reports that a book published in 1834 estimated magnetic healers operating in this city to be over 200.

> the "divinity which flows through all things" are gradually penetrated, vitality spontaneously manifests itself in every dimension of personal life ... The Swedenborgian world view depicted interaction between the physical and metaphysical orders of reality as a lawful occurrence. It only remained for adherents of various medical and religious sects to elaborate the means whereby this influx takes place. (*Ibid.*: 51–2)

As we shall see in Chapter 5, Vivekananda would redefine yoga as just one such 'Harmonial' technique detailing the "inner adjustments" necessary for approaching the indwelling deity, thus attaining "Self-realization".

But over and above Swedenborgian influences, Harmonial piety, as Hanegraaff points out,[43] also encompassed a mixture of Transcendentalist universalism, mesmerism and spiritualism. In this type of belief, spiritual composure, physical health, and even economic well-being were understood to flow from a person's rapport with the cosmos. In this context Emersonian Transcendentalism would have a pervasive influence. Emerson's central belief was that each individual possesses, apart from the conscious intellect, an inner faculty for becoming receptive to a higher power or Over-Soul. This higher power was also stated to be the final source of all regenerative and progressive action. His spirituality did not entail any specific reference to established religions, Christian, Oriental or otherwise, but an aesthetic appreciation of one's own inner connection with the fundamental laws of the universe (Fuller 1989: 35). The characteristic tendency of "Harmonial Religion", as Hanegraaff further explains, is

> to understand "the cosmos", "the universe" or "the infinite" in psychological terms. The cosmos depends upon, or is even more or less synonymous with, an immanent divine "Mind" which is the source and foundation of finite minds. Health and harmony on the level of human existence is achieved by replicating in one's own mind the harmonious perfection of the cosmic whole. Since the universe is flawless, the individual soul is flawless as well; it is only by believing otherwise (i.e. by creating an illusion of imperfection) that one disturbs the harmony and interrupts the continuity between the outer and the inner universe (1996: 494–5)

43. Hanegraaff (1996: 494; with reference to Sydney Ahlstrom).

We shall refer to this psychologized form of Harmonialism as 'Metaphysical' (capitalized; Fuller 1989: 53–65). To the defenders of Metaphysical belief "As a man thinketh, so is he" was no mere aphorism, but an incontrovertible law (*ibid.*: 62). The practical implications of this creed were fully developed by the (mainly) American constellation of groups known under the name of New Thought (Hanegraaff 1996: 484–90). It was New Thought that introduced the long-standing modern fashion of 'positive thinking'. This philosophy had as its core message that "individuals could 'take responsibility' for their situation: it told them that the only reason why external circumstances seemed to have power over them was because they *believed* that to be the case" (*ibid.*: 489). Systems of belief and healing that made more direct and exclusive reference to the mesmeric tradition, on the other hand, such as early chiropractic and osteopathy, insisted on the more immediately tangible aspects of 'harmonization', i.e. on operating a somatic realignment (however theorized and technically brought about) that would re-establish a harmonious flow of 'life force' (Fuller 1989, Chapter 4). As we shall see, yoga could easily enter into a dialogue – and did – with either psychological (i.e. Metaphysical) or somatic (i.e. mesmeric) branches of Harmonialism, due to its varied and flexible psychosomatic emphases.

Of course the American cultic milieu offered a much more varied spectrum of theories and practices than the ones outlined above: these, however, have been singled out because they were the ones that especially influenced Vivekananda in his formulation of Modern Yoga. That they should prove particularly attractive to him comes as no surprise once we know how influential Swedenborgianism, mesmerism and, even more so, Transcendentalism had been in the Bengali cultic milieu (see also Chapter 4). In a way, all that Vivekananda was coming in contact with were more advanced elaborations of beliefs that were based on, and thus confirmed, his earlier worldview.

The demand for "occult" practices at the end of the nineteenth century

There was yet another aspect of the American cultic milieu that was specific to the Western situation. We have already pointed out at the end of the last chapter how 'Egypt' and 'India' had been elected as repositories of wisdom and metaphysical knowledge by leading

Western esotericists and their followers. We have also shown how Neo-Vedāntins had appropriated these discourses for apologetic purposes. There were also more specific developments that we should be aware of. These have been studied by Godwin who summarizes them as follows:

> There seems to have been a concerted effort in the early 1870s to give out fresh doctrines to a world already familiar with spiritualistic ideas of occult phenomena and the afterlife. The new doctrines would be known collectively as "occultism", and for some years the relative merits and meanings of occultism and spiritualism would be debated. The two sects looked to different authorities and held out different goals to the aspirant. The authorities of spiritualism were the conscious spirits of the dead, and the goal was to continue one's spiritual development in the afterlife so as to become more like them. The authorities of occultism were adepts of the past, contacted mainly through their books, and living adepts who were inaccessible unless one was contacted by them. The highest goal was to attain adeptship oneself, in this life. (1994: 302–3)

First of all a clarification about terms: here Godwin uses *spiritualism* and *occultism* as emic terms. As explained in the relevant section of Chapter 1, the spiritualism to which Godwin refers (also called 'spiritism') is the one based on the nineteenth-century belief that humans can communicate with the spirits of the departed. This should not be confused with Protestant "spiritualism" and therefore, following Hanegraaff (1996: 403–4), we refer to this as modern spiritualism, without inverted commas. Similarly, Godwin talks about occultism referring to the emic term used by the groups he is discussing. As this meaning should not be confused with the central etic category of occultism used so far, the emic term that Godwin uses will be distinguished in our use by inverted commas as "occultism".

Regarding the conceptual debates between modern spiritualists and "occultists", it is beyond doubt that Vivekananda was fully aware of them: indeed he joins these debates repeatedly in his lectures.[44] It is also clear that, as a Neo-Vedāntin, he would join the "occultist" camp in which "the authorities" were past and present "adepts" and the goal was to obtain "adeptship". However, Vivekananda, in the secularizing drive that eventually led him to formulate a mixture of

44. For example, *CW* 1: 150, 157, 159, 321; *CW* 9: 88, 261, 520–1.

materialistic and psychologized Modern Yoga, sustained that such adeptship was in no way "inaccessible", but part of each human's birthright. The logical consequence of this was that the related training would start to be equated with any other type of secular training. Sister Devamata (American-born Laura Glenn; d. 1942), who became a follower of Vivekananda after attending his New York lectures in 1895–96, shows how such an assumption had become commonplace a few decades later. In 1927 she wrote in her diary: "As students in the past have gone to Paris to study art and to Germany to study music, so they will in time turn to India to acquire ... the most efficient method of developing the religious consciousness."[45]

Mention of "the most efficient method" brings us to the crux of the matter. The unprecedented development here is that the growing membership of Western cultic milieus had developed a strong craving for *practices*. In an age of swift technological growth and utilitarianism this was, of course, altogether understandable. People wanted techniques and methods to achieve more or less immediate, practical and rational goals. Increasing secularization, on the other hand, meant that lay standards were likely to be seamlessly (and unthinkingly) transposed to the religious sphere.

Godwin (1994: 346) points out how the issue of practices became a central concern of cultic milieus towards the end of the nineteenth century. The two most influential esoteric schools of the period – the Theosophical and Hermetic Societies [46] – were not providing their members with what they most wanted, namely "instruction in practical occultism". Within the Theosophical Society, for example (more interesting to us because it had strong links with Oriental teachings),

> promises had been made [for years] ... But they had come to nothing: the powers of the practical adept seemed to be limited to Madame Blavatsky. And now there were tantalizing accounts ... of the still greater powers of the Himalayan Mahatmas, which were held out as the ultimate goal of everyone. But how was one even to put one's first

45. See Sil (1997: 184) for Devamata's biographical notes and *ibid.* (p. 99) for diary entry. Of course something of what Sister Devamata foresaw actually came to pass with the 1960s' 'hippy trail' to India.
46. The Hermetic Society was founded in 1884 by Anna Kingsford and Edward Maitland, but, like other 'Hermetic' societies of the time, was not as interested in Eastern teachings as the Theosophical Society was (Godwin 1994: 333).

> step on the ladder that led to these heights? Those close to Blavatsky hoped desperately to be taken on as chelas (disciples) by one of these "great souls" (which is what *maha atma* means), but it was made clear that this privilege was almost beyond hoping for. (Ibid.: 346)

It was in this context that yoga started to attract more and more attention. We already referred to the huge success of Arnold's *Light of Asia*, which narrated the life of the Buddha in "a way that matched Victorian taste".[47] The *vox populi*, representing the intellectual and religious propensities of the time, selected this romanticized figure as one of its role models. A paragon of Protestant ethics, steeped in the unitive oceanic feeling of intuitive mysticism, doing away with abstruse theologies and ritualism and successfully applying the Victorian self-help approach to the spiritual realm, this domesticated Buddha came to represent the archetypal *yogin* in the eyes of the cultic milieu – a representation that continues to this day.[48] Vivekananda, as we saw, added his praise to the general consensus.

Vivekananda's 'turn West'

By autumn 1894, just over one year after his arrival in America, Vivekananda was well acclimatized to the local cultural temper, which he seems to have found very congenial. Several commentators, both emic and etic, remark on this change, which may be termed Vivekananda's 'turn West' to mirror the opposite and complementary ideological move of Western esotericism and occultism (see note 25, Chapter 2). Traffic on the esotericist bridge of East–West dialogue, so far taking place mainly in a West–East direction, now started to move substantially the opposite way too. But moving in this new direction required adaptation, and Vivekananda was well aware of this. We saw that the Swami's Western audiences wanted 'techniques' and 'spiritual practices' as they were bent, in good Western utilitarian fashion, on getting 'results'. Vivekananda could sympathize with them as he himself was a pragmatist,[49] and he did not see any

47. Fields (1992: 68), who adds that Arnold "succeeded because he wrote a story, and not a tract or exposition. His Buddha is part Romantic hero, part self-reliant man, and part Christ without being Christ" (*ibid.*).
48. Arnold's poem is reverentially quoted in influential Modern Yoga books such as Wood (1982 [1959]: 21–4) and, more recently, Criswell (1989: 105).
49. This term is not used in any strict philosophical sense here, but in the colloquial sense of "action or policy dictated by consideration of the immediate practical consequences rather than by theory or dogma" (Sinclair 1999: 1216).

problem in adjusting the teachings of Hinduism accordingly. As he wrote from America to his fellow monk Kali (Abhedananda) in November 1894:

> you should know that religion of the type that obtains in our country does not go here. You must suit it to the taste of the people. If you ask [Americans] to become Hindus, they will all give you a wide berth and hate you, as we do the Christian missionaries. They like some of the ideas of our Hindu scriptures – that is all ... A few thousand people have faith in the Advaita doctrine. But they will give you the go-by if you talk obscure mannerisms about sacred writings, caste, or women. (*CW* 7: 481)

Adjusting his teachings on the basis of these principles, the Swami achieved good results over the following winter (1894–95). In June 1895 he wrote to a friend that he was not going to return to India for the time being, even though his fellow monks back there were "getting desperate" for his return. He felt that he had to carry on with his Western work: "I have a seed planted here and wish it to grow. This winter's work in N. Y. [*sic*] was splendid,[50] and it may die if I suddenly go over to India" (*CW* 8: 343). Thus Vivekananda's 'turn West' shows in a complete shift in the Swami's self-chosen 'mission'. In Jackson's words:

> At the time he sailed for the United States, the swami's primary concern ... was not the propagation of Vedanta in the West but raising money to finance the humanitarian work that he planned in India ... [The] warm reception at the congress [i.e. Parliament of Religions] and during lectures in the months afterward persuaded him to launch a separate Western effort in tandem with the Indian work ... the idea of establishing Vedanta centres in the United States was an unanticipated result rather than the original intent of his Western trip. (1994: 25; cf. also *ibid.*: 28).[51]

50. Classes seem to have continued to go well: in a letter dated 25 April 1895 (*CW* 6: 306) Vivekananda refers to regular, well-attended "yoga classes" (that is, talks). In May 1895 he states that difficulties have been overcome (probably the financial difficulties referred to in *CW* 6: 308) and that "classes will go on nicely now no doubt" (*CW* 7: 489).
51. Cf. Marie-Louise Burke, who "concludes that the idea of a separate Western mission did not crystallise in Vivekananda's mind until late 1894" (quoted in Jackson 1994: 155, note 33). For etic treatments cf. *ibid.* (p. 25, partly quoted below) and Sil (1997: 154–5).

There is, however, also an inner, and arguably more seminal aspect to Vivekananda's 'turn West'. By looking closely enough, we can see the beginnings of a deeper shift from an esoteric to an occultistic worldview, thanks to which Neo-Vedānta becomes fully engaged in the shaping of New Age religion. This will create a special compatibility between these two ideological strands: the two will, as it were, develop hand in hand, overlapping in parts, but also capable of autonomous growth. Exemplarily if not exclusively embodied in Vivekananda, this deeper change was in the making over the summer of 1895, and finally came to full fruition over the winter of 1895–96.

From mid-June to early August 1895 Vivekananda ran a special retreat at Thousand Island Park. Only a few selected students were invited to this event, during which Vivekananda intended to "manufacture a few 'Yogis'" (*CW* 6: 306). Situated on an island in the St Lawrence River, the house where the group met belonged to one of the Swami's admirers. This may well have been the earliest 'yoga retreat' to take place in the West, as, according to Jackson (1994: 30), Vivekananda instructed his followers in "deep breathing and meditation". An account of the theoretical teachings given on this occasion is extant (*CW* 7: 3–104). Revealingly, we find a mixture of Sen-like religion of "divine humanity" and Metaphysical tenets, resulting in an insistence on the importance of "Self" and "Self-realization". Exemplary quotations are only too easy to find:

> It is impossible to find God outside of ourselves. Our own souls contribute all the divinity that is outside of us. We are the greatest temple. The objectification is only a faint imitation of what we see within ourselves. (*Ibid.*: 59)

> All is my Self. Say this unceasingly. (*Ibid.*: 61)

> Go into your own room and get the Upanishads out of your own Self. You are the greatest book that ever was or ever will be, the infinite depository of all that is. (*Ibid.*: 71)

> "I am the essence of bliss." Follow no ideal, you are all that is. (*Ibid.*: 74)

> Christs and Buddhas are simply occasions upon which to objectify our own inner powers. We really answer our own prayers. (*Ibid.*: 78)

> We may call it Buddha, Jesus, Krishna, Jehovah, Allah, Agni, but it is only the Self, the "I". (*Ibid.*: 88)

The first and the penultimate quotations also show signs of the New Thought view according to which we should "take responsibility" for our own situation by way of activating our mental powers. Along with these hints, we also find more direct examples of the Swami's attempts to integrate Neo-Vedānta with Metaphysical and New Thought forms of belief:

> Each thought is a little hammer blow on the lump of iron which our bodies are, manufacturing out of it what we want it to be.
>
> We are heirs to all the good thoughts of the universe, if we open ourselves to them. (*Ibid.*: 20)

> The universe is thought, and the Vedas are the words of this thought. We can create and uncreate this whole universe. (*Ibid.*: 47)

We further find in the records that the '4 yogas' model is starting to emerge as the paragon of efficient spiritual practice:

> The will can be made strong in thousands of ways; every way is a kind of Yoga, but the systematised Yoga accomplishes the work more quickly. Bhakti, Karma, Raja, and Jnana-Yoga get over the ground more effectively. (*Ibid.*: 71)

By the autumn of 1895 Vivekananda was well versed in adapting Hindu traditional lore to the requirements of the West. In an interesting letter to his onetime friend and collaborator E. T. Sturdy he gives a striking example of how he went about this. During a stay in London he had been visited by two intellectually cultivated seekers:

> both of them want[ed] to know the rituals of my creed! This opened my eyes ... It is absolutely necessary to form some ritual and have a Church. That is to say, we must fix on some ritual as fast as we can ... we shall go to the Asiatic Society library or you can procure for me a book which is called *Hemādri Kosha*,[52] from which we can get what we want, and kindly bring the Upanishads. We will fix something grand, from birth to death of a man. A mere loose system of philosophy gets no hold of mankind. (*CW* 8: 356–7)

These particular ideas did not materialize in the end. But the point is made about how eager Vivekananda was to please his followers, and

52. The "Dictionary of Hemādri": colloquial name for Hemādri's (1260–1309) *Caturvargacintāmaṇi*, a kind of encyclopaedia of ancient religious rites.

also about how sharply he realized that they needed more than a "loose system of philosophy" to hang on to. Yoga practice eventually emerged as the obvious complement.

Vivekananda's '4 yogas' model

After some trial and error the Swami succeeded in adjusting his doctrinal focus so as to satisfy his audiences: this final conceptual shift, which took place in winter 1895–96, is clearly observable when reading newspaper reports of his public addresses in chronological order from 1893 to 1900.[53] Up to early 1895 our author's main preoccupation had been to defend, explain and justify Hinduism to his American audiences. This he mainly did by presenting Brahmo-oriented Neo-Vedāntic esotericism in highly apologetic terms. Over the summer of 1895 he started elaborating and passing on more syncretic teachings and practices to an inner circle of students. Over the winter of 1895–96 these teachings, now more structured, were presented to a wider public. The second winter of successful teaching in the West and the growth of a dependable, dedicated and financially supportive following[54] also allowed (and encouraged) him to become more daring and assertive. There is also evidence that these new teachings were not only elaborated in response to his audiences' needs, but that he himself found them satisfactory and enriching.[55] The basic message was simple: a reinterpreted, simplified and modernized Vedānta was presented as the exemplary form of "Universal religion", capable of catering for all religious needs through different types of yoga.[56]

At this juncture, Vivekananda adopts Sen's "fourfold classification of devotees" (see Chapter 2). He, however, progressively re-elaborates it into what will become his '4 yogas' scheme, which from

53. See the section on "American Newspaper Reports" in *CW* 9: 429–512. Other series of newspaper reports published in Vivekananda's *Collected Works* do not reveal this pattern as they only cover periods up to April 1895 (*CW* 2) and April 1894 (*CW* 3). Other, more complete collections of newspaper reports (Basu and Ghosh 1969; Burke 1983–87) should show a similar evolutive pattern.
54. Some of his publications, including *Rāja Yoga*, were sponsored by his pupils (*CW* 8: 374–5).
55. See the comments made during the first public lecture he gave in Colombo after his return from the West (15 January 1897; CW 3: 104): "Some good has been done, no doubt, in the West, but specially to myself; for what before was the result of an emotional nature, perhaps, has gained the certainty of conviction and attained the power and strength of demonstration."
56. See Jackson's overview of the Ramakrishna movement's teachings (1994, Chapter 4).

this point onwards becomes central to his teachings.[57] In a newspaper report dated 8 December 1895 (*CW* 9: 482) we read that the Swami's universal religion is adaptable to all circumstances because it caters to all types of people: it comprises four different types of "worship" adapted to the "four general types of men ... the rational, the emotional, the mystical and the worker". By 19 January 1896 "the Swami's fundamental teachings", echoing the basic tenets propagated during the summer 1895 retreat, are reported to revolve around what is now four types of *yoga*, leading to "God-" and "Self-realization":

> Every man must develop according to his own nature. As every science has its methods, so has every religion. Methods of attaining the end of our religion are called Yoga, and the different forms of Yoga that we teach are adapted to the different natures and temperaments of men. We classify them in the following way, under four heads:
> (1) Karma Yoga – The manner in which a man realizes his own divinity through works and duty.
> (2) Bhakti Yoga – The realization of a divinity through devotion to and love of a personal God.
> (3) Rajah [*sic*] Yoga – The realization of divinity through control of mind.
> (4) Gnana Yoga – The realization of man's own divinity through knowledge.
>
> These are all different roads leading to the same center – God. Indeed, the varieties of religious belief are an advantage, since all faiths are good, so far as they encourage man to religious life. The more sects there are the more opportunities there are for making successful appeals to the divine instinct in all men. (*CW* 9: 484)[58]

It was at this time that the Swami's teachings really struck root in American soil. After the period of nomadic lecturing following the Parliament of Religions, he finally managed to establish a teaching base in New York. The faithful stenographer J. J. Goodwin joined him in the winter of 1895 and began systematically to record his teachings,[59] soon to be transformed into books. By February 1896 his first book on *Karma-Yoga* was on the market and *Rāja Yoga* was in

57. He may conceivably have started to elaborate this theme as early as May 1895, when he gave a lecture on "The rationale of yoga" (*CW* 6: 306; see full chronology (not including *CW* 9) in Williams 1974: 133–4). This text, however, is not extant.
58. An almost identical but undated passage is found in the section "Notes from lectures and discourses" in *CW* 5: 292 under the title "The goals and methods of realization".
59. See *CW* 5: 120–1, 123; *CW* 8: 370, 373. See also biographical notes in Sil (1997: 186).

the press.[60] The latter was sold out and ready to go through another edition by November of the same year;[61] *Jnana-Yoga* and *Bhakti-Yoga* would be published posthumously.

It is in *Rāja Yoga*, however, that Vivekananda's worldview takes the final leap from Neo-Vedāntic esotericism to Neo-Vedāntic occultism. We have discussed how Neo-Vedānta absorbed the three 'mirrors of secularization' (evolutionism, the study of religions, and the psychologization of religion) before Vivekananda's time. We also found that Vivekananda, while continuing to build on these foundations, took the psychologization of religion further by assimilating Metaphysical teachings into his worldview. In his final synthesis of Modern Yoga, i.e. in *Rāja Yoga*, this will continue. But beyond this, the Swami will attempt to apply the then foundational concept of mechanistic instrumental causality pervasively to his subject, thus completing the process of secularization (and occultization) of Neo-Vedānta. These developments will be analysed in some detail in Chapter 5.

Before we proceed to that, however, we must throw a final backward glance to Neo-Vedāntic doctrinal developments by discussing a central question: we saw how the ultimate aim of Vivekananda's '4 yogas' was "realization", either of "God" or of "Self". The importance and desirability of such "realization" will remain a fundamental assumption in the greatest majority of Modern Yoga elaborations. But not only is the "realization" semantic cluster fundamental in Neo-Vedānta: it will also be the main conceptual locus of overlap and identification between Neo-Vedānta and New Age religion. As we shall see in Part II, this intellectual dynamis of identification and cross-fertilization will be for the best part played out within the framework of 'alternative healing' discourses, i.e. within the framework of what will later be known as 'alternative medicine'.[62] Modern Yoga will act as a pioneering discipline in its processes of acculturation to Western occultism, to be later followed by other Indian and non-Indian traditions.[63] Because of the importance of "realization" discourses in this context, and because of their

60. Letter dated 29 February 1896 (*CW* 8: 373).
61. *CW* 6: 382; also *CW* 5: 123, which further states that the biggest buyers were India and America.
62. For a discussion of this and related terms see Chapter 6.
63. Such as, for example, Japanese martial arts and a number of Chinese traditions: acupuncture, Taiji Quan (Tai Chi Chuan) and, more recently, Qi Gong (Chi Kung) and Ayurveda.

centrality in holding Eastern and Western occultism together, we shall proceed to analyse their linguistic and semantic history in the next chapter.

4. “God-realization” and “Self-realization” in Neo-Vedānta

> We are going to enter into the domain of a new dispensation, that of science and faith harmonized...
>
> (Sen 1901: 439)

The importance of Vivekananda’s ideological and institutional contributions to modern understandings and perceptions of Hinduism has been highlighted by a number of scholars (see below). The fact that these contributions hinge on the concept of “realization” has also been pointed out. The esoterico-occultistic implications and foundations of these facts, however, still need to be made explicit. A beginning in this direction will be attempted in the present chapter and in the next.

Pervasiveness of Vivekananda’s Neo-Vedāntic influences

In the Preface to his biography of Vivekananda, Sil (1997: 11) states that the Swami is still widely perceived as “the spiritual ambassador of India to the West”, as the “most powerful inspiration behind the country’s successful nationalist struggle” and as “the most authoritative voice of Hindu India”. Rambachan, on the other hand, emphasizes the Swami’s role not only as a propagator, but also as the shaper of discourses when he writes:

> Vivekananda's influence is ... pervasive ... Not only did he largely formulate [the contemporary understanding of Hinduism], but he also gave it the language in which it is articulated. There is very little in modern Hindu, particularly Vedānta, apologetic writing that does not carry the clear imprint of Vivekananda's influence. (1994: 7)

First-person reports of how deeply the Swami affected other people's lives also abound, but one especially relevant example will suffice. The scholar and onetime president of India, Sarvepalli Radhakrishnan, one of the most successful propagators of a polished form of Neo-Vedānta in the twentieth century, was deeply influenced, along with many others before and after him, by Vivekananda's thought and example. Reminiscing about his student days he affirmed that it was the Swami's "humanistic, man-making religion that gave us courage" (quoted in King 1999: 136). As the nationalist spirit gathered momentum, the Swami's letters were circulated in manuscript form among the students, to great effect: "The kind of thrill which we enjoyed, the kind of mesmeric touch that those writings gave us, the kind of reliance in our own culture that was being criticized all around – it is that kind of transformation which his writings effected in the young men in the early years of this century" (*ibid.*).

As for Vivekananda's institutional legacy, Williams (1995a: 55) confirms that the Ramakrishna movement established by Vivekananda "has been credited with championing the cultural revival ... of modern India" and with the "purifying [of] Hindu monasticism". Reporting on the Western side of the operation, Jackson (1994: 144) states that "more than any other group, the Ramakrishna movement has become the 'official' voice of Hinduism in the West". While both these opinions may be somewhat overstated in the sense that they do not take into account dissenting or competing voices, there is no denying the pervasiveness of Vivekananda's influence on modern Hinduism and on how Hinduism came to be perceived in the West.

Centrality of the "realization" theme

As for the more theoretical aspects of Vivekananda's teachings, Rambachan highlights the centrality of the "realization" theme:

> One cannot overestimate the importance of the experience of direct perception in Vivekananda's philosophy of religion. It is this that he

signifies by the frequently used expression *realization* and that may, with good reason, be said to constitute the central and most outstanding feature of his religious thought. It is an idea that he unfailingly labors in almost every one of his lectures. (1994: 94–5)

According to Vivekananda, the foremost method to attain such "direct perception of religious truths" is through *rājayoga* practice (*ibid.*: 96). In this context, *samādhi* represents "the culmination of all the disciplines of *rājayoga*" (*ibid.*: 98). Indeed, Rambachan concludes, Vivekananda "presents *samādhi* as the only satisfactory source of *brahmajñāna*", for in his thought *samādhi* occupies "the same function and status as a source of knowledge for *brahmajñāna*, which Śaṅkara ascribes to the Vedas as *śabda-pramāṇa* (a source of valid knowledge)" (*ibid.*).

This idea of yogic experience or "realization", as defined by Vivekananda, will play a major role by becoming the standard Neo-Vedāntic translation for the two key concepts of *brahmajñāna* and *ātmajñāna*. As these two Sanskrit terms stand at the very core of much Upaniṣadic and Vedāntic thought, so their corresponding English translations as "God-" and "Self-realization" stand at the very core of the Neo-Vedāntic ideology popularized by Vivekananda. Understanding the formation of these neologisms and following their semantic transformations over time can help us to understand central aspects of Neo-Vedāntic belief.

Ultimate aims: Vedāntic and Neo-Vedāntic

Hay (1988: 72), again acting as our guide to commonplace views on modern Hinduism, states that Vivekananda became "the apostle to the world of his master's philosophy of God-realization". Is this truly what the master's teachings were about? Williams (1974: 37) seems to agree: "All that Rāmakṛṣṇa had taught converged into two principles: the realization of God and the renunciation of the world." Hay's and Williams' statements are important because they show to what extent the "realization" theme is by now considered, both popularly and academically, as an integral part of the teachings of Ramakrishna. As the latter is widely perceived to be the most representative modern Hindu holy man along with Ramana Maharshi, these are momentous statements indeed.

It is only with Vivekananda, however, that the expressions "God-realization" and "Self-realization" acquire specific Neo-Vedāntic overtones, one or the other of these expressions being sometimes emphasized to the detriment of the other. As is well known, ideologies and popular discourses are propagated on the wings of so-called 'buzzwords', the boundaries of which most of the time remain vague and the contents ill-defined. But they become 'buzzwords' precisely because, while their semantic content proves somehow very attractive and central in relation to the perceived needs of the users, they are also unspecific enough to be used as umbrella terms for quite different yearnings and programmes. This is precisely what happened with "God-" and "Self-realization". As Bharati notes,

> ["God-realization" is a] pervasive Indian-English neologism in Renaissance [i.e. Neo-Vedāntic] parlance ... its use is quite different from any British or American use of the word 'realization'. The meaning of the Indian-English term is something like 'consummation of religious experience'. Possibly, the term might first have been used by neo-Vedāntins in a semi-technical sense: if you *realize* by an act of guided intuition, that you are one with the absolute (brahman), you have *ipso facto* reached the goal of the religious life. (1970: 281, note 43)

Bharati's hunch about the expression deriving from Neo-Vedāntic milieus is indeed accurate. As we shall presently show, the "realization" terminology was in the making throughout the best part of the nineteenth century, but it finally took its current form in the entourage that gravitated around Ramakrishna, and from which Vivekananda and the influential Ramakrishna movement emerged.

Classical interpretations of *ātma-* and *brahmajñāna*

Over time, various authors have attempted to translate and contextualize in a different language (English) and mindset (modern) the central concepts of *brahmajñāna* and *ātmajñāna*. Through processes of linguistic translation and cultural transcontextualization, however, old meanings have disappeared and new ones have been created. The two Sanskrit terms themselves have a long and distinguished history in Hinduism: attaining *brahmajñāna*[1] is a goal repeatedly recommended in the *Upaniṣads*, and as such it has become a standard definition of the ultimate goal in most Vedāntic contexts. This concept has direct links with the *Vedas* and places itself centrally in both the Upaniṣadic-Vedāntic and yogic traditions. As Hardy explains:

> The Upaniṣads ... contain a large number of speculations on the One [i.e. *brahman*], along the cosmological lines of the earlier literature. And the aim is still to 'come to know it'. But the purpose of such knowledge has changed. To 'know it' now means to achieve that qualitative leap into the realm of liberation ... [T]he concept of *brahman* [now] emerges from [former Vedic speculations] as the sole survivor. This nevertheless expanded the denotation of the term far beyond what the earlier literature meant by it. Now *brahman* was not just the 'sacred' power pervading the sacrifice and the Veda itself, and not just the One out of which the many arose, but also the One into which man merges back by achieving his liberation from the cycle of rebirths (*saṃsāra*). Moreover, *brahman* is an experiential reality, available through meditation.
>
> ...The 'coming to know' itself is mentioned under different names [including *brahmajñāna*] but eventually the common and well-known term 'yoga' becomes universally used to refer to such forms of meditation. (1990: 52–3)

The earliest *Upaniṣads* (*Bṛhadāraṇyaka*, *Chāndogya*, etc.) dwelt on more mystically oriented monistic teachings, defending a special ontological relationship between *ātman* and *brahman*. A different set of interpretations, however, was already starting to appear before the beginning of the common era. In the so-called theistic *Upaniṣads* (*Śvetāśvatara*, *Muṇḍaka*, etc.), the yogic union of *ātman* and *brahman* starts to be interpreted in terms of union between individuated *puruṣa* and universal *puruṣa* or God (Falk 1986: 208–9). The full flourishing of these theories will come about in classical Vedānta with the formulation of the Advaita, Viśiṣṭādvaita and Dvaita positions, their doctrinal bias reflected in specific yogic emphases:

1. Literally "knowledge/gnosis of *brahman*" and more loosely "divine or sacred knowledge, spiritual wisdom" (Monier-Williams 1994 [1899]: 738), "divine knowledge" (Apte 1991 [1890]: 395), and "knowledge of the Absolute" or, in Neo-Vedāntic mode, "Self-realization" (Grimes 1996: 95).

> Ever since Śaṅkara put forth his system of *advaita*, Hindu philosophical and theological discussion has been a dialectical controversy within the Vedānta school of philosophy between his non-dualism on the one hand and various shades of "qualified" non-dualism (*viśiṣṭa-advaita*) or dualism (*dvaita*) on the other. On the practical religious level the two sides of this discussion have been identified with *jñāna yoga* and *bhakti yoga* respectively. (Neevel 1976: 85)

From a certain point of view, the discrepancies in teaching between Ramakrishna and Vivekananda reflect the above Dvaita-Advaita dichotomy. This would not be a major point of controversy had both teachers propagated positions consistent with the foregoing Vedāntic traditions. Indeed, due to the inclusiveness of Ramakrishna's teachings, Vivekananda's predilections may just have represented a shift in emphasis.

But the situation is not as simple as that. Not only did Vivekananda show strong leanings towards Advaita; what is much more significant is that he brought about a number of crucial doctrinal and practical changes to key traditional concepts. Of course, he was not the first to attempt novel formulations: indeed, as we saw in the previous chapters and as confirmed by Halbfass (1988, Chapter 12), such formulations were strongly called for by the nineteenth-century Indian "hermeneutic situation" from Rammohan Roy onwards. The difference with Vivekananda was that, steeped in Neo-Vedāntic esotericism, he came to combine this with avant-garde Western occultism. His physical presence and charisma, his organizational drive, an established tradition of Western interest in 'the mystic East' and the diffused *fin de siècle* anxiety were all factors that contributed to his success.[2] On a more practical and organizational level, the Swami created (thanks also to the financial support of his Western disciples) new cultural and institutional links between East and West. These have developed in very productive ways up to now, and seem to hold good potential for growth also in future – though possibly more in India than elsewhere nowadays.

2. Concerning 'the mystic East' concept, rooted in Romanticism, see Halbfass (1988, Chapters 5–8) and King (1999). Concerning *fin de siècle* gloom see Teich and Porter (1990).

Early attempts at translation and contextualization: Rammohan Roy

Let us examine some significant examples of the pre-Vivekananda tradition of attempted translations. Rammohan Roy marks an obvious beginning: the earliest modern popularizer and translator of Vedāntic teachings[3] and of selected *Upaniṣads* in both Indian vernacular (Bengali) and English, he was also the first whose English vocabulary seemed to waver and slip around this admittedly hard-to-render (in its philosophical and cultural meanings) term.

In Roberston's monograph (1995) on the famous Bengali we read that, according to Roy, "the entire literature of vedanta discusse[d] only two topics": firstly "*Brahmavidya* or *Atmavidya*, 'knowledge of the unmanifest Supreme Being' ", and secondly "sadhana 'the means' of upasana, 'worship' of the unmanifest Supreme Being" (*ibid.*: 88).[4] We may note in passing that in this radically simplified view of Vedānta we already have, at this early stage, a kind of preview of what will become the essence of twentieth-century Modern Yoga: a strong focus on "practice" justified by a theory of "realization" (whether of "God" or "Self").

Starting from these premises, Roy identified what he believed to be "the heart of vedanta", i.e. the injunction " 'Adore God alone' " (*ibid.*). Such "true worship leads to liberation (moksa) ... [as] 'He who knows God thoroughly adheres unto God' ... [and] 'whoever is endowed with knowledge of God attains God-nature' "(*ibid.*: 94). Again, we are already well on the way to "God-" and "Self-realization": *brahman* has already become "God", and 'knowing' him bestows liberation and "God-nature" onto the knower. But this was only Roy's early position – strongly theistic and somewhat simplistic, not having been worked out in too much detail – as exposed in his 1816 *Abridgement of the Vedant*. His ideas and terminology, however, were to develop over time.

We shall briefly expand on them because Roy's position was seminal with regard to later Neo-Vedāntic ideological developments. Roy's direct influence in this context is, of course, important, but we should also see him as the channel through which the concerns and

3. In his *Vedāntasāra* (1815, see Chapters 1 and 2).
4. Words within single quotation marks in extracts from Robertson (1995) are Roy's actual translations of Vedāntic texts into English.

conceptualizations of the Bengali intelligentsia of his day were voiced. It was with the support and feedback of his entourage that he addressed a number of vital issues: the gradual erosion of the relatively egalitarian, Enlightenment-informed relations with British Orientalists; the exclusivistic claims of Christianity, boosted by the West's technological might; the power that the West (and especially Britain) wielded in India and on the global stage; and the pressing need to retain a Hindu and Indian identity while accommodating the tenets of modernity.

After the publication of *The Precepts of Jesus* (1820) and the ensuing controversy, as we saw in Chapter 2, Roy shifted to Unitarian positions. This ideological battle made Roy take up a more defensive attitude and emphasize the role of an ineffable *brahman*, as opposed to his earlier, more Christian-sounding term "God". The Trust Deed of the Brahmo Samaj building, opened in January 1830,[5] seems in fact to go out of its way to avoid using the latter term, while at the same time demonstrating how firmly Christian-style ethics and morality were becoming part of Neo-Vedāntic formulations. This interesting document also shows how Roy was starting to gravitate towards forms of unstructured "spiritualism" which would greatly encourage the growth of a cultic milieu. The Brahmo Samaj building, we read, was

> [t]o be used . . . as a place of public meeting of all sorts and descriptions of people without distinction as shall behave and conduct themselves in an orderly sober religious and devout manner for the worship and adoration of the Eternal Unsearchable and Immutable Being who is the Author and Preserver of the Universe but not under or by any other name designation or title peculiarly used for and applied to any particular Being or Beings by any man or set of men whatsoever . . . and that no sermon preaching discourse prayer or hymn be delivered made or used in such worship but such as have a tendency to the promotion of the contemplation of the Author and Preserver of the Universe to the promotion of charity morality piety benevolence virtue and the strengthening the bonds of union between men of all religious persuasions and creeds. (Quoted in Farquhar 1977 [1914]: 35)

5. Roy founded a society called Brahmo Sabha in 1828, but the name was soon changed to Brahmo Samaj. It is also interesting to note that in 1815 he had already established a similar society called Atmiya Sabha which, however, stopped functioning in 1819 (Farquhar 1977 [1914]: 31). The choice of names points to the centrality of *brahman*- and *ātman*-related terminology in Neo-Vedānta.

Summing up Roy's role in the context of the present discussion we may say that he was the first to bring to prominence and explore the conceptual range of what would later be called "God-" and "Self-realization". Differently from those who were to follow, however, he was still inclined to legitimize teachings through revealed texts rather than through 'inner feeling' and inspiration as Debendranath Tagore would do after him. A kind of Neo-Vedāntic *philosophe*, Roy also sought to legitimize his religion through rationality and on the basis of "humanistic principles rather than through esoteric and metaphysical knowledge" (Godwin 1994: 314). He nevertheless actively prepared the ground for later Neo-Vedāntic esoteric speculations (albeit unwittingly) by starting to loosen Hinduism from earlier forms of orthodox dogmatism and their corresponding social structures.[6]

Subsequent attempts at translation and contextualization by Brahmo leaders and others

The next influential individual within the Brahmo intelligentsia, as we saw, was Debendranath Tagore. While he followed Roy in his belief that "original Hinduism was a pure spiritual theism, and in his enthusiasm for the Upanishads, [he] did not share his deep reverence for Christ" (Farquhar 1977 [1914]: 39) nor for the infallibility of revealed texts. He did, however, play his role in keeping the Neo-Vedāntic equivalence between "God" and "*brahman*" alive. The Brahmo Covenant is a good example of this. The Covenant was "a list of solemn vows to be taken by every one on becoming a member of the Society" (*ibid.*: 40). Drawn up in 1843, it centred upon belief in "God" and on the practice of his worship (*ibid.*). The fact that the standard ritual of formal worship elaborated by Debendranath was called *Brahmopāsana* (*ibid.*) shows how the two terms "God" and "*brahman*" were regarded as synonyms. The Bengali leader's own life and proclivities also contributed to establish the 'yogic realization mystique' as an important Neo-Vedāntic theme. This would later become a major component of the "Swadeshi Sannyasi" apologetic and nationalistic model that Vivekananda powerfully contributed to establish (see Chowdury-Sengupta 1996). As Farquhar (1977 [1914]: 40) points out: Debendranath "lived a life of constant prayer and

6. For in-depth analyses of Roy's religio-philosophical beliefs and leanings see also Killingley (1977; 1993).

worship of God; and the direct communion of the human soul with the supreme Spirit was the most salient point in his teaching".

By the middle of the nineteenth century we also find evidence of scientistic proto Modern Yoga concepts being elaborated in more secular contexts. These would have represented a more 'empirical' level of speculation *vis-à-vis* more religiously oriented Brahmo speculations. The earliest evidence traced consists of a fascinating tract by the Bengali surgeon N. C. Paul (Navīna-Chandra Pāla), first published in 1850 (Paul 1888).

This author did not employ the realization terminology we have been examining, but attempted to explain yoga in scientific and 'mesmerico-hypnotic' terms. About the latter type of explanation, for example, he stated that "The Dhyana of the Yogis is the Turya avastha of the Vedantists[7] – the ecstacy [*sic*] of the Physicians, the self-contemplation of the German mesmerists, and the clairvoyance of the French philosophers" (*ibid.*: ii). He also described various stages of yogic practice as stages of "self-trance" (*ibid.*: i–ii, 24). As for scientific explanations, he discussed the physiology and chemistry of breathing, concluding that what yogis aim to do is to exhale less carbonic acid (*ibid.*: 1–12). The two kinds of explanation are often brought together, as when Paul states that

> When the mind is abstracted from its functions [i.e. during meditation] the amount of carbonic acid is lessened. Hence the Yogis are recommended to fix their sight on the tip of the nose or upon the space between the eye-brows. These peculiar turns of the axes of vision suspend the respiratory movements and generally produce hypnotism. (*ibid.*: 3)

Apart from these more empirical speculations, however, we find that when discussing the ultimate aims of yoga he too is attempting to reach a satisfactory definition of *brahmajñāna*. When leading a fully yogic life the adept becomes "susceptible to peculiar spiritual impressions" and, after the prolonged performance of certain practices, he is "said to hold communion with the Supreme Soul" (*ibid.*: 35). At this point "The Yogi becomes full of Brahma (the Supreme Soul) ... his soul not only holds communion with the invisible, inconceivable, unalterable, omnipresent, omniscient, and omnipotent

7. See note 11, Chapter 8.

Being, but he becomes absorbed into the essence of the same" (*ibid.*: 56).

If Brahmo thinkers were gradually progressing towards the formulation of Neo-Vedāntic occultism, men like Paul show us the more materialistic, pragmatic and utilitarian sides of the Indian esoteric spectrum, already tending toward mesmeric types of speculation and cultivating an interest in alternative types of medicine and healing. We also know that these two strands of thought were in creative dialogue: the Tagore family, for example, encouraged research into the medical applications of hypnosis by supporting Dr James Esdaile's Mesmeric Hospital at Calcutta in the 1840s (Godwin 1994: 160, 180, 317). A number of other Brahmos actively cultivated and propagated the study and practice of homeopathy.[8] Eventually, physicians of the soul and physicians of the body would join forces and techniques to formulate a Modern Yoga identified much more closely, at least at first sight, with categories of 'health and healing' than with religious concerns. This secularized yoga would eventually play a major role both in Neo-Vedānta and New Age styles of religiosity.

Keshubchandra Sen is the next Brahmo leader we need to discuss. Sen further elaborated the central Neo-Vedāntic "realization" theme, albeit taking it in a different direction. Of all individuals reviewed here, Sen was the one with the strongest Christian leanings, and these were altogether of the "spiritualist" type. Through his influence, elaborations on the relationship between God and the faithful became much more firmly rooted into English, Christian and esoteric semantic modes, while Sanskritic conceptualization faded into a distant background. Under such conditions, radical conceptual shifts from the standards of classical Hinduism were relatively easy to operate. Hence what Vivekananda will later reappropriate under the label of "God-" and "Self-realization" would already have been charged with strong Christian and esoteric values. This defining trait, also retained in the Neo-Vedānta of the Ramakrishna movement, will

8. "Many [Brahmo] doctors in the late nineteenth century went abroad to study homeopathy" (Kopf 1979: 111). More research into the overlaps between Neo-Vedānta, Indian medical sciences and esoterico-alternative forms of healing may bring to light further examples of this type of dialogue. In any case, the fact that such an 'esoteric' medical system has been fully accepted as 'orthodox' in India from quite early on is in itself revealing in the context of the present discussion. For an interesting overview of the practice of Homeopathy in nineteenth-century Bengal (and a discussion of related research methodologies) see Arnold and Sarkar (2002).

prove, perhaps unsurprisingly, very appealing to unchurched or dissenting Christian milieus.

As the first fully-fledged Neo-Vedāntic esotericist, Sen introduced the modern reading of individualistic "God-realization" as 'direct perception', a concept that will become pivotal in Vivekananda's understanding of "realization". This is clearly expressed in two lectures, delivered in 1875 and 1880 respectively (Sen 1901: 194–241, 394–442).[9] In the first one Sen states that "The great question in which all Hindu devotees are anxiously interested is whether the soul has seen the Lord. Have you perceived Him? is what they ask each other" (Sen 1901: 205–6).[10] Sen then goes on to appropriate for Neo-Vedānta the central "spiritualist" tenet of the Divine Spark, by affirming that "the Hindu mind" is eminently receptive to this inner spiritual reality. To "the primitive Hindu mind", he states, the "idea of perceiving the In-dwelling Spirit, far from being foreign, is eminently native" (Sen 1901: 207). As for his verdict on scripture, his arguments resemble the ones that Vivekananda will later echo in even more secularized form:

> Is the word of God a book? No. It is spoken, not written ... God speaks to every one of us, and we hear his thrilling voice in the soul ... [Scriptures] are only instructive narratives of what the Lord said and did in the lives of prophets and saints ... To each man, saint or sinner, the Holy Spirit speaks directly as the In-dwelling Teacher. (*Ibid.*: 208–9)

In the 1875 lecture this is still a matter of "spiritual perception":

> Seeing and hearing, these are my testimonies. The eye and the ear are my witnesses; I mean the eye and ear of the soul ... Our ideas of the Divinity are not abstract and intellectual, but are based upon direct and intuitive knowledge. Our faith in God is not so much a conception as a spiritual perception. We see him as a present Reality, a living Person, with the mind's eye. (*Ibid.*: 204–5)

By 1880, however, as the approaching occultization of esotericism brings the "clashing worldviews" of science and traditional belief

9. Similar ideas are already found in Sen's thought as early as 1859 (see Sen 1938: 21–2, 62–5).
10. Cf. the future Vivekananda's anxious questioning of his peers and teachers in the same way, as he himself relates (*CW* 4: 179).

into an uncomfortable partnership, the difference between 'natural' and 'spiritual' vision is starting to become blurred. The seemingly Spencerian arguments that Sen musters are highly reminiscent of how Vivekananda will defend his theories a quarter of a century later. "Between God-vision and the spirit of science in the nineteenth century, there is no discord, but rather concord. The scientists of the present ardently love unity", Sen (*ibid.*: 405) affirms. And while all "physical, mental, and moral energies are traceable to one primitive force" which "all scientific men . . . are seeking" (*ibid.*: 407, 408), the answer is already known to some: "This mysterious primary force, underlying all secondary forces," Sen tells us, "I unhesitatingly call God-force" (*ibid.*: 409).

To this, as it were, energetic Neo-panentheism, Sen adds romantically charged deistic and vitalistic images,[11] and these are said to grant us revelatory visions: "vision[s] in which we directly *realize* God-force" (*ibid.*: 414, emphasis added). As Vivekananda will also teach later, science was starting to confirm religion, to make it accessible: "in these days science has killed the distance – in the physical world by steam and electricity, and in the spiritual world by introspection and immediate vision" (*ibid.*: 416). Thus the "long ladder" that led to "God's sanctuary in days gone by" has all but disappeared: "Instead of many steps there is but one step from earth to heaven. One step from mind and matter to God; one step now from the muscles and the nerves, from the eye and the ear to God" (*ibid.*: 417).

"God's sanctuary", under the circumstances, is made not only more readily, but also more widely available: "To every humble believer, to every man and woman who believes in the Living God, He reveals Himself in these days" (*ibid.*: 431). This is "the domain of a new dispensation, that of faith and science harmonized" (*ibid.*: 439), or also "the philosophy of God-vision in modern times. It is a vision in which Divinity and heaven are *realized* together" (*ibid.*: 426, emphasis added).

As we progress towards the end of the century, the language of 'realization' gets closer to what will eventually become standard expressions. Yoga is by now routinely regarded as a practice to be

11. The universe as a clock, the root nourishing the tree, the mother suckling the little infant (Sen 1901: 412–15).

taken up by all, rather than as a subject of purely scholarly interest or specialist religious endeavour.

We should, of course, remember that, from 1875 onward, the Theosophical Society was very active in popularizing these ideas (Bevir 1994). After it relocated to India (1878), it also started to play an important role in the cultural life of the subcontinent. We shall only mention one example here, directly relevant to the popularization of 'spiritual realization' terminology. In his exposition of *Rāja-Yoga* (1890) the Indian Theosophist Manilal N. Dvivedi[12] explains that the Vedānta is dedicated to "explaining the nature of *Brahma* and the method of realising it" (Dvivedi 1890, Part I: 50). Various Vedāntic doctrines, he continues, concur in "declaring *mokṣa* to consist in the realization of the unity of *Brahma* and *Jiva*" (*ibid.*). In his textual commentary he also explains that it is the ultimate, eternal "*Ātman* ... which is the thing to be understood and realised" (*ibid.*, Part II: 2). The ultimate aim of yoga, he concludes, is "realising the Absolute" (*ibid.*, Part II: 40, 41).[13]

Ramakrishna and his interpreters: the elaboration of a *sampradāya*

At this point we return to the question of Ramakrishna's teachings: are they really the same as those propagated by Vivekananda and by the Ramakrishna movement? We shall single out the *jñāna*/realization discussion in order to attempt an answer.

As previously mentioned, a number of good critical works discussing Ramakrishna, Vivekananda, their relations and their entourage have initiated a more realistic appraisal of both men, and of their historical and hermeneutic situation after decades of glorification and mythicization.[14] We rely on these sources for our discussion. In Chapter 3 we argued that the circumstances of Vivekananda's initiation were highly unorthodox, and also that he was much more a modern tormented seeker than a self-possessed 'natural' renouncer. A comparison of his and Ramakrishna's, position with regard to *jñāna*/

12. Also a delegate (representing Hinduism) at the 1893 Chicago Parliament of Religions (Chowdhury-Sengupta 1998: 24–5; Sil 1997: 159).
13. Also this neologism, "realising the Absolute", will eventually be adopted in Neo-Vedāntic and New Age discourses.
14. See notes 38 and 40, Chapter 1 and note 3, Chapter 3.

realization casts doubts on the reconcilability of their teachings. We know that Vivekananda prioritizes (his interpretations of) Advaitic *ātma-* and *brahmajñāna* as ultimate Vedāntic aims, and that he theorizes that these liberation-granting experiences can only, or at least optimally, be achieved through a *samādhi* attained by way of *rājayoga*. We also know from his own and others' reports, that he himself struggled for most of his life to achieve such states, which he seems to have attained, if at all, only on rare occasions.

Biographical accounts of Ramakrishna, on the other hand, are replete with well-documented reports of recurrent *samādhi* experiences. These came to him so naturally and frequently, indeed, that he had to learn to control and contain them by way of orthopractical knowledge gathered from at least two different teachers (a female tantric ascetic called Bhairavī Brāhmaṇī and the Advaita *sannyāsin* Totapuri). But apart from *experiencing* these states, how did he actually evaluate them from the point of view of religious doctrine? Neevel throws some useful light on this question:

> We wish to clarify Rāmakrishna's position in its relation to Śankara's *kevalādvaita* ("absolute non-dualism") and its path of *jñāna*. This issue is a confused one because Rāmakrishna often talks as if he accepted *kevalādvaita*, and his disciples have emphasized his seeming acceptance. The key to understanding Rāmakrishna's formal acceptance of *kevalādvaita* is to note that this acceptance is given under very strict conditions. Rāmakrishna sees two "realms" or frames of reference in which *kevalādvaita* and *jñāna yoga* are valid – realms which in both cases are totally removed from the state of man as he now exists in the world.
>
> The first theoretical context in which Rāmakrishna recognized the validity of *kevalādvaita* was the purer age or *yuga* that existed long ago before the world degenerated to the present corrupt *Kali yuga*. (1976: 87)

We shall soon see that Vivekananda contradicts this tenet in his teachings. But the second theoretical context has more interesting implications from the point of view of our discussion. Here, Neevel explains, Ramakrishna felt that

> the teaching that "Brahman alone is real and the world is illusory; I have no separate existence; I am that Brahman alone" is relevant only

> in and for the moment when one is merged in *nirvikalpa samādhi*[15] ... Only in this state is it valid for one to view the world as illusion; only in this state is it valid for one to feel that he is Brahman. As soon as the jñāni returns to a level of normal consciousness, as soon as he has enough sense of individuality or "body-consciousness" to utter the word "I" so that he can say aloud "I am Brahman," what he says is no longer true and valid. It is as a matter of fact dangerous for the jñāni and for those who listen to him (*Ibid.*: 88)

Ramakrishna himself stated this position in no uncertain terms:

> "I am He" – this is not a wholesome attitude. If anyone attains this idea before he has overcome the consciousness of the physical self, great harm comes to him, his progress is retarded and by and by he is dragged down. He deceives others and deceives himself as well, in utter ignorance of his woeful plight. (*Ibid.*: 89)[16]

Coherently with the above position, Ramakrishna was adamant in sustaining that Advaita was not a suitable teaching for householders (i.e. non-renunciates) and for those who "identify themselves with the body". These individuals should rather cultivate a *bhakti*-like religiosity:

> ...for those who lead a householder's life, and those who identify themselves with the body,[17] this attitude of "I am He" is not good. It is not good for householders to read Vedānta or the *Yogavāsishtha*. It is very harmful for them to read these books. Householders should look on God as their Master and on themselves as His servants. They should think, "O God, You are the master and Lord, and I am your servant." People who identify themselves with the body should not have the attitude of "I am He". (Gupta 1984 [1942]: 593)

15. *Nirvikalpa samādhi* indicates the highest stage of *samādhi* in Vedāntic terminology, i.e. when it occurs "without distinct and separate consciousness of the knower, the knowable and the process of knowing" (Aranya 1983: 465).
16. Neevel (1976: 59) quotes this from *Gospel of Shri Ramakrishna (According to M., a son of the Lord and disciple)* or *The Ideal Man for India and for the* World, Part II (Madras, The Brahmavadin Office, 1907 [1897]), pp. 70–2).
17. This important point is rarely emphasized in the relevant literature, which tends instead to focus on the (usually exclusively male) householder/renouncer polarity: the category of those who "identify themselves with the body" is a much more comprehensive one than that of "householders". It may well include women, unmarried males of all ages, and those (struggling, failed or possibly 'part-time') renouncers who fit the description.

This, however, is in stark contradiction with Vivekananda's (and Brahmo) teachings, propounding that everyone should seek *samādhi*-based *ātma-* and *brahmajñāna*, and that enlightenment and liberation (*mokṣa*) are theirs by birthright. Talking about *samādhi* in the context of his *rājayoga* teachings, Vivekananda says:

> All the different steps in Yoga are intended to bring us scientifically to the superconscious state, or Samadhi. Furthermore, this is a most vital point to understand, that inspiration is as much in every man's nature as it was in that of the ancient prophets. These prophets were not unique, they were men as you or I; they were great Yogis. They had gained this superconsciousness, and you and I can get the same. They were not peculiar people. The very fact that one man ever reached that state, proves that it is possible for every man to do so. Not only is it possible, but every man must, eventually, get to that state, and that is religion. Experience is the only teacher we have. (*CW* 1: 185)

And regarding the universality and 'naturalness' of this experience the Swami further states:

> The [religious] teachers all saw God; they all saw their own souls ... and what they saw they preached. Only there is this difference, that by most of these religions, especially in modern times, a peculiar claim is made, namely, that these experiences are impossible at the present day; they were only possible with a few men, who were the first founders of the religions that subsequently bore their names. At the present time these experiences have become obsolete, and, therefore, we have now to take religion on belief. This I entirely deny. If there has been one experience in this world in any particular branch of knowledge, it absolutely follows that that experience has been possible millions of times before, and will be repeated eternally. Uniformity is the rigorous law of nature, what once happened can always happen. (*Ibid.*: 126–7)

As we notice, this passage contradicts both conditions set by Ramakrishna for the acceptability of Advaita: the *Kali Yuga* variant and the 'overcomer/body-identified' variant. Vivekananda's rendition of yoga, as we shall see in more detail in the next chapter, also thoroughly naturalizes and secularizes this discipline. Here yoga becomes a science based on 'natural laws', or a 'spiritual technology' for attaining *samādhi*. Perhaps unsurprisingly under such circumstances Patañjali's *Yoga Sūtras* (or, more precisely, Patañjali's *aṣṭāṅgayoga*) are perceived as a sort of DIY manual of practice. As

Vivekananda affirms, "The science of Raja-Yoga proposes to put before humanity a practical and scientifically worked out method of reaching this truth" (*CW* 1: 128).

With time, these transformed semantic and contextual meanings were grafted onto the existing *jñāna*/realization terminology, eventually gaining widespread acceptance. Popularization was also achieved through the ongoing production of publications and other activities of the Ramakrishna movement. Among the more influential texts we may quote the English translations of Gupta's *Kathāmṛta* (1978; 1984) and Vivekananda's *Collected Works*, but many more tracts have been produced over the years in which this terminology abounds.

There are also, however, interesting differences of emphasis within the Ramakrishna movement itself, and these are reflected in the *jñāna*/realization language used in these texts. The first important difference is that, overall, the two translations of Ramakrishna's sayings (Gupta 1978 [1907]; 1984 [1942]) insist more on "God-realization" than on "Self-realization" if compared with Vivekananda.[18] Secondly, Gupta's translation is closer to the spirit of the Bengali (and hence of Ramakrishna), while Nikhilananda's version makes many more concessions to the teachings of the Ramakrishna movement (as opposed to Ramakrishna himself).[19] And of course Vivekananda's teachings, as we saw, contradict Ramakrishna's on some important counts.

Gupta, Vivekananda and Nikhilananda all, however, similarly translate (or use) the "realization" terminology by way of overlapping terms or synonyms (it is difficult to decide which). An in-depth analysis of some central texts[20] shows that the most common include:

> For *brahmajñāna*:
>
> knowing, attaining or "realizing" →
>
> God, Brahman, the Absolute, Knowledge, God the Absolute, Infinite Being, Supreme Being, Universal Soul

18. Jackson's comparison of the movement's teachings as expressed in 1904 and in 1950 (1994: 68–9) could, however, be interpreted to suggest a noticeable, if not drastic, shift towards a "Self-realization" emphasis. This could partly be explained by the fact that Jackson studies the American (rather than the Indian) situation. Generally speaking, it would be interesting to see what a more in-depth analysis of Ramakrishna movement literature (English and Indian) would show in this respect.
19. For a critique of existing translations see Kripal (1995) and Sil (1997: 12).
20. Gupta (1978; 1984) and Vivekananda's *Collected Works*.

For *ātmajñāna*:
knowing, attaining or "realizing" →
the soul, the Self, the Higher Self

The same cluster of words and meanings also became an integral part of New Age religion from early on, thanks to the ideological overlap between New Age religion and Neo-Vedāntic occultism during their formative phases (end of the nineteenth century/beginning of the twentieth). This semantic cluster has therefore become common currency throughout the English-speaking world, at least in circles receptive to esoteric and occultistic discourses.

Interestingly, but perhaps not surprisingly, we also find a similar dynamis and/or tension between the two expressions "God-" and "Self-realization" in New Age contexts. An emphasis on the "God-realization" theme usually indicates a (relatively) more conservative understanding of theological and religious questions. Conversely, an insistence on "Self-realization" tends to indicate more radically esoterico-occultistic, and hence secularized, interpretations of religious traditions.

Following what has been said above it may be difficult for us to believe that Ramakrishna's teachings were as "spiritualistically" oriented as Vivekananda makes them out to be: "This is the message of Shri Ramakrishna to the modern world", the Swami tells us,

> "Do not care for doctrines, do not care for dogmas, or sects, or churches, or temples; they count for little if compared with the essence of existence in each man, which is spirituality . . . Show by your lives that religion does not mean words, or names, or sects, but that it means spiritual realisation . . ."
>
> . . . my Master's message to mankind is: "Be spiritual and realise truth for yourself" . . . The time has come for renunciation, for realisation; and then you will see the harmony in all the religions of the world . . . (*CW* 4: 187)

The above summary would be a much more fitting tribute (in all senses) to Keshubchandra Sen than to Ramakrishna. The Bengali holy man should instead be seen as an example of the non-individualistic 'true mystic': steeped and in some way also lost within his own tradition, but at the same time supported by it. Sen and Vivekananda, on the other hand, are perfect representatives of Neo-Vedāntic esotericism: they had to grapple with the spirit in a thoroughly secularized world, and they were forced to seek the metaphysical within because the metaphysical without had dissolved from the extended social culture.

PART II

Modern Yoga Theory and Practice

> The traditional orientation of society and of religion was the afterlife, but there is a basic incongruity between consumer society and afterlife concerns ... Consumer society demands the rejection of the 'culture of postponement' ... Instead, there must be immediate access to direct experience, for which neither socialization nor learning are really necessary. ... It is wholly characteristic for new religious movements to facilitate mobility, quicker ways to the spiritual top, that cut through the encrustations of ritual, institutionalization, intellectualism, and the whole apparatus of scholarship that religions tend to accrete. Thus the instancy and the urgency are not in themselves new, but their combination with intense subjectivism, rejection of the culture, and the preoccupation with the self is new.
>
> (Wilson 1979: 100–1)

5. Vivekananda's *Rāja Yoga* (1896): Modern Yoga formulated

> ...out of bewildering Yogi-ism must come the most scientific and practical psychology.
>
> (Swami Vivekananda *CW* 5: 104–5)

Chapter 4 should have made it clear that the concept of "realization" is the keystone of Neo-Vedānta's *orthodoxy*. Modern Yoga, on the other hand, and more specifically *rājayoga* as defined by Vivekananda, is the keystone of its *orthopraxis*. "Realization" is in fact stated to be eminently personal and experiential. Once the relatively simple tenets of Neo-Vedāntic orthodoxy have been assimilated and accepted, therefore, orthopraxis becomes all-important. We shall now examine how these elements of theory and practice are developed in Vivekananda's *Rāja Yoga*.

Rāja Yoga: style, structure and overall contents

Rāja Yoga (see Figure 10) is divided into two parts. Part I is a record of talks delivered by Vivekananda in New York during the Winter of 1895–96 and stenographed by Mr J. J. Goodwin. It is not clear whether Part II, described by Vivekananda himself as "a rather free translation of the aphorisms (Sutras) of Patanjali, with a running commentary" (*CW* 1: 122) was also originally delivered as a series of talks. The style of the text suggests that this is probably the case.[1] We know, however, that the whole of *Rāja Yoga* was reworked by Vivekananda himself before publication (*CW* 8: 373).

We must remember that Vivekananda's success at the Parliament of Religions turned him overnight into a major authority on Indian religions and into an ideological leader. As in the case of the missionary work he was to elect as his own – to preach Indian spiritual knowledge to the West – keeping up these roles meant delivering numerous public addresses. Not the thorough scholar at the best of times, and now doubtlessly under constant pressure to deliver talks and lectures, he mainly delivered these impromptu and with little preparation.[2] Therefore his style (in *Rāja Yoga* as elsewhere) is very uneven and in turn discursive or expository, conversational or declamatory.

Despite such shortcomings *Rāja Yoga*, as we saw, became very popular. The book is still kept in print by the Ramakrishna movement, and is profusely available in both cheaper and more expensive editions. Its message was what many in cultic milieus worldwide had been waiting for: a flexible set of teachings that would meet their craving for exotic but nevertheless accessible and ideologically familiar forms of practical spirituality.

Essentially, this book represents Vivekananda's attempt to understand and interpret the Classical Yoga of Patañjali and a selection of *haṭhayoga* teachings on the basis of the beliefs that he shared with his cultic milieu followers. The fact that his beliefs were remarkably eclectic made Vivekananda's task difficult: he brought to bear on his yoga elaborations very different systems of thought: from traditional Hindu lore to elements of Western science (mainly physics, psychology, anatomy and physiology); from modern philosophy

1. There are in fact several passages containing direct forms of address such as: "For instance, most of you ladies play the piano ..." (*ibid.*: 240).
2. See his own description of his lecturing method and his comments on writing (*CW* 6: 293):

> As for lectures and so forth, I don't prepare them beforehand. Only one I wrote out, which you have printed. The rest I deliver off-hand, whatever comes to my lips – Gurudeva [i.e. Ramakrishna] backs me up. I have nothing to do with pen and paper ... They ask me here to write a book. Well, I think I must do something that way, this time. But that's the botheration; who will take the trouble of putting things in black and white and all that!

(especially empiricism and idealism, but with no precise reference or adherence to any school or thinker) to the Neo-Vedāntic esotericism of the Brahmo Samaj and Western occultism (especially influences from American Harmonial Religion, including mesmerism and Metaphysical beliefs). The result is a rather impressionistic and sometimes disjointed mixture of ideas. However, a number of general patterns emerge if one studies the text carefully, gathering isolated statements and recomposing them under common headings.

Vivekananda's reinterpretation of yoga (i.e. Modern Yoga) is predominantly based on the most practice-oriented section of the *Yoga Sūtras*, the so-called *aṣṭāṅgayoga*.[3] Part I of *Rāja Yoga* is an exposition of *aṣṭāṅgayoga* itself, and while Part II treats the whole of the *Yoga Sūtras*, Vivekananda's core interpretation of yoga is still based on *aṣṭāṅgayoga*.

Following the canonical division of *aṣṭāṅgayoga* into *bahiraṅga* and *antaraṅga* sections,[4] Vivekananda's teachings may be divided into what we shall call the *Prāṇa* Model and the *Samādhi* Model, and while these two models overlap and interact to some extent, they will be examined separately for heuristic purposes. The first one, more prominently expounded in Part I, draws more heavily from haṭhayogic teachings, proposes a cosmology in which *prāṇa* (as understood by Vivekananda) plays a central part, describes soteriological aims and methods in terms of power and control over 'gross' and 'subtle', 'internal' and 'external' aspects of the cosmos, and predicates the achievement of freedom or liberation by way of an 'accumulation' or 'concentration' of *prāṇa*, which will speed up the adepts on their evolutionary path towards the ultimate goal. Vivekananda's interpretation of these teachings is heavily influenced by the mesmeric beliefs popular in North American milieus at the time.

In Part II of *Rāja Yoga*, on the other hand, the *Samādhi* Model is more prominent: 'mind' plays a central role, and the influence of Metaphysical ideas and Functionalist psychology is strong. Here Vivekananda construes yoga in terms of the mind undertaking a

3. "The yoga of the eight limbs" (*YS* II. 28 to III. 8), comprising *yama* ("restraints"), *niyama* ("observances"), *āsana* (yogic "posture"), *prāṇāyāma* ("regulation of breath"), *pratyāhāra* ("sense withdrawal"), *dhāraṇā* ("concentration"), *dhyāna* ("meditation"), *samādhi* ("enstasy").
4. Respectively "external limbs" (the first five; see *YS* II. 28–55) and "internal limbs" (the last three; see *YS* III. 1–8).

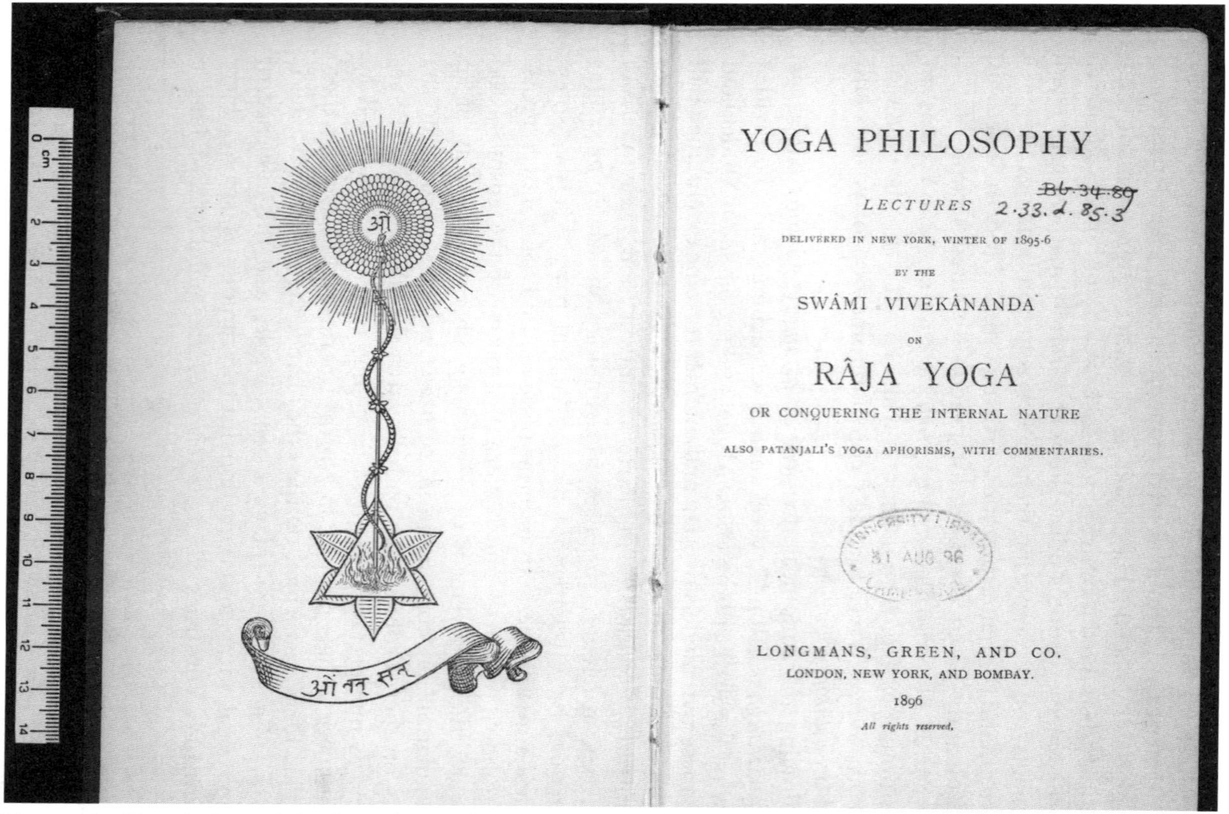
YOGA PHILOSOPHY

LECTURES 2.33.d.85.3

DELIVERED IN NEW YORK, WINTER OF 1895-6

BY THE

SWÂMI VIVEKÂNANDA

ON

RÂJA YOGA

OR CONQUERING THE INTERNAL NATURE

ALSO PATANJALI'S YOGA APHORISMS, WITH COMMENTARIES.

LONGMANS, GREEN, AND CO.

LONDON, NEW YORK, AND BOMBAY.

1896

All rights reserved.

Figure 10 Frontispiece of the first edition of Swami Vivekananda's *Rāja Yoga*. From Vivekananda, S. (1896) *Rāja Yoga: Conquering the Internal Nature*. Longmans, Green and Co., London, New York and Bombay. (By permission of the Syndics of Cambridge University Library)

proprioceptive[5] journey back to "the source of intelligence" through various levels of meditative practice. Each individual mind is part of the "universal mind", he postulates, and by accessing higher or "superconscious" states (*samādhi*) each of us can tap into the omniscience of the universal mind and attain ultimate gnosis. This has profound transformative effects on the adept, eventually bringing to the fore his or her forgotten almighty, omniscient, and divine nature.

Apart from the two models just described, we also find that Vivekananda occasionally shifts to a third mode of thought, which we shall call Neo-Advaitic. While both *Prāṇa* and *Samādhi* Models are 'weak this-worldly' in orientation,[6] the Neo-Advaitic mode is radically otherworldly. According to it, only when all powers and attainments are left behind (a renunciation on which Vivekananda insists repeatedly but with minimum elaboration), only then will the adept be able to reach an altogether transcendent state. This corresponds to the last stage of *samādhi* and leads to realization of an advaitic state of total identification with *puruṣa*, "the only 'simple' that exists in this universe" (*CW* 1: 287) or the "One existing as many" (*ibid.*: 133).

In schematic form, these are the ways in which Vivekananda presents *aṣṭāṅgayoga* in his *Rāja Yoga*. These teachings still form the conceptual foundations of Modern Yoga, even though they have been developed in a number of different ways and directions from the beginning of the twentieth century onward.

An emanationist cosmology

As Vivekananda was attempting to formulate teachings suitable to Western cultic milieus, *Sāṃkhya-Yoga*'s emanationist philosophy

5. Proprioception, a term usually applied to somatic experience, refers to "The extraction and use of information about . . . one's own body." It "concerns stimuli arising within, and carrying information about, one's own body" (Honderich 1995: 652). Due to the pervasive materialistic assumptions of Modern Yoga (about which see below), I will employ it also to describe psychological experience.

6. 'Weak this-worldly' may mean "either a better 'this-world' located on our earth, or such an existence located in 'higher' realms. Most typical of the last variety is the view that, although this world is not perfect, it is to be valued positively as a means for reaching the higher realities beyond" (Hanegraaff 1996: 116).

must have seemed highly compatible with the Neoplatonic thought currents underlying much Western esotericism and occultism. The more practical prescriptions of Classical Yoga also represented an attractive feature. That Vivekananda would adopt these teachings for his revivalistic elaborations makes perfect sense. As other occult sciences such as alchemy, astrology and magic were being revived and transformed under the secularizing influence of nineteenth-century ideas, so too was yoga. While Vivekananda played a major role in this process, he also capitalized on the interest in Indian religions generated by the academic study of religion and, even more so, by the popularization of Oriental ideas carried out by occultist groups such as the Theosophical Society.

In *Rāja Yoga* all three soteriological Models (*Prāṇa, Samādhi* and Neo-Advaitic) outlined above are developed (albeit not in full and not always coherently) against a common emanationist background. As Vivekananda affirms, "we are the outcome and manifestation of an absolute condition, back of our present relative condition, and are going forward, to return to that absolute" (*ibid.*: 195). The cosmic dynamis consists of "only going out to a distance, and coming back to the centre from which [we] started" (*ibid.*: 196). Vivekananda further explains that the unmanifested state is higher than the manifested, a view that, he suggests, is held by all religions in the world: "The idea is that [man's] beginning is perfect and pure, that he degenerates until he cannot degenerate further, and that there must come a time when he shoots upwards again to complete the circle" (*ibid.*: 197). Indeed, our author insists, "What is commonly called life is but an embryo state" (*ibid.*: 199), thus "the sooner we get out of this state we call 'man' the better for us" (*ibid.*: 198). This is because our true nature is divine or Godly: "man is God, and goes back to Him again" (*ibid.*: 197), or again, "Each soul is potentially divine. The goal is to manifest this Divinity within … " (*ibid.*: 257).

Rāja Yoga follows *Sāṃkhya-Yoga* cosmology in postulating an original duality of *puruṣa* and *prakṛti*. A sentient but actionless *puruṣa* causes by his mysterious influence the manifestation of all the forms implicit in *prakṛti*, the dynamic and creative matrix of all manifestation. Beyond this point, however, *Rāja Yoga*'s cosmology becomes quite different from the *Sāṃkhya-Yoga* one. The latter is well known[7] and will only be briefly summarized here: *Sāṃkhya-*

7. A good summary is found in Michaël (1980: 29–47).

Yoga postulates the existence of three *guṇas* (literally "threads", meaning primordial qualities) as composing *prakṛti*. It is the perfect equilibrium of these that the *puruṣa* disturbs by way of its mysterious influence, thereby initiating a cycle of manifestation. Different combinations of these three *guṇas* are found throughout the resulting emanational chain, consisting of a series of 23 further *tattvas* ("thatnesses", the basic categories or fundamentals composing the cosmos) as emanates of *prakṛti*.[8] These are hierarchically arranged along several different cosmological levels and guṇic lines of manifestation.[9] Differently from what Vivekananda proposes, this is a static cosmological model based on correspondences, with symbolic and analogic relations linking the various levels of manifestation. It is a logical construct rather than a historical or evolutionary one. It is not progressive, but eternally self-repeating, cyclically reproducing the same pattern through alternating phases of manifestation or emanation (*sṛṣṭi*) and reabsorption or dissolution (*pralaya*).

Three guṇas vs. two evolutes

But instead of a static cosmos formed by the interplay of the three *guṇas*, what we find in *Rāja Yoga* is an evolutionary cosmos based on the interplay of *prāṇa* and *ākāśa*.[10] These two are stated to be the very first emanates of *prakṛti* (*CW* 1: 147), and this couple, rather than the guṇic triad inherent in *prakṛti*, is said to compose the dynamis through which all further manifestation comes into being:

> By what power is this Akasha manufactured into this universe? By the power of Prana ... [At the beginning of each cycle of manifestation] out of this Prana is evolved everything that we call energy ... [or] force. It is the Prana that is manifesting as motion; it is the Prana that is manifesting as gravitation, as magnetism ... as the actions of the body, as the nerve currents, as thought force ... The sum total of all the forces in the universe, mental or physical, when resolved back to their original state, is called Prana. (*Ibid.*: 147–8)

8. *Puruṣa* and *prakṛti* bring the total number up to 25.
9. The number of these varies depending on the type of analysis used. Standard subdivisions are in series of four or seven.
10. Because the *guṇas* play such a prominent part in the *Yoga Sūtras* (and in Hindu philosophy and religion at large), it would have been difficult for Vivekananda not to mention them at all. So they are mentioned on occasion (i.e. in the sections where he discusses *YS* I. 16, II. 19, 52), but they are not made to play a significant role in cosmological or soteriological terms.

> At the end of a cycle the energies now displayed in the universe quiet down and become potential. At the beginning of the next cycle they start up, strike upon the Akasha, and out of the Akasha evolve these various forms, and as the Akasha changes, this Prana changes also into all these manifestations of energy. (*Ibid.*: 148)

According to *Rāja Yoga*, all of the *tattvas* developing from *prakṛti* are composed of *ākāśa*: "With the exception of the Purusha all of these are material . . . between the intellect [*buddhi*] and the grosser matter outside [*mahābhūtas*] there is only a difference in degree" (*ibid.*: 135; see also *ibid.*: 147).

Prāṇa and *ākāśa* are thus postulated to produce the whole of the manifested universe by way of their interaction. The whole cosmos remains, however, a unified, if stratified, "ocean of energy" and of "matter" (*ibid.*: 149, 151, 156, 159, 256). The only difference between various forms and components of the cosmos is their state (or rate) of vibration: the closer to their ultimate *prakṛti* source, the finer the vibration; the further away, the grosser:

> Think of the universe as an ocean of ether, consisting of layer after layer of varying degrees of vibration under the action of Prana; away from the centre the vibrations are less, nearer to it they become quicker and quicker; one order of vibration makes one plane. (*Ibid.*: 158)

Vivekananda's Naturphilosophie

One may wonder at this stage why Vivekananda places *ākāśa* and *prāṇa* in such prominent positions when they are not at all central in the classical *Sāṃkhya* scheme: in the latter, *ākāśa*, far from being the first evolute of *prakṛti*, is one of the last, while *prāṇa* is not even one of the 25 *tattvas*.[11] The answer lies in the fact that the Swami was elaborating his own *Sāṃkhya-Yoga*-based *Naturphilosophie*.

As we saw, Sen's proto Modern Yoga was already fully esotericized but only vaguely 'scientific'. His references to 'science' were used more for literary effect than for logical argumentation. Vivekananda, on the other hand, brings in 'scientific' elements much more vocally and visibly, although hardly more coherently. This is clearly seen

11. *Prāṇa* is, however, mentioned in the *Sāṃkhya Kārikā* (XXIX) as "breath".

when we examine some of the implications of his '*prāṇa* and *ākāśa*' theme. The way he conceptualizes these terms is as follows:

	Prāṇa	*Ākāśa*
in the *Prāṇa* Model	energy	matter
	force	existence
	power	ether[12]
in the *Samādhi* Model	thought	mind[13]

The top line of translations shows that Vivekananda was trying to match *Sāṃkhya-Yoga* cosmology with the cosmology of contemporary physics, the latter being concerned with "matter and energy with the aim of describing phenomena in terms of fundamental laws" (Walker 1997: 826). In *Rāja Yoga*, our author tries to apply this basic approach to *Sāṃkhya-Yoga* cosmology by focusing on *prāṇa* and *ākāśa* and translating them (linguistically and, in tentative fashion, conceptually) as "energy" and "matter" respectively, and by affirming that they interact on the basis of recurring and knowable "natural laws". This, however, is as scientific as the model gets. For the rest, Vivekananda's Modern Yoga constructs are thoroughly esoteric, hence his theories soon become *Naturphilosophie* rather than 'science'. His universal laws of "mechanical causality", for example, rather than obeying the laws of Newtonian physics, operate along the lines of more arcane correspondences between microcosm and macrocosm. Human beings, furthermore, can and should learn to control these laws in order to use them for their own 'progressive' purposes:

> According to the Raja-Yogi, the external world is but the gross form of the internal, or subtle. The finer is always the cause, the grosser the effect. So the external world is the effect, the internal the cause ... The man who has discovered and learnt how to manipulate the internal forces will get the whole of nature under his control. The Yogi proposes to himself no less a task than to master the whole universe, to control the whole of nature ... He will be master of the whole of nature, internal and external. The progress and civilisation of the human race simply mean controlling this nature. (*CW* 1: 132–33)

12. *Prāṇa* synonyms, respectively: *CW* 1: 147, 148, 146; *ākāśa* synonyms, respectively: *ibid.*: 210, 147, 151.
13. *Ibid.*: 150, 210 (thought), and *ibid.*: 151, 210 (mind).

In a philosophical sense, this goes back to the Enlightenment 'naturalization' of man and of the cosmos. Gellner (1993: 11ff.) explains how in pre-industrial, pre-scientific Western civilizations, there was a tendency to view the human being as "half-angel, half-beast", a vision that created much anguish in individuals because of the tensions implicit in such polarity. But the same vision, Gellner continues,

> also provided an idiom and an explanation for all the forces within man which were opposed to the higher and purer elements. However much the Lower Aspects of our nature might have been reprobated, their very existence was not denied...
>
> However, with the coming of modernity, the total dualistic picture, of which divided man was a part, lost its authority. The twin currents of empiricism and materialism destroyed it, and replaced it with a unitary vision both of nature and of man. Henceforth, nature was to be one single system, subject to invariant and neutral laws, and no longer a stratified system whose ranked levels in nature, society and man were to symbolize and underwrite our values. If materialism/mechanism is a great leveller and unifier, so is empiricism: at its root is the idea that all things are known in basically the same way, and nothing can have a standing greater than the evidence for its existence, and evidence is assembled and evaluated by men. Thus, obliquely, through the sovereignty of public evidence, all authority, sacredness, absoluteness are gradually eliminated from the world. (*Ibid.*: 12–13)

Vivekananda, like many other occultists, tries to avoid the bleakness of this picture and at the same time to salvage the "natural laws" of the Enlightenment with their materialist and empiricist principles. "There is no supernatural," he affirms, "but there are in nature gross manifestations and subtle manifestations" (*CW* 1: 122). As for empiricism, he assures us that the "one universal and adamantine foundation of all our knowledge [is] direct experience" (*ibid.*: 126).[14] The centrality of experiential epistemology in religious as in other matters is continuously reiterated not only in *Rāja Yoga*, but throughout Vivekananda's literary corpus, and is directly linked, as we saw in Chapter 4, to his understanding of "Self-realization".

In Vivekananda's more extreme moments, all of the cosmos is 'naturalized', and the result is a stark dualism of 'spirit' and 'matter'

14. See also the opening sentence of *Rāja Yoga*: "All our knowledge is based on experience" (*ibid.*: 125).

with nothing in between, 'soul' or 'psyche' having been compounded either into matter (in both *Prāṇa* and *Samādhi* Models, but through a sort of 'materialistic panpsychism' in the latter) or into 'spirit' (in the Neo-Advaitic theme). In one particular case, however, this naturalization/materialization becomes so pervasive that it is carried through to the 'spiritual' plane itself, as the following quotation demonstrates:

> Every form in this world is taken out of the surrounding atoms and goes back to these atoms. It cannot be that the same law acts differently in different places. Law is uniform. Nothing is more certain than that. If this is the law of nature, it also applies to thought. Thought will dissolve and go back to its origin. Whether we will it or not, we shall have to return to our origin, which is called God or Absolute. We all came from God, and we are all bound to go back to God. Call that by any name you like, God, Absolute or Nature, the fact remains the same. (*ibid.*: 196–7)

Here 'God', the 'Absolute' and 'Nature' are seen as equivalent: Vivekananda's affirmations, carried through to their logical conclusions, must also imply that "God" and the "Absolute" are made of "atoms". This, however, is an extreme example of philosophical materialism, and not representative of *Rāja Yoga* as a whole.

Starting from such a 'disenchanted' platform, Vivekananda goes on to reinterpret and fill out Sen's proto Modern Yoga scheme by assimilating a number of powerful esoteric motifs, as we shall presently see in our discussion of the *Prāṇa* and *Samādhi* Models. Not surprisingly, the results of mixing the cosmological approaches discussed above with these traditional themes is a typically occultistic "syncretism between esotericism and science, correspondences and causality" (Chapter 1).

The *Prāṇa* Model

In Part I of *Rāja Yoga* we read that "wherever any sect or body of people is trying to search out anything occult and mystical, or hidden, what they are doing is really this Yoga, [i.e. an] attempt to control the Prana" (*ibid.*: 159). Contrary to Vivekananda's intention, this passage is more revealing of his own beliefs than explanatory of what "occult" and "mystical" schools were actually doing. Obviously our author identified with these groups and their practices even though he believed that they only held a partial truth. Faith healers, he states for example, use a kind of *pratyāhāra*[15] to train their patients to "deny misery and pain and evil" (*ibid.*: 171). Both faith healers and hypnotists, he asserts, make use of this technique, but it is wrong for them to do so as such practices should always be self-directed and not imposed by others, as in the latter case they can be dangerous (*ibid.*: 172). Our author nevertheless places faith healers at the top of a hierarchy of medical practitioners, which also includes homoeopaths (in middle position) and allopaths (at the bottom; *ibid.*: 154–5). We further read that there are

> sects in every country who [*sic*] have attempted this control of Prana. In this country [USA] there are Mind-healers, Faith-healers, Spiritualists, Christian Scientists, Hypnotists, etc., and if we examine these different bodies, we shall find at the back of each this control of the Prana, whether they know it or not ... It is the one and the same force they are manipulating, only unknowingly ... it is the same [force] as the Yogi uses, and which comes from Prana. (*ibid.*: 149–50)

Vivekananda even recommends some of these techniques himself: "Always use a mental effort, what is usually called 'Christian Science', to keep the body strong" (*ibid.*: 139), he instructs, and: "Tell your body that it is strong, tell your mind that it is strong" (*ibid.*: 146). He also describes mesmeric practices affirming that there is no reason that they should not work (*ibid.*: 153–4), and concludes that also spiritualism is "a manifestation of Pranayama" (*ibid.*: 157).

Prāṇa *as vitalistic element*

It is obvious from these and other passages that both Vivekananda and his audiences were deeply engaged in forms of alternative medicine, in healing and in related occultistic concerns. As we saw in Chapter 3, various forms of Harmonialism, Metaphysical belief and mesmeric practice were widespread in the USA at the time. These ideas surely played a part in inspiring Vivekananda to select the Sanskritic concept of *prāṇa* to perform the same function. Hellenberger summarizes the four basic principles of mesmerism or, more

15. "Gathering towards oneself", sense withdrawal; the fifth limb of *aṣṭāṅgayoga*.

precisely, of the healing system based on "animal magnetism" as follows:

> (1) A subtle physical fluid fills the universe and forms a connecting medium between man, the earth, and the heavenly bodies, and also between man and man. (2) Disease originates from the unequal distribution of this fluid in the human body; recovery is achieved when the equilibrium is restored. (3) With the help of certain techniques, this fluid can be channeled, stored, and conveyed to other persons. (4) In this manner, "crises" can be provoked in patients and diseases cured. (Quoted in Hanegraaff 1996: 430–1)

Due to the fact that Vivekananda reinterprets *aṣṭāṅgayoga*, and especially so *prāṇāyāma*, in the light of mesmeric theories, we find direct links to these tenets in *Rāja Yoga*. After what has been said about his evaluation of Harmonial beliefs this is hardly surprising. Vivekananda's mesmeric adaptations of yoga are, however, particularly important in the context of the present discussion as they have remained foundational in Modern Yoga speculations, especially so in the case of more somatically oriented types of practice. Let us examine how the four basic principles of mesmerism quoted above are applied in *Rāja Yoga*.

Vivekananda's interpretation of *prāṇa*, or rather of the "omnipresent, all-penetrating" (*CW* 1: 147) dyadic combination of *prāṇa* and *ākāśa*, mirrors his *naturphilosophisch* attempt to represent the concept of the mesmeric fluid in the 'scientific' terms of the physical sciences, and to prove at the same time that such knowledge had already been attained in ancient India. His insistence that "[t]he whole universe is a combination of Prana and Ākāsha" (*ibid.*: 223)[16] is revealing in this context both of his mesmeric convictions and of the materialistic ways in which he interpreted them. His view of the *prāṇa-ākāśa* cosmic substratum is in fact much closer to a kind of materialistic vitalism than to the 'force' of physics. In this our author was of one mind with Franz Anton Mesmer himself, for whom, as Podmore remarks, "the Magnetic system [was] purely a question of matter and motion" (quoted in Hanegraaff 1996: 434).

16. See also: the whole cosmos is "an infinite ocean of Prana" (*ibid.*: 149), and an "infinite ocean of matter [i.e. *ākāśa*]" (*ibid.*: 151; see also 156, 158, 159, 256).

A great advantage of the mesmeric theory was its conceptual simplicity and polyvalence:

> Since the same "fluid" could be interpreted as either spiritual or material, it [was] not surprising that elements of mesmerism were adopted by various individuals and movements for very different reasons. Mesmerism was embraced by a whole range of illuminist and occultist movements ... as a theory which could serve to unify esotericism and modern science...
>
> [The attraction of this system] was due in large part to its essential simplicity: an invisible fluid connects all parts of the universe, whether "spiritual" or "material", and this fluid is the universal key to health and harmony. (Hanegraaff 1996: 434, 435)

When, therefore, our author identifies *prāṇa* with "the vital force in every being" (*CW* 1: 150, 153) we should be aware that he is employing one of the expressions by which the mesmeric fluid was commonly known in his day (Fuller 1989: 44).

Before we go on to discuss the second principle of mesmerism, a further occultistic connection should be highlighted. While Vivekananda was most likely among the first to put forward explicitly the term *prāṇa* as a candidate for full-blown mesmerico-cosmological assimilation, speculations along these lines had already been in evidence before his time, and are indeed likely to have influenced his own elaborations. For example, we saw how, throughout the last quarter of the nineteenth century, the Theosophical Society was playing a leading role in 'making the West turn Eastward' (Bevir 1994). Writing as early as 1877 the Society's founder Helena Petrovna Blavatsky "portrayed Hinduism as a mystical religion that encouraged people to turn inwards and find the divine within themselves", and "made India the centre for the natural magic which occultists traditionally associated with their cosmological schemes" (*ibid.*: 764). As part of her ongoing defence of India as the source of a natural magic which should be adopted to compensate for the limited view of mainstream science, she more specifically wrote:

> Nothing can be more easily accounted for than the highest possibilities of magic. By the radiant light of the universal magnetic ocean, whose electric waves bind the cosmos together, and in their ceaseless motion penetrate every atom and molecule of the boundless creation, the

> disciples of mesmerism – howbeit insufficient their various experiments – intuitionally perceive the alpha and omega of the great mystery. Alone, the study of this agent, which is the divine breath, can unlock the secrets of psychology and physiology, of cosmical and spiritual phenomena: (*Isis Unveiled* 1972 [1877], I: 282, as quoted in Bevir 1994: 754–5).

Whether at this time Blavatsky and her colleagues were attempting to homologize this mesmeric "divine breath" with the Sanskritic *prāṇa* or with a different pneumatic concept we have not attempted to establish. By 1893, however, such theorizations had become relatively more specific: the Theosophist Srinivasa Iyangar, for example, in his English translation of the *Haṭhayogapradīpikā*'s *Jyotsnā* (commentary by Brahmānanda) points out that "'breath' does not mean the air taken in and breathed out, but the Prāṇa, i.e. the magnetic current or breath" (Iyangar 1994: 22).[17] To draw even more specific connections between 'magnetism', 'divine breath' and '*prāṇa*', and to construct a whole cosmology around these ideas would not have been too far fetched at this stage, and this is precisely what Vivekananda proceeded to do. Exploring other areas of ideological overlap between Vivekananda's thought, Neo-Vedāntic esotericism and Theosophical speculation would surely be a productive exercise.

Prāṇa *as healing agent*

The second basic principle of mesmerism postulates the unequal distribution of the 'vital fluid' ('*prāṇa*' in Vivekananda's case) as etiological agent, thus entering the domain of more practical speculation and actual application of these beliefs in daily life. Mesmeric interpretations of everyday phenomena are found in several passages of *Rāja Yoga*.[18] As usual in this type of discourse, however, there is special emphasis on health and healing. Vivekananda's views in this context are not very different from those of his occultist predecessors

17. The text consulted is a revised and corrected edition. Without consulting the original 1893 edition we cannot be certain that this was the original wording. The antiquated turn of phrase, however, suggests that this is likely.
18. It is through a transmission of "vital force" that people influence each other in various ways (strengthening, weakening, healing or controlling others; *CW* 1: 154, 155, 172–3); charismatic leaders "can bring their Prana into a high state of vibration" (*ibid.*: 155); etc.

and contemporaries, the main variant being the name given to the fluidic element:

> Sometimes in your own body the supply of Prana gravitates more or less to one part; the balance is disturbed, and when the balance of Prana is disturbed, what we call disease is produced. To take away the superfluous Prana, or to supply the Prana that is wanting, will be curing the disease. That again is Pranayama – to learn when there is more or less Prana in one part of the body than there should be. The feelings will become so subtle that the mind will feel that there is less Prana in the toe or the finger than there should be, and will possess the power to supply it. (*CW* 1: 155–6)

A complete materialization of the concept of *prāṇa* is evident in this passage: *prāṇa* is stated to be an altogether material, perceivable substance, responding to physical laws (albeit 'subtle' ones) in controllable fashion.

Another passage relates the same principles to *āsana* practice. Vivekananda does not give much importance to this aspect of yoga, but the little he does say is very much along the lines of what somatically oriented forms of Modern Yoga[19] will develop in the following decades. The reference to 'nerve currents' is, of course, to one of the main manifestations of *prāṇa*:[20]

> The next step [of *aṣṭāṅgayoga*] is āsana, posture. A series of exercises, physical and mental, is to be gone through every day, until certain higher states are reached. Therefore it is quite necessary that we should find a posture in which we can remain long ... We will find later on that during the study of these psychological matters a good deal of activity goes on in the body. Nerve currents will have to be displaced and given a new channel. New sorts of vibrations will begin, the whole constitution will be remodelled, as it were. But the main part of the activity will lie along the spinal column, so [one should sit erect]. You will easily see that you cannot think very high thoughts with the chest in. (*Ibid.*: 137–8)

As far as the *Prāṇa* Model is concerned, it is obvious that Vivekananda resolves the mind-matter problem in a thoroughly materialistic way.

19. What will be defined as Modern Postural Yoga in the next chapter.
20. See, for example: "It is the Prana that is manifesting as the actions of the body [especially breathing], as the nerve currents, as thought force" (*ibid.*: 147–8).

Prāṇāyāma *as healing technique*

Turning now to the third basic principle of mesmerism, regarding how to channel, store and convey the all-important *prāṇa*, we look at how *prāṇa* is regulated according to the *Prāṇa* Model, viz. through *prāṇāyāma*. Vivekananda starts to describe the mechanism of *prāṇa* regulation through *prāṇāyāma* by saying that we need to regain the (now lost) [21] control of our own individual *prāṇa* (*ibid.*: 152–3). We begin to do this by controlling its most obvious manifestation in the human body – breathing – with the help of which we "slowly travel towards the most subtle until we gain our point" (*ibid.*: 152). This involves gaining further control of other, more subtle workings of *prāṇa* in the body (*ibid.*: 153), the basic sequence being:

> breath control
> → leads to control of nerve currents
> → which in turn leads to control of thoughts (*ibid.*: 143–4),
>
> or
>
> breath observation
> → leads to awareness of nerve currents
> → and of the motions of the mind (*ibid.*: 144).

This will result in many positive changes in the practitioners, including developing an ability to heal themselves and others, clearing "[a]ll the sickness and misery felt in the body" (*ibid.*: 153), and increasing willpower (*ibid.*: 155). When practitioners start practising concentration and meditation they will also be "intensifying the power of assimilation" (*ibid.*: 157) and become capable of "concentrating the Prana" (*ibid.*: 156). By 'fuelling' themselves with more *prāṇa* (*ibid.*: 157) they will be able to proceed more swiftly along the evolutive ladder, typified by Vivekananda in his customarily eclectic style as stretching from "fungus" to "God" (*ibid.*: 156). As practitioners control subtler and subtler levels of *prāṇa*, they will bring themselves to "quicker" states of "vibration", and this will lead them to *samādhi*: "All this bringing of the mind into a higher state of vibration is included in one word in Yoga – Samadhi" (*ibid.*: 159).

21. In Harmonial/New Thought fashion Vivekananda states that our control is lost because of conditioning (*ibid.*: 129); because "We have become automatic, degenerate" (*ibid.*: 245); because we are not sufficiently "discriminating" i.e. "sensitive" (*ibid.*: 153, 144).

"[L]ower states of Samadhi" grant visions of subtle reality; the "highest grade of Samadhi is when we see the real thing, when we see the material out of which the whole of these grades of beings are composed" (*ibid.*). We thus see how, at the level of practice, the *Prāṇa* and the *Samādhi* Models develop into each other.

We find many references to this kind of endeavour in *Rāja Yoga*, but in the following one the principles of this process are set out especially clearly:

> We do not know anything about our own bodies ... Why do we not? Because our attention is not discriminating enough to catch the very fine movements that are going on within. We can know of them only when the mind becomes more subtle and enters, as it were, deeper into the body. To get the subtle perception we have to begin with the grosser perceptions. We have to get hold of that which is setting the whole engine in motion. That is the Prana, the most obvious manifestation of which is the breath. Then, along with the breath, we shall slowly enter the body, which will enable us to find out about the subtle forces, the nerve currents that are moving all over the body. As soon as we perceive and learn to feel them, we shall begin to get control over them, and over the body. The mind is also set in motion by these different nerve currents, so at last we shall reach the state of perfect control over the body and the mind, making both our servants. Knowledge is power. We have to get this power. So we must begin at the beginning, with Pranayama, restraining the Prana. (*Ibid.*: 144)

Here we see how, in his effort to validate his interpretations of yoga by the standards popularly accepted in the West, Vivekananda draws elements not only from physics, but also from empiricist epistemology, then (as now) widely influential. The centrality of experience as the only true source of knowledge leads him to anatomize the yogi's internal journey, and to describe (and teach it) in highly individualistic proprioceptive terms. The 'subtle' physiology of Vivekananda's *Prāṇa* Model, it should be stressed, is not intended to be read symbolically as in the case of *haṭhayoga*,[22] but to be interpreted literally.

22. See Bharati (1992: 291) on the classical approach to such intellectual constructs: "this yogic body [composed of *cakras* and *nāḍīs*] is not supposed to have an objective existence in the sense the physical body has. It is a heuristic device aiding meditation, not any objective structure; the physical and the yogic body belong to two different logical levels."

It is our lack of training which prevents us from being aware of our 'subtle' physiology, not its lack of ontological status. Indeed, when describing "Psychic Prana" and related *kuṇḍalinī* teachings (*CW* 1: 160–70), Vivekananda implicitly argues that modern anatomy and physiology are discovering what the yogis already knew, i.e. the anatomy and physiology of the nervous system.

An equation between "knowledge", "power" and "control" underlies Vivekananda's proprioceptive recommendations for practice: if one becomes aware, feels, and perceives gross and subtle energy movements within oneself (or the progression of perception in the *Samādhi* Model), then one will come to know and control them fully – so goes the logic of the text. Further still, if one controls one instance (usually one's own *prāṇa*, one's own body), then one will control all (all *prāṇas*, all bodies).

> ...he who has grasped the Prana has grasped all the forces of the universe, mental or physical. He who has controlled the Prana has controlled his own mind, and all the minds that exist. He who has controlled the Prana has controlled his body, and all the bodies that exist... How to control the Prana is the one idea of pranayama. (*Ibid.*: 149)[23]

It is in such overt but unsupported postulations that magic correspondences of microcosm and macrocosm are activated in Vivekananda's system. There is nothing especially new in the postulates themselves, as he follows the same *siddhayoga* and *haṭhayoga* traditions about which White says:

> In the monistic or pneumatic perspective of the yoga-based Indian gnoseologies, it is ultimately breath, breathing in and breathing out, that unites the microcosm and the macrocosm (indeed, ātman can be translated as "spirit" or "breath, re-spir-ation")... It is for this reason in particular that breath control plays such a paramount role in the entire yogic enterprise. (1996: 46–7)

What is different in Vivekananda (but common to other occultists) is his purporting to be in line with the latest discoveries of science. And while his attempts to integrate worldviews based on correspondences

23. See also: "The causes [of this universe] being known, the knowledge of the effects is sure to follow" (*CW* 1: 165).

and on instrumental causality were logically untenable, they were nevertheless successful at popular level. Similar conceptual filters will be applied to yogic theory and practice as Vivekananda interprets the *Yoga Sūtras* and elaborates the *Samādhi* Model, only the inner journey in this case will be described in psychological terms, rather than in anatomical and physiological ones.

Samādhi *as psychological "superconsciousness"*

This brings us to the last principle of mesmerism, concerning 'healing crises'. Hanegraaff (1996: 438–9) explains that the 'crisis' postulated by Mesmer as part of his system was replaced by Mesmer's influential follower de Puységur (1751–1825) with what became known in those days as "induced somnambulism". Such new and more psychologically oriented approach was used for the same therapeutic and experiential purposes as Mesmer had done with his 'crises', the system eventually developing into what we now know as hypnotism. As this type of research grew, so did the interest, especially on the part of the emerging science of Functionalist psychology and its successors, in the variety and nature of hypnotic and other altered states of consciousness. Such states, but self-induced and referred to as "superconsciousness" and "Self-realization",[24] Vivekananda will define as the key locus not of a healing 'crisis', but of a self-validating and life-transforming (and hence, ultimately, existentially healing or soteriological) religious experience.

The *Samādhi* Model

The *Samādhi* Model continues Sen's motif of "spiritual empiricism", but follows more closely than Sen did the Patañjalian model of meditative introspection found in the *antaranga* section of *aṣṭāṅgayoga*, comprising *dhāraṇā*, *dhyāna* and *samādhi*. The internal journey of the practitioner, however, is not interpreted, as Patañjali does, in terms of an ahistorical process of purification and involution towards a state of radically transcendent liberation. It is described instead in terms of evolutive realization of human potential. Strongly influenced by the New Thought style of Metaphysical teachings that

24. *CW* 1: 180, 185, 213, 233 ("superconsciousness"), and *ibid.*: 304 ("self-realisation"), 264 ("realisation of the Self").

pervaded the American cultic milieu to which he had acculturated (Chapter 3), Vivekananda reinterprets Patañjali's *saṃyama* in psychological terms: *samādhi* is defined as a going 'back to the source of intelligence', or back to the "immanent divine 'Mind' which is the source and foundation of finite minds" (Hanegraaff 1996: 494–5). Thus, Vivekananda posits, "the potential god [which is in man] becomes manifest" (*CW* 1: 293). Echoes of Patañjali's ultimate model of radical transcendence (*kaivalya*) are occasionally found in the form of the Neo-Advaitic component, and testify to the author's attempts to integrate the Advaitic tradition he admired so much into his yoga framework. As we shall see, however, they are not very prominent.

The influence of Metaphysical beliefs

We saw with regard to the *Prāṇa* Model that Vivekananda reinterprets *Sāṃkhya-Yoga* cosmology in occultistic terms. The bottom part of the *prāṇa* and *ākāśa* scheme of translations discussed on page 157 shows that he assimilates meditative practices in the same framework by translating *prāṇa* as "thought" and *ākāśa* as "mind". "Thought is the finest and highest action of Prana" (*ibid.*: 150), he affirms in this context, and "when the action of Prana is most subtle, this very ether [*ākāśa*], in the finer state of vibration, will represent the mind" (*ibid.*: 151). Even though we are in the 'finer' regions of the cosmos, the emanational chain is still the same, with the two main evolutes causally interacting to form grosser and grosser forms of manifestation. A key Metaphysical element, however, is powerfully brought in by reinterpreting the classical concept of *puruṣa* in a way that closely resembles occultistic elaborations of the Emersonian Over-Soul.

It is true that on occasion Vivekananda follows the Classical Yoga scheme by representing the *puruṣa* as altogether transcendent, "beyond the whole of nature", "not material at all", and "entirely separate, entirely different" from *prakṛti* (*ibid.*: 251). Most of the time, however, the same *puruṣa* is understood anthropocentrically in terms of what we may call 'idealist panpsychism'. It is both the deepest ontological core of human beings *and* the ultimate spiritual source vivifying and pervading the whole of the cosmos: "It is the real nature of man, the soul, the Purusha [whose] freedom is percolating through layers of matter in various forms, intelligence, mind, etc. It is its light which is shining through all" (*ibid.*: 254).

Vivekananda is still struggling to match Harmonialist and *Sāṃkhya-Yoga* cosmological frameworks at this stage, and at times pronounces contradicting statements. We find, for example, that "purusa", "mind" and "prana" are stated to be all similarly "omnipresent" and vivifying the cosmos,[25] thus seemingly holding the same roles and equal status. This is more coherent with the ultimately materialistic vision of the *Prāṇa* Model. We also read, however, that the Yogi's mind "is one bit of the universal mind" (*ibid.*: 281–2). The latter statement is more akin to what will emerge as the core teaching of the *Samādhi* Model, viz. the rationale on which most of Vivekananda's meditation-related teachings will be based. This postulates the primacy of a creative "universal mind" in which all human beings may partake by way of the 'subtle' layers of their mind. Once the 'natural' laws regulating these subtler layers are known, they can be controlled. These laws, Vivekananda continues, are as yet undiscovered by Western science, but are well known to yogis, who master them to perfection and are therefore able to realize fully the human potential which is dormant in all of us. The development of this dormant potential is presented by Vivekananda in terms of '*kuṇḍalinī* arousal'. In a passage summarizing a number of recurrent themes he states:

> Some day, if you practise hard, the Kundalini will be aroused ... [then] the whole of [your] nature will begin to change, and the book of knowledge will open. No more will you need to go to books for knowledge; your own mind will have become your book, containing infinite knowledge. (*Ibid.*: 168–9)[26]

At this point anything becomes possible. If such laws are not known, the mind "can only work through the nerve currents in [the] body, but when the Yogi has loosened himself from these nerve currents, he can work through other things" (*CW* 1: 282), i.e. tap into the creative cosmic levels of the "universal mind".

Vivekananda would eventually postulate this core teaching expli-

25. Cf. the following statements: "not only [man's] soul [*puruṣa*] is omnipresent, but his mind also, as the Yogi teaches" (*ibid.*: 281), while *prāṇa* is defined as "the infinite, omnipresent manifesting power of this universe" (*ibid.*: 147).

26. We may note in this context that it was through the publication of *Rāja Yoga* that the concept of *kuṇḍalinī* was first popularized in the West. Taylor was obviously not aware of this fact and therefore states (1996: 148) that this concept was first popularized by Avalon in his *The Serpent Power* (1918).

citly in a lecture delivered in 1900. Here 'mind' (instead of *puruṣa*) is brought forward as 'prime mover' and "sum total of all minds":

> Matter cannot be said to cause force nor [can] force [be] the cause of matter. Both are so [related] that one may disappear in the other. There must be a third [factor], and that third something is the mind. You cannot produce the universe from matter, neither from force. Mind is something [which is] neither force nor matter, yet begetting force and matter all the time. In the long run, mind is begetting all force, and that is what is meant by the universal mind, the sum total of all minds. Everyone is creating, and [in] the sum total of all these creations you have the universe – unity in diversity. (*Ibid.*: 506, square bracket editing in original)

Within the framework of this 'psychologized' cosmos, in the 'creative' and evolutionary thrust of which (as New Thought affirmed) each of us can partake, meditative yoga is redefined as a technique allowing us to 'attune ourselves' to the 'universal mind' and hence partake of its perfection and power. In this context, "All manipulations of the subtle forces of the body, the different manifestations of Prana, if trained, give a push to the mind, help it to go up higher, and become superconscious" (*ibid.*: 150).

The influence of Functionalist psychology

This "superconsciousness", as already hinted at the end of our discussion on the *Prāṇa* Model, is defined in psychological terms partly inspired by William James' Functionalist psychology. James and Vivekananda were relatively well acquainted as they gravitated in the same intellectual circles.[27] Indeed, James was asked to write a preface for *Rāja Yoga*, but his contribution never materialized (see *CW* 9: 85). This author is usually regarded as the founding father of Functionalist psychology. As Hanegraaff explains, this school of thought emerged from about 1890 against a background of Emersonian idealism and

> held that psychology must not be concerned with what consciousness *is* but with what it *does* (i.e., with its functioning). Beyond that, however, functionalist theories typically adopted the more specific

27. See Vivekananda's humorous report on "a congress of cranks" which both he and James attended (*CW* 6: 436–8).

premises of "romantic evolutionism" within a broadly Transcendentalist framework:

> Approaching Darwin's developmental-evolutionary theory armed with the romantic philosophies of Hegel, Schelling and eventually Bergson, the functionalists robbed Darwinian biology of its reductionist sting. Henceforth all discussions of nature – even when couched in scientific terms – could be interpreted as descriptions of the concrete processes whereby an immanent divine force progressively unfolds its creative potential. By implication, psychology is essentially a special instance of a distinct metaphysical interpretation of reality. Psychological descriptions of human nature, though framed in the language of secular science, could yet be understood as defining the structures that allow us to participate in nature's upward surge. (1996: 491, quoting Fuller)

It is in this sense that Vivekananda brought together *Sāṃkhya-Yoga* theories and elements of Functionalist psychology. Interpreting them as closely related areas of knowledge and of empirical experimentation, Vivekananda discusses *Sāṃkhya-Yoga* in terms of Empiricist theories of perception (*CW* 1: 134–5, 200–1), which he defines as "psychology" (*ibid.*: 135). He also equates "religion", "metaphysics" and "psychology" as similarly dealing with "the inner nature of man" (*ibid.*: 131, 225). Thus the Swami joins the intellectual current of secularization which was shaping the forms and language of the psychologization of religion. One of the central exponents of this current was James:

> When William James interpreted the unconscious as humankind's link with a spiritual "more", he gave shape to a peculiarly modern spirituality. James' vision of the unconscious depths of human personality as at once psychological and spiritual made it possible for modern Americans to view self-exploration as spiritually significant and religious experience as psychologically profound. (Fuller, as quoted in Hanegraaff 1996: 492)

James also defended an epistemology of "radical empiricism", which conceded "no a priori or preconceived limits to what constitutes a 'fact'", thus accepting "the entire field of consciousness including its margins or fringes as basic datum to the psychological sciences" (Hanegraaff 1996: 492). James "compared this field of consciousness to a light spectrum, of which we ordinarily perceive only small fractions while the rest remains 'unconscious'. The upper or higher reaches of the unconscious could, however, be studied in such phenomena as telepathy, clairvoyance, religious experience or trance states" (*ibid.*).

It is here that we find the most direct borrowing on the part of Vivekananda, who similarly uses the metaphor of the light spectrum to explain his understanding of "consciousness", and of our ability to access its various levels (*CW* 1: 198, 158, 213). As our eyes are not aware of the lower and higher frequencies of the light spectrum, but only of the middle band to which our sight is attuned, he reasons, so we are normally aware only of our middle "plane of thought":

> There is ... instinct or unconscious thought, the lowest plane of action ... There is again the other plane of thought, the conscious ... The mind can exist on a still higher plane, the superconscious. When the mind has attained to that state, which is called Samādhi – perfect concentration, superconsciousness – it goes beyond the limits of reason, and comes face to face with facts which no instinct or reason can ever know. (*Ibid.*: 150)

James' psychological speculations as expressed in his seminal textbook *The Principles of Psychology* (1890) must have played an inspirational role in Vivekananda's modern reinterpretation of meditation and *samādhi*. Applying James' approach to psychology based on "looking into our minds and reporting what we there discover",[28] Vivekananda prescribed the same formula for his religio-psychological "science of yoga": we need to get to know "the internal nature of man", he affirmed, by "observing the facts that are going on within" (*CW* 1: 129).

Psychological proprioception as practice

Following on from the proprioceptive method used in the *bahiraṅga* practices, Vivekananda adopts a similar approach for the *Samādhi* Model. This time, however, it will be a matter of becoming aware of the workings of our mind, and of attaining "superconsciousness", rather than of learning to feel and control 'pranic currents'. As in the case of the *Prāṇa* Model, also the *Samādhi* Model will go on to

28. *The Principles of Psychology* (1890), quoted in Gregory (1987: 650).

become one of the most productive and influential in Modern Yoga circles. A brief description of it runs as follows:

> The Yogi proposes to attain that fine state of perception in which he can perceive all the different mental states. There must be mental perception of all of them. One can perceive how the sensation is travelling, how the mind is receiving it, how it is going to the determinative faculty,[29] and how this gives it to the Purusha. (*Ibid.*: 136)[30]

This, however, is not easy to do because, Vivekananda explains in keeping with New Thought tenets, due to societal conditioning "we have been taught only to pay attention to things external ... hence most of us have nearly lost the faculty of observing the internal mechanism" (*ibid.*: 129). The only way to carry out this type of observation is through the "method" of "concentration" (*ibid.*: 130),[31] and the "instrument" used for carrying out this exercise is "the mind itself" (*ibid.*: 129) – it is a case of "mind studying mind" (*ibid.*: 131). This concentration has an intrinsic epistemological potential, our author explains, as it will take us inwards "to the basis of belief, the real genuine religion. We will perceive for ourselves whether we have souls ... whether there is a God in the universe or more.[32] It will all be revealed to us" (*CW* 1: 131).

Vivekananda is never monolithic in his interpretations, but the main message of *Rāja Yoga* is that yoga is a deeply transformative practice. Culminating in the experience of "Self-realization", Vivekananda's *Rāja Yoga* allows us to cultivate what in New Age terms would be described as 'Personal Growth' and to attain our 'higher potential': "when a man goes into Samadhi, if he goes into it a fool, he comes out a sage ... his whole character changed, his life changed, illumined" (*ibid.*: 180–1), Vivekananda affirms. Or again: "perfection is man's nature, only it is barred in and prevented from taking its proper course ... Those we call wicked become saints, as soon as the bar is broken"; "when knowledge breaks these bars, the god becomes

29. One of the ways in which Vivekananda translates *buddhi* (*CW* 1: 135, 200).
30. Because of Vivekananda's epistemological reliance on perception, he at times cannot avoid turning *puruṣa* into the 'ultimate perceiver': see "The soul itself [*puruṣa*] is the centre where all the different perceptions converge and become unified" (*ibid.*: 255).
31. The term is also used to translate *samādhi* (*ibid.*: 291).
32. Interestingly, *CW* 1 reads "more" here (*ibid.*: 131), while a pocket edition of *Rāja Yoga* (Himalayas: Mayavati, 1994: 10) reads "none".

manifest" (*ibid.*: 292, 293).[33] Vivekananda's 'gods', 'sages' and 'saints', however, should not be mistaken for the categories of Hindu or Christian doctrine and theology usually referred to by these names: Vivekananda's 'divinity' is rather a state of advanced human development, a further evolutive condition in which the potential of humanity is truly fulfilled. "The progress and civilisation of the human race simply mean controlling this nature" (*CW* 1: 133), Vivekananda states. Ultimately, he reminds us along the lines of other New Thought authors, we are in charge of our own destiny:

> The man who thinks that he is receiving response to his prayers does not know that the fulfillment comes from his own nature, that he has succeeded by the mental attitude of prayer in waking up a bit of this infinite power [i.e. *kuṇḍalinī*] which is coiled up within himself. (*Ibid.*: 165)

There is no question of supernatural achievements here (*ibid.*: 122), but just of accessing our true power and nature, which we have forgotten through identification with our lower modes of consciousness.

The Neo-Advaitic component

Vivekananda does not seem to notice that what he describes as the "superconscious" state sounds much like the siddhic condition that, when in Neo-Advaitic mode, he categorically affirms should be shunned in order to attain final liberation. When in this mode, in fact, our author takes a much more otherworldly and transcendent approach to the question of the ultimate human state, and predicates transcending the human condition altogether:

> There is no liberation in getting powers. It is a worldly search after enjoyments, and ... all search for enjoyment is vain; this is the old, old lesson which man finds so hard to learn. When he does learn it, he gets out of the universe and becomes free. (*Ibid.*: 211)

"It is only by giving up this world", he affirms elsewhere, "that the other comes; never through holding on to this one" (*ibid.*: 247; see

33. For an extended refutation of such claims see Bharati (1976, Chapter 4).

also 285–6). But this position is hardly elaborated or discussed: it is rather stated than argued in *Rāja Yoga*, and it is really secondary to the overall argument and thrust of the text. Indeed, at times it appears to contradict the main flow of the book, as in the instance where the two opposite ultimate goals (*mokṣa* and a siddhic state) are mentioned in the same passage: "... the aim, the end, the goal of all this [yoga] training is liberation of the soul. Absolute control of nature, and nothing short of it, must be the goal" (*ibid.*: 140). An analysis of the text suggests that, all in all, Vivekananda recommends the 'divinization' or rather 'full evolution' of the human being, and only adds suggestions of radical transcendence more as a reflection of cultural habit than as necessary parts of the overall argument.

Yogic experience in classical Vedānta

So we see that Vivekananda recommends yoga, and in particular (what he calls) *rājayoga* as the best, at times even the only, technique or rather 'science' apt to lead us to a self-validating "realization" experience, the only locus where true religion may be found. We also know that throughout his life he repeatedly invoked Vedānta, and especially Śaṅkara's Advaita, as a validating source for his teachings. We cannot, of course, fully discuss such momentous claims here. We can, however, briefly compare Vivekananda's message with what Śaṅkara and Rāmānuja, the two main Vedāntic authorities, thought about yogic experience or perception (*yogipratyakṣa*). About Advaita's main exponent we read:

> ... Śaṅkara does not invoke any extraordinary "psychological events" and he does not try to validate the truth of non-dualism by referring to "visionary" or "mystical" experiences of extraordinary persons. Instead, he reflects on the nature of self-awareness and immediacy, as it is present even in ordinary life, and he tries to find in it what the Upaniṣads teach explicitly. However, he insists that without the guidance of revelation [*śruti*] such reflection would not be able to uncover the true, i.e. non-dual nature of "experience" and the self. He projects absolute *anubhava*, i.e. *brahmānubhava* or *brahmabhāva* as a soteriological goal, which is by definition transpersonal and transworldly. He never refers to such "experience" as an actual worldly occurrence which could be used as empirical evidence for the truth of non-

> dualism. There are no worldly "empirical data" for what transcends the horizon of worldly cognition. (Halbfass 1988: 390; also see *ibid.*: 302–3)

This must suffice to show that Vivekananda's empirical approach to the validity of yogic experience, stressing the attainment of "superconsciousness" and of self-validating forms of revelation, is at great variance with Śaṅkara's.

As for Rāmānuja,[34] he too is far from regarding yogic experience as a valid source of religious knowledge. To extract just a couple of essential passages from Lester's book on the subject:

> Rāmānuja affirms that dogma defines practice in three ways which bear on our concern:
>
> (1) He affirms that scripture is the source of knowledge of Brahman and yogic perception is not. In fact, he affirms that yogic perception is not at all a source of knowledge; rather, it is simply a vivid imagination of an object due to intense concentration upon that object.
>
> (2) He affirms that gaining right knowledge of the nature of the real – right theological orientation – from scripture is fundamental to the pursuit of release [*mokṣa*].
>
> (3) He rejects the Yoga School's view of the nature of the soul and of the Lord (Īśvara). This is the one and only direct comment which Rāmānuja makes on the Yoga school; yet it is sufficient to indicate that Rāmānuja will structure Patañjalian-type Yoga strictly in terms of his theistic doctrine; for he says, 'The nature of the meditation in which the Yoga consists is determined by the nature of the object of meditation...' (1976: 133–4)
>
> In *dhyāna* the mental faculties have been focused exclusively on the Supreme Person – not with a view to making the object more and more abstract until an objectless state is attained, but with a view to generating devotion towards the Supreme person. *Dhyāna* is simply remembrance and its result is an entirely subjective vision. Rāmānuja simply omits *samādhi* – *dhyāna* goes on and on resulting only in ever greater devotion, ever more vivid imagination. (*Ibid.*: 140–1)

Validation of Vivekananda's position from the Viśiṣṭādvaita teacher is therefore also out of the question.

34. From whose tradition Vivekananda draws heavily in his treatment of *Bhakti-Yoga* (CW 3: 29–100).

The *Yoga Sūtras*: a *rājayoga* textbook?

One last but central question needs to be examined before we conclude this chapter. In *Rāja Yoga*'s Preface we find an important affirmation: "The aphorisms of Patanjali are the highest authority on Raja-Yoga, and form its textbook" (*CW* 1: 122). We must question the identification of *rājayoga* with the *Yoga Sūtras* of Patañjali. This identification, unlike the identification of *aṣṭāṅgayoga* with *rājayoga*, is not documented in the classical tradition and must therefore be considered a modern accretion.[35]

The Theosophical Society seems again to have been the first group to propagate this idea. Writing in 1880–81 Blavatsky made a general distinction between an 'inferior' *haṭhayoga* and a 'superior' *rājayoga*, affirming that the former was only based on physical practices whereas the latter "train[ed] but [the] mental and intellectual powers" (Blavatsky 1967: 463). She then proceeded to identify this superior *rājayoga* semi-explicitly with Patañjali's yoga (*ibid.*: 466–7) and, explicitly, with "what is termed in our day 'hypnotism' or self-mesmerisation" (*ibid.*: 458). Finally, she affirmed that the only true practitioners of *rājayoga* were "Śankara's Dandis of Northern India" (*ibid.*: 462). Now the name Daṇḍins ("those who have a staff", *daṇḍa*) designates the four orders among Śaṅkara's Daśanāmī monks who are drawn exclusively from the Brahaminical caste (Ghurye 1995 [1953]: 71–2). Hence they represent the choice intellectual element of a monastic order traditionally associated with high intellectual endeavours. As such, their area of expertise and authority would be, if anything, in the field of *jñānayoga*. Blavatsky, however, amalgamates *rājayoga*, Patañjali's yoga, Vedāntic *jñānayoga* and "self-mesmerisation" by stating, effectively, that they are one and the same thing.

The influential American Theosophist W. Q. Judge (1889: vi–vii) continues along similar, if less eclectic, lines. In his "interpretation" of the *Yoga Sūtras* he also states that yoga consists essentially of *haṭhayoga* and *rājayoga* and he identifies Patañjali's teachings with *rājayoga*, if only half-explicitly. The Indian scholar and Theosophist Dvivedi, finally, affirms that Patañjali covers both "*Hatha*-(physical) and *Rāja*-(mental) *Yoga*" (1890, I: 49), and that both aim at suspending "the action of the mind" (*ibid.*, I: 50). He also explicitly

35. For a list of classical references see Philosophico Literary Research Dept. (1991: 245).

identifies *rājayoga* with the classic Patañjalian formula *yogaścit-tavṛttinirodhaḥ* (*YS* I. 2) at least once in his work.[36] With *Rāja Yoga* and other texts Vivekananda and the Ramakrishna movement went on to sanction and popularize similar ideas.[37]

The misidentification between Vivekananda's *rājayoga* and the *Yoga Sūtras* of Patañjali is very revealing in the present context as it betrays a cognitive confusion which causes a typically esoteric variety of yoga (further occultized by Vivekananda and his followers) to be understood not only in terms of mainstream yoga, but as the most important and universally applicable form of yoga.

This compounding of Classical Yoga and *rājayoga* is so widespread nowadays that it is usually taken for granted, at least in esoteric circles.[38] Contemporary evidence suggests that, a century down the line from the publication of Vivekananda's *Rāja Yoga*, this erroneous notion has been completely assimilated into Modern Yoga culture, and beyond it into a 'global' community of seekers. Thus if occultistic definitions of yoga have gained enormous ascendancy in Modern Yoga circles this will in good part be because the full authority of the *Yoga Sūtras* has been mistakenly attributed to them. The same process has, conversely, greatly contributed to create a widespread *un*awareness of how many links branch out from the highly condensed structure of Patañjali's text (and from the attached commentatorial literature) to radiate and connect at many different chronological, textual and performative levels throughout the Hindu tradition. It is only because of such unawareness that Modern Yoga exponents can claim that "Yoga is not a religion, it is a way of life."[39] While the *Yoga Sūtras* are a highly sophisticated intellectual compendium providing a synthetic and semantically layered overview of

36. He refers to "... the method of *vṛttinirodha* or *Rājayoga*" (Dvivedi 1890, II: 14), but also, in perfect proto New Age fashion, states that "true *yoga* or *Rājayoga*" is attained "when the microcosm becomes attuned to the macrocosm", which will "make experience full of that harmony and bliss which is the inevitable result of unity with nature" (*ibid.*, I: 37).

37. Apart from Vivekananda's own texts, see, for example, the definition that the influential Swami Nikhilananda (in Gupta 1984 [1942]: 1043) proposes in a Glossary entry: "*Rājayoga* – The famous treatise on yoga, ascribed to Patañjali; also the yoga described in this treatise."

38. Many Modern Yoga texts equate the *Yoga Sūtras* with *rājayoga*: the Theosophist Ernest Wood, for example, does so in the very popular *Yoga* (Wood 1982 [1959]: 82, 98, 168; see especially page 188 where he refers to the *Yoga Sūtras* as "this *rāja-yoga* manual").

39. Or, 'a philosophy', 'a tool', etc. Statements of this type are a leitmotif in Modern Yoga literature; see, for example, the titles chosen by Pillai (1986) and Devdutt (1997).

all main types of yoga, within the conceptual universe of Modern Yoga the *Sūtras* find themselves demoted to representing only a very limited range of (usually occultized) haṭhayogic practices.

All the changes that we have discussed in the preceding chapters may be seen to have led to a paradigmatic shift in the ways in which yoga is popularly perceived nowadays: from the classical *Gītā* model of the three yogas (*bhakti*, *jñāna* and *karma*, the whole including, but also tempering, more esoteric forms of practice),[40] we have come to Vivekananda's '4 yoga' model, in which *rājayoga* is not only put on a par with the classical threefold subdivision of yoga, but actually portrayed as superior to all other forms. As Vivekananda himself states:

> The goal is to manifest this Divinity within, by controlling nature, external and internal. Do this either by work, or worship, or psychic control, or philosophy – by one or more or all of these – and be free. This is the whole of religion. Doctrines, or dogmas, or rituals, or books, or temples, or forms, are but secondary details. (*CW* 1: 257)[41]

40. Ramakrishna refers to three yogas (Gupta 1984 [1942]:467–8), and so does Vivekananda in *Karma-Yoga* (*CW* 1: 25–118), composed before *Rāja Yoga*.
41. This passage, rightly selected as representative of the whole of Vivekananda's *Rāja Yoga* message, is quoted at the beginning of many editions of the text, for example Vivekananda (1994) and *CW* (1: 124). The list of four in the second sentence refers of course to the '4 yogas' as interpreted by the author and, in the light of the foregoing discussion, it is significant that he uses "psychic control" to signify *rājayoga*.

6. Twentieth-century developments of Modern Yoga

Health is religious. Ill-health is irreligious.

(B. K. S. Iyengar *YV*: 10)

As we saw in the preceding chapter, the crucial conceptual shift operated by Vivekananda is as follows: from a Sen-like romantically interpreted 'science of yoga' leading one to an 'intuitive' vision of God Vivekananda moves towards a technologically interpreted 'science of yoga' aimed at 'reattuning' the practitioner to the cosmos. This should lead adepts to 'realize' their own true nature, which is essentially spiritual. The contradiction in terms implicit in the statement that our true *nature* is *spiritual* is an integral part of this definition, and is rooted in the conceptual and terminological history of Modern Yoga. It is implicit in the shift from an esoteric, still relatively enchanted "spiritualism" to a thoroughly secularized, rationalistic and occultistic one. In both views, however, the yogic experience is considered as the central, indeed the only real core of religion, all other aspects of religion being "but secondary details" (*CW* 1: 257).

Thus Vivekananda represents the epitome of the religious crisis of the late nineteenth century, as undergone by Neo-Vedāntins: eagerly absorbing the new knowledge and ways of life, but inwardly feeling a heart-rending nostalgia and longing for the old traditional forms.

This would lead many Neo-Vedāntins to a tortured, passionate and dedicated first-hand search for a new truth. In this sense Vivekananda's vision, while bringing to bear the core elements of 'alternative medicine' (see below) to his redefinition of yoga, was still explicitly and not only implicitly religious. The publication of *Rāja Yoga*, sanctioning and giving body to these teachings, immediately started something of a "yoga renaissance" both in India and in the West.[1] Not much research has been done on Modern Yoga so far (see Introduction), but most emic and etic discussions agree that Vivekananda had a pervasive influence on its development.

An early article by Jackson (1975) is especially interesting in this context. It examines "one singular manifestation of the *fin de siècle* Oriental vogue, the New Thought movement's discovery of ancient Indian thought" (*ibid.*: 525) on the basis of American textual material. Here the author reports how Vivekananda and his co-workers "made a profound impression upon members of the New Thought movement" (*ibid.*: 529), who felt "a strong attraction to yoga" (*ibid.*: 534). Jackson also points out that they "seem to have been searching for practical and concrete methods of coping with their daily physical, psychological and spiritual problems" (*ibid.*). This can, of course, be seen as a variation on the "demand for 'occult' practices" theme discussed in Chapter 3. Jackson's material, however, also provides revealing – and more specific – evidence with regard to *Rāja Yoga*'s popularity and direct influence in these milieus. Even though Jackson does not mention the book at all, his analysis of primary sources ranging from the last years of the 1880s to the first decade of the twentieth century shows that immediately after 1896, New Thought discussions shift from a general interest in "yoga" to more specific elaborations on "four types of yoga – Karma, Bhakti, Raja and Jnana", and that "Raja Yoga" is recommended as the best of the four types of practice (*ibid.*: 534–5). As already mentioned in Chapter 3, Vivekananda himself pointed out that the book had been an instant success both in India and in North America (*CW* 5: 123; *CW* 6: 382; *CW* 8: 486). Based on its ongoing popularity to date we can confidently assume that *Rāja Yoga* has been very influential indeed.

As for a revival of yoga in India, we have as evidence the creation

1. A commemorative plaque found in the grounds of the Yoga Institute at Santa Cruz, Bombay (see below), welcomes visitors by proudly announcing that they find themselves at: "the heart of modern yoga renaissance" (see Figure 1). The age of the Institute, also inscribed on the plaque, is updated every year.

of the two earliest Indian Modern Yoga institutions: the Yoga Institute at Santa Cruz, Bombay (established 1918), and the Kaivalyadhama Shrimad Madhava Yoga Mandir Samiti at Lonavla (established 1921), roughly half way between Bombay and Poona. Both of these institutions remain influential to this day, training teachers, running camps and retreats, offering yoga therapy, publishing affordable books and pamphlets, and generally propagating various aspects of Modern Yoga in India and abroad. They owe their creation, at least in part, to Vivekananda: their founders' common *guru*, Śrī Madhavadasji of Malsar, had in fact been very receptive to the Swami's message.[2]

Space constraints prevent us from looking at the first fifty years of Modern Yoga in detail, though we will propose an interpretative typology of Modern Yoga based on the developments which took place during this period (see below). As studies of Modern Yoga stand at this point in time, this may actually prove to be a more useful analytical tool than a detailed history would be.[3] Before going on to this, however, we need briefly to discuss the ways in which 'alternative medicine'[4] is connected with New Age forms of religiosity. It is in fact in these areas of endeavour and theorization that the Modern Yoga renaissance stimulated by Vivekananda will become fully acculturated in the West.

Alternative medicine and New Age religiosity

After elaboration under rapidly secularizing Western conditions, Modern Yoga came to be described more and more as an inward, privatized form of religion. Its association with emerging forms of alternative medicine developed accordingly. We shall attempt to

2. Author's interview with Dr Jayadeva Yogendra, son of the founder and current head of the Yoga Institute, 2 July 1994, unpublished. Regarding these institutions see Alter (2000, Part II and, especially, forthcoming).
3. Ceccomori (2001) does cover the history of this period, and while her work focuses mainly on the French situation, several of the Modern Yoga schools and teachers she discusses also have bases and/or followers in English-speaking countries.
4. Also referred to nowadays as 'complementary' and 'integrative' medicine. It is worth noting here that these three appellations have appeared one after the other since the late 1970s, the latter one becoming established only towards the end of the 1990s (see, for example, ElFeki 1999: 143). Their implicit and explicit semantic content signals the differing ways in which these therapeutic approaches have been perceived and propagated: namely, as progressively more acceptable and compatible with mainstream medicine.

review some of the possible ritual and symbolic values of these phenomena in the concluding chapter. All that we need to point out at this stage is that the various concerns relating to Modern Yoga as found within the field of alternative medicine had, by the 1960s, started to develop characteristic theories and practices. By this stage, contact with the metaphysical, the transcendent or the sacred, if at all envisaged, is affirmed to take place almost exclusively through one's interiority, and on the basis of one's own personal 'spiritual work', one's seeking or, most of all, 'practice'. This process is understood to be part of the natural evolutionary development of each human being, a development that can be fostered and accelerated by way of specific forms of practice.

These developments contribute, throughout the 1960s, 1970s and 1980s, to the "astonishing resurgence of healing systems that overtly embrace a metaphysical notion of causality" (Fuller 1989: 91). With the emergence of a self-conscious New Age movement in the mid-1970s, they crystallized in one of the five main trends of New Age religion (as discussed by Hanegraaff 1996, Chapter 2), i.e. the one concerning itself with 'healing and personal growth',[5] to a brief analysis of which we now turn.

New Age healing...

As Fuller (1989: 5) points out, healing "is a profoundly cultural activity. Labeling a disease and prescribing treatment express a healer's commitment to a particular set of assumptions about the structure and properties of physical existence." Indeed, different types of medicine conceptualize states of health and non-health in different ways. In the present context it will be useful to employ a standard distinction used by medical anthropologists between 'bio-medicine' on the one hand and 'holistic medicine' on the other.[6] The former is what is understood as today's mainstream medicine; the latter encompasses non-mainstream approaches to medicine, as well as various forms of folk and religious healing, and pre-modern approaches to health and well-being. Holistic medicine thus described tends to comprise

5. The other four trends are: Channelling, New Age Science, Neopaganism and the concept of 'New Age' (in a restricted and in a general sense) (see Hanegraaff 1996, Part One).
6. As formulated here, the distinction combines elements from the work of Helman (1994), Young (1982) and McGuire (1985).

> Naturalistic systems [which] conform above all to an equilibrium model; health prevails when the insensate elements in the body, the heat, the cold, the humours of *dosha*, the yin and yang, are in balance appropriate to the age and condition of the individual in his natural and social environment. When this equilibrium is disturbed, illness results. (Foster and Anderson, as quoted in Hanegraaff 1996: 45)

As such, this type of medicine regards non-health as illness, meaning a person's perceptions and experiences of certain socially disvalued states including, but not limited to, disease. It concerns itself with the complex social, psychological and spiritual condition of the sick person, and constitutes the proper domain of healing, with healers as practitioners. The emphasis here is on healing as a holistic practice, while preventive medicine and health-oriented lifestyles are also actively promoted.

Biomedicine, on the other hand, concerns itself with disease seen as a biophysical condition: it regards conditions as abnormalities in the structure and/or function of organs and organ systems. It refers to pathological states whether or not they are culturally recognized. Medical practitioners are concerned with curing these conditions once they arise, mainly relying on an allopathic pharmacopoeia and on surgical interventions to effect their cures. Medical and paramedical professionals, as well as hygienists and health counsellors of various types, are generally expected to work according to this model. Biomedicine *cures disease* whereas holistic medicine *heals illness*.

As one might expect, the New Age aligns itself with the more traditional and holistic forms of medicine; it is more concerned with the business of 'healing' than with that of 'curing', even though it is receptive to suggestions from modern science and, most of all, from psychology (*ibid.*: 46).

. . . and personal growth

As Hanegraaff explains, metaphysical alternative healing systems encompass, along with physical and psychological notions of healing, also religious concerns which similarly attempt to "give answers and prescriptions for dealing – either practically or conceptually – with human weakness and suffering" (*ibid.*: 44). Concepts of ultimate religious attainment (Christian salvation; Hindu *mokṣa* or "liberation"; etc.) may thus be seen as radical forms of 'healing'. In the case of New Age religion, this notion of ultimate 'making whole' is understood in terms of personal growth:

> In a general sense, "personal growth" can be understood as the shape "religious salvation" takes in the New Age movement: it is affirmed that deliverance from human suffering and weakness will be reached by developing our human potential, which results in our increasingly getting in touch with our inner divinity. Considering the general affinity between salvation and healing, the close connection between personal growth and healing in the New Age Movement is hardly surprising in itself. It is important to note, however, that therapy and religious "salvation" tend to merge to an extent perhaps unprecedented in other traditions. (*Ibid.*: 46)

As will be noted, the above quotation could equally well apply to the Neo-Vedāntic aim of "Self-realization". This is why "realization" terminology abounds in New Age discourses: on the basis of the linguistic background discussed in Chapter 4 this flexible terminology is perfectly suited to describe the attainment of ultimate personal growth and of maximum "human potential". While the Sanskrit *jñāna* terminology attempts to describe through analogic categories the unitive, supra-discursive insights accessed on occasion by human beings, the English versions of these expressions have come to represent a much more anthropocentric and mechanistic view of these experiences. This is especially evident as, with the emergence of the New Age movement in the mid-1970s, the 'realization' focus progressively shifts from "God-" to "Self-realization".[7] We shall analyse this trend in more detail in Chapter 7. For the moment, however, we need to fill in the picture with regard to overall developmental trends in Modern Yoga.

7. Note, for example, the following field observation: a *YS* translation by Prabhavananda and Isherwood (1953) was widely used in Modern Yoga circles throughout the 1970s and early 1980s. By the end of this period, however, Modern Yoga practitioners started objecting to its title, *How to Know God*. It was in fact widely felt that yoga led to knowledge of 'Self', not of 'God', and that this title was therefore inappropriate. Quite apart from the book's contents, its title was regarded as a major drawback, especially when this text was considered for inclusion in teacher training courses' reading lists (own field data).

Towards a typology of Modern Yoga

This will be done by introducing a typology of Modern Yoga as found in English-speaking milieus worldwide and by subsequently discussing the developmental phases of Modern Yoga in the latter half of the twentieth century. Many groups claim to be practising or teaching yoga, but what do they mean exactly? While each group interprets and uses yogic teachings in unique ways, having an idea about overall orientations can help to clarify a number of basic issues, such as which aspects of practice any particular school may stress, or the amount of personal involvement that is likely to be expected from a new follower. A visual outline of the typology is shown in Table 3.

Some general comments about the overall structure of this typology will be in place here. After Vivekananda's 1896 formulation, Modern Yoga developed into various schools dedicated to body-mind-spirit 'training', which we shall call Modern Psychosomatic Yoga (MPsY). During this period a number of followers, emulators and intellectual heirs of the Swami carried on cultivating and extending the doctrines he had formulated. Within a couple of decades, further specialization had occurred, with some schools putting greater stress on the cultivation of physical practices, and others on the cultivation of more mental ones. More specifically, Modern Postural Yoga (MPY) developed a stronger focus on the performance of *āsana* (yogic postures) and *prāṇāyāma* (yogic breathing), while Modern Meditational Yoga (MMY) mainly relied on techniques of concentration and meditation.

Typically, both MPY and MMY stress the orthoperformative side of participation within a limited 'classroom' or 'session' type framework. This may extend to special courses and retreats for the more committed or advanced practitioners. Relatively pure examples of MPY schools are Iyengar Yoga and the so-called Astanga Yoga of Pattabhi Jois. Relatively pure examples of MMY groups found in Britain are (early forms of) Transcendental Meditation (TM)[8], the centres established by Sri Chinmoy and some modern Buddhist groups (regarding the latter see note 27, Chapter 2).

From the doctrinal point of view both MPY and MMY tend to limit themselves to very basic and polyvalent suggestions concerning the religio-philosophical underpinnings of their practices. Committed

8. More recently, TM seems to have been veering towards Denominational forms (see below).

Table 3 Typology of Modern Yoga

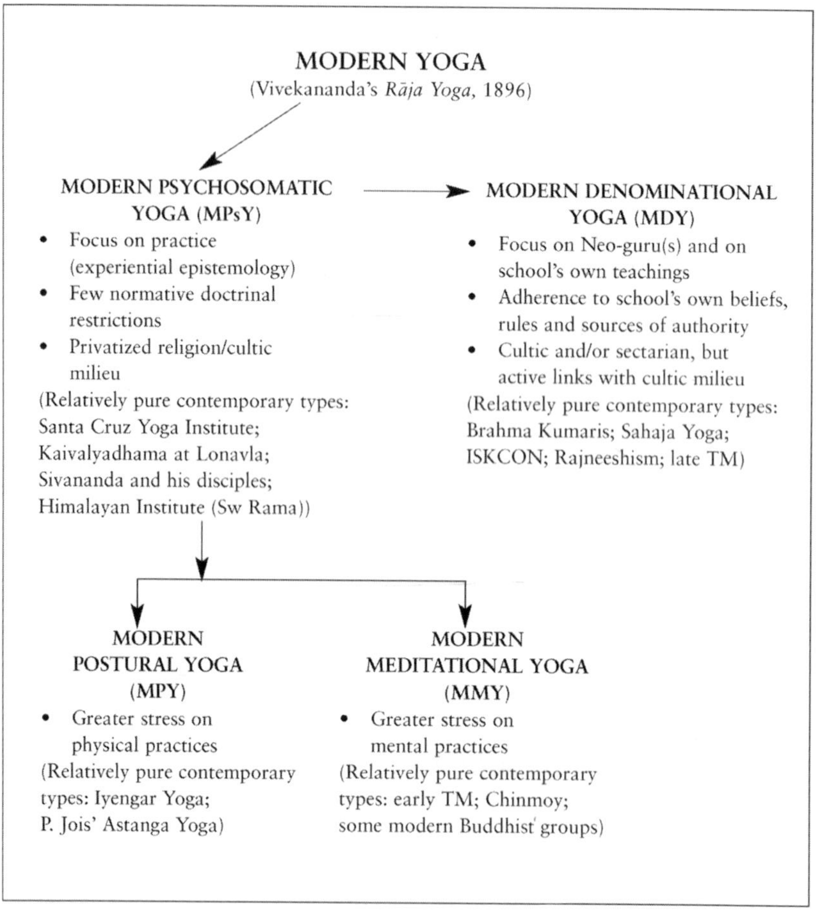
MODERN YOGA
(Vivekananda's *Rāja Yoga*, 1896)
MODERN PSYCHOSOMATIC YOGA (MPsY)
• Focus on practice (experiential epistemology)
• Few normative doctrinal restrictions
• Privatized religion/cultic milieu
(Relatively pure contemporary types: Santa Cruz Yoga Institute; Kaivalyadhama at Lonavla; Sivananda and his disciples; Himalayan Institute (Sw Rama))
MODERN DENOMINATIONAL YOGA (MDY)
• Focus on Neo-guru(s) and on school's own teachings
• Adherence to school's own beliefs, rules and sources of authority
• Cultic and/or sectarian, but active links with cultic milieu
(Relatively pure contemporary types: Brahma Kumaris; Sahaja Yoga; ISKCON; Rajneeshism; late TM)
MODERN POSTURAL YOGA (MPY)
• Greater stress on physical practices
(Relatively pure contemporary types: Iyengar Yoga; P. Jois' Astanga Yoga)
MODERN MEDITATIONAL YOGA (MMY)
• Greater stress on mental practices
(Relatively pure contemporary types: early TM; Chinmoy; some modern Buddhist groups)

engagement in intellectual reflection and evaluation of their own heritage is not especially encouraged, and often lacking. The doctrinal aspects of the teachings are mostly rudimentary, the general underlying assumption being that understanding will come through first-hand experience rather than from intellectual deliberation. As in Vivekananda's *Rāja Yoga*, the key epistemological presuppositions are experiential here, and practitioners are mostly left to make sense of the received theories and practices, and of how these should be fitted into their lives, on the basis of their own rationalizations. The latter, as fieldwork data show, are generally shaped by the religio-philosophical assumptions characteristic of New Age religion.

By and large, most MPsY schools group themselves in the type of associative forms that sociologists of religions define as 'cultic'. As we saw in Chapter 1, this means that they tend to be individualistic and loosely structured (especially as far as sources of authority are concerned), they place few demands on members, they are tolerant, inclusivist, transient, and have relatively undefined social boundaries, fluctuating belief systems and relatively simple social organizations.

Modern Denominational Yoga (MDY), on the other hand, was a later development that seems to have got fully underway only during the 1960s with the appearance of more ideologically engaged Neo-Hindu *gurus* and groups that incorporated elements of Modern Yoga teachings. While retaining active links with the cultic milieu from which many of their recruits come, these groups have more marked sectarian tendencies: collectivist and more tightly structured, they make more demands on members, and have more stable belief and organizational systems which often result in more intolerant and/or exclusivist attitudes than is the case with MPsY. MDY groups draw from the whole range of Modern Psychosomatic, Postural and Meditational forms of yoga in whichever way suits them. Contrary to MPsY and its sub-branches, however, they have not been instrumental in shaping, defining and elaborating more 'mainstream' forms of Modern Yoga theory and practice, and yoga is not their primary concern.

As with all typologies, the one just discussed also fails to mirror the complexities of real-life situations and must therefore be understood as a heuristic device. Modern Yoga types will and do overlap when observed in the field.[9] As one would expect, however, there is an especially strong level of compatibility between Postural and Meditational groups as the two sets of practices can easily be seen as complementary. It should also be stressed that the present typology does not include those Indian schools of Modern Yoga active only in India and through the medium of local languages.[10] It does, however, include those Indian schools that rely mainly on the English language for the diffusion of their teachings, and which also have centres, or at least significant contacts, abroad.

9. Such overlaps are further discussed, though not extensively, in De Michelis (1995).
10. These have developed their own specific discourses and social structures and, in some cases, close links with Indian political and socio-religious movements. For studies in this area see Alter (1997 and forthcoming).

The development of Modern Postural Yoga: 1950s to date

Having explained the ways in which various sub-groups of Modern Yoga differ, we shall now proceed to draw a historical sketch of the main developments of MPY from about 1950 onward. Specific examples will be drawn from the British situation, but, as mentioned earlier, overall patterns will be found to be rather similar throughout the English-speaking world.

With regard to types of MPY, the two most influential schools in Britain are Iyengar Yoga (after the name of its founder, B. K. S. Iyengar), which started to be propagated in Britain from 1954, and the British Wheel of Yoga (BWY), established in 1962 by Western individuals interested in yoga. Since the early 1990s, Pattabhi Jois' Astanga Yoga (and its offshoots) has also been gaining in popularity, aided in part by the highly visible acrobatic and aesthetic qualities of its practice. Considering that the BWY acts as an umbrella organization validating a number of smaller schools (for example Viniyoga Britain and the Scottish Yoga Teachers Association), it is estimated that these schools currently provide about 80 to 85 per cent of the Postural Yoga teaching currently taking place in the UK, with Jois' style being smaller and less institutionalized than the other two. The leftover 15 to 20 per cent of the teaching is carried out by individuals or centres teaching other styles of yoga independently, such as Sivananda Yoga, Dru Yoga, and so on (own field data).

Though very different in many respects, the British Wheel of Yoga grew alongside the Iyengar School and in somewhat parallel ways. Precise statistics are not available, but fairly detailed data provided by the schools themselves in 1993 suggest that in terms of numeric and geographical spread the two institutions were on a more or less equal footing at the time.[11] Since then, the 1995 recognition of the BWY as

11. For numbers and other data relating to Britain see below.

Continental Europe also has lively Modern Yoga communities. Modern Yoga was suppressed in East European countries before 1989, but after this date it has attracted substantial public interest and support (own field data). All in all, however, per capita density of practice is likely to be lower on the continent than in Britain. Across Europe, density is also likely to be greater in urban areas (informed guesses based on own field data).

Concerning the USA, a Roper poll commissioned by *Yoga Journal* (a popular North American Modern Yoga magazine) in 1994 revealed that "over six millions (about 3.3 per cent of the population) practice [*sic*] yoga . . . [C]lose to 17 million more – or about 1 in 10 – are 'interested in yoga,' although they haven't tried it yet" (*Yoga Journal* Editors 1994: 47).

ruling body for yoga by the British Sports Council (Iyengar Yoga and the BWY were the only two schools competing for the title) has strengthened its position in Britain. Possibly in part as a result of this defeat, British Iyengar Yoga underwent something of a management crisis during the latter half of the 1990s. It seems, however, to have emerged from it undamaged and with renewed dynamism (own field data).

Current fieldwork data still suggest that the two schools wield a comparable amount of influence in yoga circles. Iyengar Yoga benefits from wider international representation, and more Iyengar than British Wheel students engage in yoga on a full-time basis, thus becoming active agents of propagation. Furthermore, this school has a unified system of practice which makes it potentially more adaptable to the requirements of other professional bodies, especially in the fitness and medical domains, whether alternative or conventional.

The BWY, on the other hand, has gained important national status through its association with the Sports Council, has a more flexible and varied, if at times somewhat unfocused, approach to practice, and gives more scope to theoretical speculation in its teaching and teacher training courses. It can also accredit smaller schools of yoga, which are then grouped under its aegis. All these characteristics are likely to attract as much interest and commitment, in Britain, as Iyengar Yoga does.

Most of the longer-established Postural Yoga schools in the UK have gone through similar developmental phases from the 1950s onwards. These are: Popularization (1950s to mid-1970s), Consolidation (mid-1970s to late 1980s) and Acculturation (late 1980s to date). Briefly, these three phases may be characterised as follows:

Popularization: 1950s to mid-1970s

- The earlier slow spread turns to fast popularization: numerous schools and teachers (Indian and non-Indian) appear on the scene.
- Substantial media attention is given to yogic disciplines: numerous popular books and some successful television programmes facilitate the circulation of information on the subject.
- Yoga classes become popular: some are run by Adult Education authorities, others are run privately by teachers.
- The wave of "hippy" travel to India peaks: it leads many to more or less in-depth contact with yogic practices and ideas.

- *GURUS*: As the schools are smaller, interaction with teachers tends to be more frequent and personal. In some cases, custom-made teachings can be imparted. The charismatic qualities of the teachers can be deployed to full advantage. Sociological, economic and psychological conditions are ripe for the more sectarian MDY groups to develop.
- *FIGURES*: In 1970 Howard Kent, a well-known figure in British yoga circles,[12] conducts a survey of Postural Yoga practitioners in the UK: he estimates that there are about 30,000 (Kent 1993: 15).

Consolidation: mid-1970s to late 1980s

- Many schools and teachers fall into oblivion, but popularization is achieved. The surviving schools start a process of consolidation consisting in the establishment of more substantial and permanent institutional structures or in expanding the existing ones. Teacher training courses are standardized and teaching qualifications are awarded.
- The surviving schools achieve a certain degree of maturity, which reflects in the progressive development of distinctive practices: a number of schools show increased levels of specialization and technical elaboration. Below the Indian-inspired terminology and imagery, religio-philosophical elaborations of MPY schools align themselves more and more with, and in turn reinforce, those of the New Age movement. Reflecting this trend, which assimilates Modern Yoga to alternative medicine concerns, the main UK yoga magazine changes its name from *Yoga Today* to *Yoga and Health* (late 1980s).
- The schools start to explore in more depth, and to standardize the various possible practical applications of yoga: sports and keep-fit; stress management; medical therapy and prevention (both physical and psychological); perinatal yoga; yoga for children, the elderly and the handicapped; yoga practice for convicts; yoga as applied to creative artistic expression (such as dance or photography); etc.
- *GURUS*: Indian teachers tend to be honoured and revered, but, because of the growing size of the schools, contacts with them become more impersonal and diluted. Differentiations between

12. Howard Kent founded the Yoga for Health Foundation at Ickwell Bury, Biggleswade, Bedfordshire (UK) in 1976.

core members and more marginal followers emerge and are sometimes reflected in institutional hierarchies. More complex and stratified power dynamics develop within the groups.

Acculturation: late 1980s to date

- Several institutions grant official or unofficial recognition to yoga schools. The BWY is recognized by the Department for Education as awarding body for vocational qualifications (1992), then by the Sports Council as the ruling body for yoga practice in the UK (1995). Postural Yoga is accepted by many as a useful form of complementary medicine: it is not rare for GPs to recommend it on a number of accounts. The British Health Education Authority describes and recommends Postural Yoga practice in its leaflets promoting keep-fit routines and healthy lifestyles.[13]
- The schools reorient themselves along the lines suggested by feedback received from participants, the public and society at large (perceived needs, commercial considerations, standards required for official recognition, etc.): this brings about an increased professionalization of yoga teaching, a stronger tendency towards technical specialization, standardization and/or institutionalization, and renewed efforts to cover efficiently and propagate the more immediately practical applications of the practices. This is reflected in the appearance of many specialized publications.[14] It also results in further secularization as far as the more 'public' face of MPY is concerned. Religio-philosophical elaborations along esoterico-occultistic New Age lines nevertheless continue to be standard in most MPY milieus.
- *GURUS*: Some of the leading MPsY Western teachers of the new generation establish their leadership more on grounds of high-level professionalism and technical specialization than of 'spiritual' charisma or religious knowledge. Explicit or implicit criticism of Indian-style *gurus*, at times perceived as authoritarian,

13. See, for example, two booklets published by the Health Education Authority itself (1990; 1995). In the first one yoga is recommended as a convenient form of exercise because "There are lots of [yoga] classes available" (1990: 21), while the second mentions yoga as form of exercise suitable for all (1995: 9, 10).
14. Some examples: medical and therapeutic, Schatz (1992); stress control and prevention, Lasater (1995); yoga for pregnancy, Freedman and Hall (2000); senior yoga, Stewart (1995); everyday keep-fit, Friedberger (1991); yoga for children, Stewart and Phillips (1992).

emerges in some cases. Even though the *guru-śiṣya* model is often referred to, what one finds at grassroots level is more akin to client–professional or client–therapist relations, with only a tinge of 'spiritual pupillage' overtones.

- *FIGURES*: On the basis of data provided to the Sports Council by the two major Postural Yoga schools it has been worked out that in the year 1992–93 yoga practitioners attending classes in Britain were likely to be in the region of 120,000, showing an increase of about 300 per cent from 1970 (own field data). If one were to include people who practise Postural Yoga on their own or in classes run by other schools and people who practise other types of yoga, including MMY or specific forms of MDY, the total would be much higher. At the beginning of the twenty-first century the popularity of Modern Yoga – now thoroughly acculturated – is showing no sign of abating.[15]

The Iyengar School of Modern Postural Yoga

The interpretative theories discussed so far will now be put to the test by being applied to the Iyengar School of Yoga. As of today (2003), Iyengar Yoga is arguably the most influential and widespread school of Modern Postural Yoga worldwide.[16] It has a growing international network of centres dedicated to the teaching of the Iyengar method and to the training of teachers. Its expertise in postural practice is respected across Modern Yoga milieus worldwide,[17] and Iyengar Yoga-inspired teachings (often mixed with others to a greater or lesser extent)[18] are also propagated outside of the Iyengar network

15. Hasselle-Newcombe (2002: 1) reports a set of statistics which are of special relevance in this context: a "Lexis-Nexis [Internet] search for 'yoga' in UK Newspapers" revealed that in 1980 there were 0 occurrences, followed by 25 in 1985, 104 in 1990, 403 in 1995, 1,567 in 1999, 2,546 in 2000 and 3,675 in 2001. The years between the quoted ones (the original source tabulates results year by year) show a steady, regular increase, and half way through 2002 the total was already significantly higher than half of the 2001 total (*ibid.*).
16. Iyengar Yoga is practised in most developed and urbanized milieus worldwide, and especially so in English-speaking areas: from Australia to the Americas, from India to Japan, in East and Western Europe, as well as in smaller cultural enclaves such as white South Africa and Hong Kong.
17. Though over the years, and especially so in the past, this style of MPY has been criticized for the allegedly fierce and at times challenging teaching style of some of its representatives.
18. Though this is frowned upon in 'purist' Iyengar Yoga circles.

proper. This MPY school also boasts a substantial literary output authored by at least three subsequent generations of teachers (Iyengar himself, his pupils, his pupils' pupils). Furthermore, it propounds a remarkably homogeneous system of theory and especially of practice (orthoperformance), a fact that becomes especially apparent when this style is compared to other schools of Modern Postural Yoga such as the BWY.

The Iyengar School has been chosen as the ideal case study on grounds of wealth of written sources and of orthoperformative coherence. Iyengar Yoga schools and centres worldwide also have a relatively unified administrative nature insofar as all teaching qualifications are ultimately sanctioned by the central Iyengar Yoga Institute in Pune, India. The availability of historical records, of explicit theoretical formulations and of orthoperformative standards against which developments, variations, dissent and other elaborations can be measured allows the analyst not only to clarify issues concerning the school itself, but also, by comparison, the ones relating to a wider range of Modern Postural Yoga schools.

The present analysis is mainly (but in no way exclusively) based on knowledge of this school as operating in Britain and in India. Many of the considerations and results that will transpire, however, may be said to apply to Iyengar Yoga practitioners and institutions worldwide and, in different ways and with some (more or less substantial) degree of adaptation, also to other MPY and MPsY schools.

B. K. S. Iyengar: his life and work

Iyengar was born of a Brahmin family in 1918 at Bellur.[19] He grew up in the highly nationalistic atmosphere of the Indian Independence struggle, and, while he never became involved in politics, he did identify with contemporary Neo-Hindu values and discourses, especially at the level of social and ethical orientation. At the more specific religious level, however, he always remained deeply attached to his religion of birth, South Indian Śrīvaiṣṇavism. Yoga became part of his life from early on: one of his older sisters married their fellow Śrīvaiṣṇava Tirumalai Krishnamacharya. Under fortuitous circumstances, this man became Iyengar's yoga *guru*.

Krishnamacharya (1888–1989) was a man of letters and an

19. Kolar district, now part of Karnataka State (*ILW*: 3).

accomplished scholar. But while he held degrees in various branches of Indian Philosophy[20] from six different Indian universities (Dars 1989: 6) and wrote numerous books in different languages (*Viniyoga* Editors 1989), the teaching that most affected his life was the training he received in the Himalayas for over seven years from the age of twenty-eight onwards. His own yoga school and family tradition report that for the duration of that training he resided with his teacher Rama Mohana Brahmachari at the foot of Mount Kailash, near Lake Mānasarovar in Tibet. Upon leaving his teacher, Krishnamacharya was asked to take a vow which committed him to "teach and even preach yoga, but avoid making any professional use of his knowledge or his diplomas in all the other branches of knowledge he had studied" (*ibid.*: 5, author's translation).

Iyengar lived with his brother-in-law from the age of sixteen up to the time he moved to Pune, to become himself a professional yoga teacher, three years later (1934 to 1937). It was also from Krishnamacharya that he received his *upanayana* initiation in 1935. These were crucially formative years, during which Iyengar learnt not only through direct instruction as any pupil does, but also and maybe even more importantly through example, observation and the experiences provided by full-time residence in Krishnamacharya's household. In those days Krishnamacharya had just started running the *yogaśālā* ("yoga hall") at the Palace of the Wodeyar family, the Mahārājas of Mysore, which he ran from 1933 to 1950. He had previously taught yoga at the Mysore Sanskrit Institute.

The Mysore princely family is known for having skilfully played its hand in the complex politics of growing nationalism (Manor 1977, Chapter 1). What is less well known is their long-standing patronage of yoga (Sjoman 1996), and their ongoing interest in, and support of, the East–West esoteric dialogue. Apart from running the Mysore *yogaśālā* and liaising with other Modern Yoga institutions in the subcontinent, the family also encouraged and sponsored influential figures such as Vivekananda (Williams 1974: 55–7), the writer of esoteric bestsellers Paul Brunton (Godwin *et al.* 1990: 14–15), and Swami Yogananda of *Autobiography of a Yogi* fame (Yogananda 1950), whom Iyengar met at the Mysore Palace (*ILW*: 14).

20. His titles are listed above his portrait in Iyengar's *Light on Yoga* (1984: 7), as follows: "*Sāmkhya-yoga-Śikhāmani*; *Veda-kesari*; *Vedāntavāgīśa*; *Nyāyāchārya*; *Mīmāmsa-ratna*; *Mīmāmsa-thīrtha*" (transliteration as per original text).

We mentioned Indian Modern Yoga institutions at the beginning of this chapter: the Yoga Institute at Santa Cruz, Bombay and the Kaivalyadhama Shrimad Madhava Yoga Mandir Samiti at Lonavla. While the Yoga Institute's profile currently comes very close to that of a community-cum-further-education and retreat centre, from its beginning Kaivalyadhama was (and is) especially committed to integrating the scientific (quantitative and empirical) and the speculative-scholarly study of yoga.[21] Krishnamacharya was sent by the Mysore Palace to observe this institution's work as early as 1934 (*ILW*: 8, 14). While he never attempted to emulate Kaivalyadhama's scientific approach, he did integrate Western physical fitness and training techniques in his practice and teaching, following in this a modern tradition already established by his princely sponsors (Sjoman 1996).

Iyengar's yoga practice developed at first within this framework, and after he moved to Pune the elaboration of what was by then becoming his own style of yoga was partly stimulated by, partly formulated in reaction to, what he knew to be happening at the Lonavla and the Bombay institutes (*ILW*: 49–51; Cushman 1997: 91). If we consider that he was also interested in the teachings of Swami Sivananda of Rishikesh (*ILW*: 55), who wrote many books on yoga and was very influential in Modern Yoga circles,[22] it will become apparent that Iyengar combined within himself influences from all the main early formulations of MPY. In due course we shall also hear about other influences, which only came to fruition later in his life.

A key, early collaborator should, however, be mentioned here: Iyengar's friend and supporter Dr Gokhale, MD, who also facilitated his relocation from Mysore to Pune. It was under his influence that Iyengar started using Western medical sciences in order to explain and propagate his style of yoga. The following quotation relates, in Iyengar's own words, how this came about. It also highlights his lack of theoretical training:

21. Though its laboratories and testing facilities are now very out of date, and the sort of funds that would be necessary to carry out state-of-the-art scientific experimentation do not seem to be forthcoming (own field data). About these two institutions see Alter (2000, Part II; and, especially, forthcoming).
22. For studies on Sivananda, his historical context, the Modern Yoga movement he established, and the ways in which some of his disciples developed his teachings see Strauss (1997; 2000; 2002a; 2002b; 2003).

> Doctor V.B. Gokhale ... was a great help to me. He used to give talks, and I used to give demonstrations. Because I could not speak on yoga, and I was not knowing philosophy. He said "The body is known to me. You leave it to me, I will explain very accurately. And you do the poses." Well, it was a really good combination ... and while he was explaining I started getting the anatomical words, which helped me a great deal to develop my subject. (Quoted in Cushman 1997: 158)

Popularization

The ten years after Iyengar moved to Pune (up to 1947) were a period of intense practice and just as intense financial hardship, but he eventually managed to establish himself as a well-respected yoga teacher in 1947. He held a number of regular yoga classes, gave private instruction, and also performed yoga demonstrations for audiences belonging to important professional bodies and institutions. By 1953 he had become instructor to the likes of J. Krishnamurti (more about this below), Jayaprakash Narayan, the "great Jain guru" Shri Badrankarji Maharaj and the violinist Yehudi Menuhin. The latter would also be instrumental in introducing him to Europe, to which Iyengar would travel for the first time in 1954, then again in 1956, when he also visited the USA.[23] But the first nucleus of regular British Iyengar Yoga practitioners was only created in 1960, again following a teaching invitation from Yehudi Menuhin. Beatrice Harthan, a member of this early group, explains how this came about, and how events progressed from that date:

> During [his 1960 visit] the Asian Music Circle made arrangements for a small group of people to be taught Yoga by Mr. Iyengar ... The small group grew in numbers with members from different parts of London. From this time on Mr. Iyengar came from India every year to teach an ever-growing number of students. His pupils started teaching... (Harthan 1987: 37)

Then, in 1966, Iyengar's *Light on Yoga* (or *LOY*; see Figures 11 and 12) was published. An instant bestseller, it immediately became the standard reference work on *āsana* practice in Modern Yoga circles all over the world. From the point of view of practice, two things made this book outstanding: (1) the thorough, step-by-step, DIY type of instruction, and (2) the obvious proficiency of the author in the

23. For these and more biographical details see *GY* (pp. 30–4).

practice, teaching and practico-therapeutic applications of *āsanas* as revealed, respectively, by the book's numerous photographs, by its instructions and practice plans, and by the suggested condition-related treatment programmes. In the mind of the public, this book came at times to complement, but more often to supersede two earlier, very popular publications which had been used as practice manuals or reference books by a growing number of practitioners: Theos Bernard's *Hatha Yoga* (1982 [1944]) and Swami Vishnudevananda's *The Complete Illustrated Book of Yoga* (Vishnudevananda 1988 [1960]).

On the institutional and teaching level, *LOY* turned out to be a milestone not only for the growth of the Iyengar School, but also for the development of MPY at large. As far as the Iyengar School was concerned, it sanctioned and gave huge diffusion potential to the vigorous kind of instruction and training that Iyengar had already started carrying out in person in India and in the West. As for MPY, it brought the performance and teaching of *āsana*, on which MPY relied so heavily, to new, impressive standards of completeness regarding range of postural variation and performance proficiency. These standards, furthermore, were for the first time presented so as to stand up to international scrutiny and appreciation. Bernard's book, while well researched and presented, was not acculturated enough to gain bestseller status. Swami Vishnudevananda's manual came closer to having a more general appeal, but the author's performance of *āsanas* lacked the qualities of precision, skilfulness and artistry that propelled Iyengar to fame in the West.[24] And while neither Vishnudevananda nor Iyengar shone at handling the written word, Iyengar received much stylistic and editorial help from professionally competent pupils and well-wishers.[25]

LOY's publication was instrumental in establishing Iyengar as a yoga teacher of international standing and repute. Indeed, the practice and the teaching of *āsana* have always been Iyengar's real passion. There are good reasons for this. First of all, *āsana* practice changed the course of his life by transforming him from a sickly

24. Vishnudevananda (1988 [1960]) is nevertheless still recognized as an MPY classic, while its postural shortcomings have been redressed in the Sivananda School's more recent manual *The Book of Yoga* (Sivananda Yoga Centre 1993 [1983]). See De Michelis (1995) for a more detailed comparison of various MPY schools' postural techniques.

25. See *ILW* (pp. 427–32), *GY* (p. 18), *LOYSP* (pp. xx–xxi).

youth into a healthy and strong young man (*GY*: 1; *ILW*: 3, 8). Secondly, the practice and teaching of *āsana* became his profession early on in life. He started teaching when he was sixteen years old, and, as an orphan of humble family with no other qualifications, he had no career prospects worth mentioning. Thirdly, his personality had a strong artistic and theatrical component. This led him to attempt to join a famous dance troupe at one point (*ILW*: 29–30), and to try to apply the concept of art fairly extensively in his interpretation of yoga.[26] While he never became a dancer, he would eventually excel by single-handedly enthralling live audiences worldwide. This he did by performing hundreds of "yoga demonstrations" consisting of seamlessly interlinked sequences of *āsanas*, some highly acrobatic, which he would present along with a captivating running commentary without ever getting out of breath or betraying any strain.[27] Throughout his career Iyengar has remained a master of postural performance with great stage presence.

Consolidation

After the death of his wife Ramamani in 1973, Iyengar had only one focus left in his life: yoga (*ILW*: 79). Ramamani died shortly after conducting the purificatory *pūjā* for the land on which the future Iyengar Yoga Institute would stand, and the institution was eventually named after her.

The Ramamani Iyengar Memorial Yoga Institute (RIMYI) opened its doors at Pune in December 1975. This was a momentous event for the Iyengar movement: the school's founder had now a purpose-built base from which to propagate his teachings, and where pupils from all over the world could come to study and train. This was especially important as, despite a certain amount of recognition within India, the Iyengar method was mainly successful in the West[28] or, to be more specific, in English-speaking countries and communities. Before 1975 "early enthusiasts [had] muddled along" by following Iyengar

26. See especially *AY*, but this is a recurring theme in Iyengar's work (though in no way pervasive).
27. Some of these performances are recorded on film and video.
28. In a 1988 speech Iyengar lamented that "outstanding people are kept standing out in our country" (*GY*: 18). Since then, Iyengar's merits have been recognized much more widely in India. Most recently (2002) he has been the recipient of two prestigious awards: The Padma Bhushan conferred by the Indian government to individuals who have excelled in their field, and an honorary Doctorate in Literature from the Tilak Maharastra Vidyapeeth (*Iyengar Yoga News* 2002: 16).

to his varied travel destinations, or by undergoing instruction in his cramped family residence.[29] More generally, the spread of Iyengar Yoga benefited from the explosion of interest in physical exercise prompted by the 'fitness revolution' of the latter part of the 1970s (Stirk 1988: 12): at this time MPY started to be seen by even more people as a safe and balanced way to keep fit and improve well-being.

Another pervasive influence was that of New Age religion, which, around the mid-1970s, had become a self-conscious 'movement' (Chapter 1). We have repeatedly noted that Modern Yoga and New Age religion developed in parallel and often intertwining fashion. This topic, and its effect on Iyengar Yoga theory and practice, will be discussed in more depth in the following chapter. All that will be pointed out now are the visible effects that these influences have had on the more institutional aspects of Iyengar Yoga. These are exemplarily represented by the first (and key) official aim of the RIMYI:

> 1. To promote yogic education and impart yogic instruction for the development of and integration of human personality in all its aspects, physical, mental and spiritual, in accordance with the techniques evolved and developed by the Director, Yogacharya B.K.S. Iyengar, and as followed by associate Directors Miss Geeta and Mr. Prashant.[30]

As we see, New Age concepts of healing ("integration") and personal growth ("development") are by this stage of primary importance in Iyengar Yoga, as in most other forms of MPY, while reference to the personalized 'techniques' or 'tools' so dear to modern esotericists and occultists are also well in evidence.

Significantly, the official aims of the RIMYI are also adopted or integrated as part of the 'Aims and Objectives' of other official Iyengar Yoga institutes and centres worldwide. The London Iyengar Yoga Institute, for example, which has played a prominent role in the

29. See Harthan (1985: 15); also see photographs in Perez-Christiaens (1976: between pages 96 and 97).

30. "The aim and objects of the Ramamani Iyengar Memorial Yoga Institute" as widely reproduced, including in the *Members' Handbook* of the B. K. S. Iyengar Yoga Teachers' Association (BKSIYTA 1992: 19). Geeta and Prashant are Iyengar's eldest children and, as the wording of the document clearly indicates, they too are expected to follow closely in their father's footsteps. They have certainly done so throughout the Consolidation period, but new potentialities for power configurations have slowly started to emerge in the mid- and late 1990s. From the late 1990s, Iyengar's daughter Geeta has taken over most of the international commitments that would in the past have been carried out by her father (own field data).

history of the school, opened in 1983. It has "pledged to ensure that only Yoga teaching in a pure form according to the method of B.K.S. Iyengar takes place on [its] premises", and teachers are further "required to practise and promote the work taught at the Ramamani Iyengar Memorial Yoga Institute in Pune" (Iyengar Yoga Institute 1988: 16).

The B. K. S. Iyengar Yoga Teachers' Association (BKSIYTA; established 1977) shows a similar pattern of allegiance to Pune. Its mandate is to co-ordinate communication among teachers, "[t]o assess applicants for Teaching Certificates, and to issue certificates .... [which] are those of the Ramamani Iyengar Memorial Yoga Institute".[31] The Association also maintains "a national register of approved teachers" and "a list of approved teacher-training courses" (BKSIYTA 1992: 16). Its Constitution specifies that the BKSIYTA is "affiliated" to the Pune "Parent Institute", and that Iyengar is its President. Its foremost aims are: "a. To spread the teaching of Yogacharya B.K.S. Iyengar and to maintain the teaching standard set by him", and "b. To support the aims and objects of the Parent Institute" (*ibid.*).

The key elements that would allow the consolidation process to unfold and, eventually, to progress towards full Acculturation were now in place: a network of institutionally structured and efficient training centres gravitating around the unquestioned authority of a charismatic leader, and a system of accreditation that would in due course produce the power structures of the Iyengar movement and its teaching hierarchies.

The Consolidation phase also sees a flourishing of Iyengar or Iyengar Yoga-related texts (i.e. written by senior pupils, admirers, or people otherwise inspired by Iyengar's work).[32] Of all the books published in these years, however, *Light on Prāṇāyāma* (or *LOP*; 1983 [1981]; see Figure 13) is the most authoritative. In *LOY* Iyengar

31. The awarding of the very first official Iyengar Yoga Teacher Certificates (to some of Iyengar's South African students) took place in October 1975. The issuing of such certificates is another clear sign that the Consolidation period was starting.

32. At least twenty have come this writer's way without doing any special search or carrying out specific enquiries, and surely there must be several more. Just to mention the ones cited in this book: Perez-Christiaens (1976); *LOP* [1981]; Smith and Boudreau [1981]; *AY* [1985]; *ILW* [1987]. A concise edition of *LOY* was also first published during the Consolidation period (in 1980) thus making this seminal text even more widely available.

had interpreted the yoga tradition in careful, tentative and impersonal fashion. In *LOP*, however, older influences finally come to the fore, namely the early contacts he had with Indian representatives of Neo-Vedāntic esotericism. Judging by his biography and by his style of writing and address, among the most formative ones are Sivananda of Rishikesh and, most of all, Jiddu Krishnamurti.

From a chronological point of view these influences were exercised well before the Consolidation period. Up to 1975, however, Iyengar was mainly busy elaborating and propagating his style of yoga *practice*. It was only after *LOY*'s success, the establishment of the RIMYI and the attainment of professional and personal maturity that these influences could emerge. We know that Iyengar read Sivananda's books, attended some of the lectures that he gave in Pune in 1950 and tried, unsuccessfully, to meet him (*ILW*: 55). Sivananda, however, bestowed on him the title of 'Yogi Raja' ("King of Yoga" or Yoga Master) in 1952, after seeing a photographic album of Iyengar's *āsanas*, which the latter had sent him as a present (*ibid.*: 57).

As for Krishnamurti, he was probably the one who exerted the greatest, if so far unacknowledged, intellectual influence on Iyengar: Iyengar had in fact personal and protracted contacts with him. As is well known, Krishnamurti was the Theosophical Society's chosen messiah. In the event, however, he rejected this role and went on to deconstruct systematically the whole concept of the authority of the teacher, although, somewhat ironically, he had to accept his new-found role of cultic milieu *guru*. He was bred (if not quite born) within the esoterico-occultist milieus that we have highlighted as formative to Modern Yoga, and he made the most of his knowledge and background. Iyengar – a totally different kind of person, but, as already noted, a sensitive and receptive one – must have learned much about the unwritten laws regulating esoteric milieus from his new-found pupil and friend.

Iyengar was thirty when he met Krishnamurti in 1948. The latter was giving a three-month long series of discourses in Pune. Iyengar attended most of them, and at some point a common friend introduced the two men. Iyengar showed his yoga poses to Krishnamurti, then asked to see his *āsana* practice and, tactfully, corrected it. Krishnamurti requested that Iyengar teach him yoga,[33] and tuition "continued for the next 20 years" (*GY*: 31, under 1948; *ILW*: 49). At

33. *ILW*: 48 and *GY*: 31. *GY*: 14, however, states that the two met in 1946.

first Iyengar did not realize that Krishnamurti was internationally famous: "As I did not read books or papers, I was not aware of personalities or world events", but he now witnessed how his fellow South Indian had a substantial following, numbers of which came to his talks (*GY*: 14; *ILW*: 48). According to Iyengar himself, Krishnamurti taught him to think more independently:

> . . . I learnt something from him. I should not be disturbed or swayed by the opinions of others. For example, Yogis all over the world criticised me for doing physical Yoga . . . [But] I do not do yoga for other people's comments. Let them criticise as long as they like. I do for the sake of doing and am keen to evolve in my practices. I am not keen to justify that what I do is right . . . (*GY*: 14–15)

This would indeed have been momentous input for a man struggling (like most Neo-Hindus in particular and countless modern individuals in general) between the contradicting dictates of 'tradition' and 'modernity'. The two men "used to discuss together, and developed an intimate relationship", and for periods of time, while travelling and teaching, they also shared the same quarters (*ibid.*: 15). Iyengar was mildly critical of Krishnamurti's 'deconstructionist' style of address, feeling that it may "convey a negative meaning for a lay person" (*ibid.*). In at least one instance, however, he openly admits to having been inspired by Krishnamurti's talks for the language he would use in his teaching (*ibid.*), and his rhetorical style is at times curiously reminiscent of Krishnamurti's own.

It would seem quite safe to assume that Krishnamurti played a considerable (if unconscious) part in changing Iyengar's mentality so that he would feel free – and motivated – to switch from his earlier mixture of traditionalism and Neo-Hindu ideas to more de-traditionalized, cultic milieu style theories and elaborations. The fact that Iyengar had familiarized himself with the culture of the Anglo-Indian cultic milieu within which Krishnamurti operated probably also paved the way for easier, more successful relations with Menuhin when he met him in 1952, as well as with the many Western students with whom he would eventually associate. Without such cultural input and individual contacts, Iyengar Yoga may not have flourished in the same way it has done.

Acculturation

And flourish it did. By 1990 the Mehtas, senior British Iyengar Yoga teachers, could report that "[Iyengar] has several million students all over the world following his method. There are Iyengar Institutes and centres in the UK, Europe, Australia, Canada, Israel, Japan, New Zealand, South Africa and the USA, as well as India" (Mehta, S. *et al.* 1990: 9; see also *GY*: 105–26). Like a number of other Modern Yoga groups, Iyengar Yoga was becoming fully 'globalized' by the 1990s. This went hand in hand, unsurprisingly, with a process of acculturation. We shall briefly look at two aspects of this phenomenon: the participation of the British Iyengar Yoga movement in the process of selection of a 'ruling body' for yoga on the part of the UK Sports Council, and Iyengar's support of the professionalization of MPY teaching not only as a way to make a living, but as a comprehensive way of life.

By the 1990s MPY had undoubtedly become part of everyday British life, and was regarded, at least by some, as a fairly mainstream leisure activity or as a form of 'sport' rather than as an esoteric or religious pursuit.[34] This was recognized by the Sports Council, which proposed to elect a national ruling body for yoga. Interestingly, a previous attempt to do so (in the 1970s) had failed: obviously MPY was not ready to gain such a degree of official recognition.

As the time to discuss with the Sports Council approached, British Iyengar Yoga groups started to devise a common strategy. The Light on Yoga Association (LOYA) was set up in 1988 to co-ordinate the work of existing Iyengar Yoga institutes and centres, and to promote the formation of new ones throughout the country.[35] One of the main motivations behind its foundation, however, had been the need to

34. For example, I had occasion to carry out brief unstructured interviews with Cambridge University first-year students interested in taking up the practice of yoga in 1996, 1997 and 1998. In many instances their parents had been (or were) yoga practitioners, which is why they were thinking of taking up yoga at all. They regarded yoga (that is, MPY) as an essentially health- and wellbeing-related pursuit and, tellingly, several of them were surprised at finding out that yoga was an acquired taste in the West, and that it originates from India.

    It will also be noted that MPY associations were listed under 'sports' in University of Cambridge Student Societies' directories throughout the second part of the 1990s. Such a categorization never elicited any surprise or comment from the general public or from more or less committed practitioners of MPY.

35. LOYA and BKSIYTA have since merged into a unified association. The latter was launched in June 2003 under the name Iyengar Yoga Association of the United Kingdom, or IYA (UK).

establish a national institution which could compete with the British Wheel of Yoga (BWY) in the bid to become the Sports Council's recognized ruling body. This prompted the creation of a substantial number of Iyengar Yoga Institutes throughout the UK. While the very first British Iyengar Yoga Institute had opened in Manchester in 1972, quite independently of this later acculturation drive, by 1988 the number of Institutes in Britain had risen to three, and by the mid-1990s there were twelve (Ward 1994: 8–9). After a protracted negotiations (1991 to 1995) with the Sports Council and the BWY, however, the BWY eventually won the battle, and was recognized as the British ruling body for Yoga by the Sports Council (under the sub-heading of 'Movement and Dance') in August 1995. Despite not having gained official recognition, this process had strengthened the foundations of the movement within the UK: now Iyengar Yoga could present itself as an institution with a coherent national profile.

Over time, national networks, centralized teacher training procedures and more or less formalized adaptations to local conditions have become of central interest to Iyengar Yoga institutions worldwide. Such endeavours allow them not only to survive, but to grow and develop. B. K. S. Iyengar, in his own way, has been responding to these trends. The story of his life shows that he is in no way business minded or greedy. He does, however, support the professionalization of yoga, and has attempted, in the light of his own experiences, to define an ethos of yoga teaching as a way of life. A number of senior Iyengar Yoga teachers met during fieldwork confirmed that they follow Iyengar's lines here, thus justifying their profession to themselves and to society at large.

We find this concept clearly expressed in Iyengar's *Light on the Yoga Sūtras of Patañjali* (or *LOYSP* 1993; see Figure 14), a translation and commentary of the central text of Classical Yoga, and the most important text of the Iyengar school in the Acculturation period.[36] Here Iyengar attempts what may be regarded as a quintessentially Neo-Hindu manoeuvre, viz. to combine Western concepts of professional development, the Brahmo Puritan ethic of self-support, and the classical Hindu scheme of the four *varṇas* (social "classes") – though with the ultimate intent to adapt MPY practice and teaching to polyvalent, globalized conditions. In the relevant passage Iyengar

36. Iyengar's latest book was published in 2001 (Iyengar 2001). Rather than establishing any new trend, it is best described as an expansion and updating of *LOY*-type themes.

states that the pupil who begins the practice of his style of MPY "has to sweat profusely in body and brain to get a grasp of it ... This is *śūdra dharma*." Then comes *vaiśya dharma* "when one consciously sets out to accumulate experience in order to teach, so as to earn a living". This will be followed by "*sādhana* ... of the *kṣatriya*", when one builds up courage and expertise, strives to develop the art and "gains the authority to share one's knowledge and experience". Finally, if one achieves union with the "Universal Spirit (*Paramātman*), and surrenders to Him in word, thought and deed, one is a *brāhmaṇa* in yogic *sādhana*" (*LOYSP*: 267).

We see from the developments described above how MPY (Iyengar or otherwise) was progressively adapted to the spirit of modernity and secularization. In the next chapter we will look more specifically at parallel developments in Iyengar Yoga theory and practice. This will be done through analysis of textual evidence.

7. Theory and practice of Iyengar Yoga

When one rests on the vision of the soul, divinity is felt in this empirical state.
(B. K. S. Iyengar *LOYSP*: 26)

Iyengar's Modern Yoga trilogy

This chapter is based on an analysis of Iyengar's three main books on yoga: *Light on Yoga* (or *LOY*; 1966), *Light on Prāṇāyāma* (or *LOP*; 1981) and *Light on the Yoga Sūtras of Patañjali* (or *LOYSP*; 1993).[1] This trilogy may be considered paradigmatic for the purposes of showing the characteristics and ideological range of Modern Postural Yoga (MPY) as it evolved through the three developmental phases described in the previous chapter. All three books contain the three main conceptual frameworks found in most MPY elaborations, but, significantly, emphases and the ways they are expressed change through different periods. The three elements are (a) the Neo-Vedāntic layer, (b) the Harmonial (Metaphysical and mesmeric) layer, both of these layers appropriating elements of *haṭhayoga*, and (c) the more personal religio-philosophical approach added on by each teacher.

In Iyengar's case the Neo-Vedāntic layer is mainly found in the social and ethical, this-worldly orientation of his teachings, and in the occasional attempts to link them to 'scientific' knowledge, theories or similes. The Harmonial layer is the conceptual filter used to interpret and to elaborate practices, and because practices ('techniques', 'sys-

1. See Figures 11–14 for reproduction of pages.

tems') are so prominent in MPY, this layer is very prominent. As time goes by, Iyengar's Harmonial interpretations align themselves more and more with the New Age leanings of his pupils' milieu. Finally his more personal contribution is an element of mainstream devotionalism and theism, deriving from the diffused religiosity of his native background, which makes him very receptive to the teachings of the *Bhagavad Gītā*. This includes, importantly, the *Gītā*'s rendition of the concept of yoga, quite different from the ways in which yoga is interpreted in the *Yoga Sūtras*.

With regard to differences of emphasis over time, we see that *LOY* (1966) is, quantitatively speaking, pre-eminently practical and generally humble in tone. It is also rather cautious and impersonal in its exposition of theoretical doctrines and beliefs. Essentially, *LOY* absorbs the surrounding Neo-Vedāntic ethos, and retransmits it. The only difference from other yoga books is that Iyengar has been working hard and in peculiarly focused fashion at practising and teaching *āsanas* for over three decades and he is, as it were, reporting on this work.

In *LOP* (1981) what has emerged as the Iyengar style of Yoga, i.e. a modernized form of *haṭhayoga*, is assimilated to occultist Harmonial thinking, now in the New Age version of healing and personal growth philosophy. The marriage of *haṭhayoga* and Harmonial thinking that Vivekananda had tentatively initiated now becomes an accomplished fact, and the standard form of MPY. In this sense too, apart from the more tangible institutional sense described in the previous chapter, we witness a progressive consolidation of this discipline.

Completing his trilogy of MPY classics, Iyengar publishes *LOYSP* in 1993. As we saw in the previous chapter, this is the key book of the Acculturation period, a time of further expansion but also of new challenges and internal revisions. For Iyengar himself, now entering his seventies, this is also a natural time of reflection and of searching deeper into the subject to which he has dedicated his life. *LOYSP* is a bold attempt to co-ordinate and bring together the somewhat divergent and definitely diverse MPY ideological strands delineated above. As in *LOP*, the New Age presuppositions and the "Self-realization" theme are quantitatively most apparent in this text. These tenets are essential to the justification and shaping of a fully acculturated Iyengar Yoga, which now proceeds to assimilate the meditative *saṃyama* disciplines into its orthopractical scheme. The theistic and devotional approach, based on Iyengar's native Śrīvaiṣṇavism, however, emerges as the one closest to his heart. Interpreted through the Neo-Vedāntic filter – also part of Iyengar's original background – this approach emerges in what we may call a Neo-Śrīvaiṣṇava form. But, mindful of the "modern disquietude concerning traditional religious authority" (Fuller 1989: 119–20), Iyengar refrains from forcing his convictions on anyone. Thus he tones down this more traditional theistic and devotional theme, and fits it at the margins and in (important) interstitial spaces of the text.

Apart from providing interesting evidence in relation to the development of the Iyengar School and to modern and contemporary forms of yoga, this trilogy provides us with fascinating insights about the ways in which religious practices and beliefs are moulded by the human beings through which they are transmitted, the transmitters in turn being moulded by specific historical and cultural circumstances. In order to appraise better the conceptual steps involved in such transformations, let us now turn to a more detailed examination of these texts and of their relation with Iyengar Yoga theory and practice.

Light on Yoga (1966): the Popularization period

As already stated, the centrepiece of Iyengar Yoga is the theory and practice of *āsana*. *Āsana* was Iyengar's way into yoga, and it has remained his speciality. As an American travel guide to 'spiritual India' states, Iyengar

> is probably the most famous hatha yogi in the world. For thousands of students the photographs of him in *Light on Yoga* – his illustrated Bible of yoga postures – are the ultimate standard for asana practice. And his precise, scientific approach to alignment and form have revolutionized the way yoga is taught in the West. (Cushman and Jones 1999: 221)

By the time *LOY* came to be written, Iyengar had invested much time and energy in what he had come to regard as his mission: the popularization of yoga.[2] *LOY*'s huge commercial success only strengthened his resolve in this direction. As far as the *practice* of Iyengar Yoga is concerned, compared to what went on earlier in the world of MPY, *LOY* played a major role in standardizing and demystifying (from a Western or Neo-Vedāntic point of view) the practice of Postural Yoga.

LOY was written, essentially, in DIY-manual form. We saw that this type of textual approach, based on the modern 'self-help' ethos, had become increasingly successful among the American and more generally English-speaking public from the first part of the nineteenth century onward. Iyengar further succeeded in presenting the topic of yogic *āsanas* in a thoroughly modern way thanks to the use of medical and anatomico-physiological models. As he himself states, his main aim in *LOY* is "to describe as simply as possible the āsanas ... and prāṇāyāmas ... in the new light of our own era, its knowledge and its requirements" (*LOY*: 13). Importantly, *LOY* (along with Iyengar's "Yoga Demonstrations") also created in the Western public an awareness of the acrobatic and artistic potential of postural practice. These developments opened up spaces for the aesthetic appreciation of *āsanas*, something quite novel in the field of yoga. *LOY*'s popularity played a major role in raising postural practice standards to higher levels of performance: Iyengar's manual became the acknowledged point of reference in the sense that no MPY practitioner or school could afford to ignore its existence.

MPY practice as psychosomatic self-help

The most notable and MPY-specific developments in *LOY*, however, take place under the influence of medical, physical culture and fitness applications. These are not (yet) theorized as fully-fledged interpretations of yoga, but are expanded and elaborated in such a way that MPY starts to emerge as the ultimate system of psychosomatic self-help. Yoga can then be seen as a comprehensive tool for self-improvement and healing, potentially suitable for self-ministration in total autonomy from institutional and societal control, purely on the basis of individual choice, taste or need.

LOY comprises three main parts, plus appendices, a glossary and

2. In a 1977 feature, for example, he stated: "When I was first introduced to the West in 1954 by Yehudi Menuhin, I began to sow the seeds of Yoga and today I am proud to say those seeds have grown into a forest ..." (*ILW*: 84).

an index. Part I consists of a theoretical introduction (see next section), Part II, covering about four-fifths of the book, is dedicated to *āsana* (see below), while Part III gives a brief outline of *prāṇāyāma* techniques, a subject that Iyengar will develop in much greater depth in *LOP*. Part II on *āsana* is further complemented by Appendix I, giving the details of a graded *āsana* course covering all the postures described in the book, and by Appendix II, giving a list of "Curative Āsanas for Various Diseases". Here Iyengar's exposition of postural practice is detailed, systematic and comprehensive enough not only to satisfy, but to impress Western audiences. He presents each *āsana* as follows (see also Figures 11 and 12):

(a) NAME: the Sanskrit name of the posture is given and the meaning of the words, the symbolism of the name and sometimes the related mythology are explained. A brief description of the pose is usually given. Each *āsana*'s difficulty is represented by a starred number from 1 to 60, 1 being the simplest.
(b) TECHNIQUE: this section provides a step-by-step description of each *āsana*'s execution. Detailed anatomical movements and breathing patterns are specified. Typical mistakes or limitations often encountered by beginners are pointed out and addressed.
(c) EFFECTS: the physical, physiological and psychological effects of each pose are described. Curative and preventive effects are also listed. Variations of the posture may be prescribed for beginners or for specific conditions. Cautions are given specifying when a posture should not be practised. Quotations from yogic texts and theoretical explanations may be given either under (a) or (c).
(d) ILLUSTRATION(S): each pose is illustrated by one or more photographs.

Throughout most of Part II of the book, Iyengar substantiates the value and effectiveness of *āsanas* in pure MPY style by discussing their effects mainly in terms of Western medical knowledge and fitness training. One pose "relieves backaches and neck sprains" (*LOY*: 64), while another "cures impotency and promotes sex control" (*ibid.*: 173). We find out that "by doing [a certain] posture the abdominal organs are exercised and gain strength" (*ibid.*: 266), or that "[t]he minor muscles of the arms will be developed and toned by the practice of [another] pose" (*ibid.*: 282). Specific fitness needs are also addressed: a certain pose "is recommended for runners" (*ibid.*:

330 *Light on Yoga*

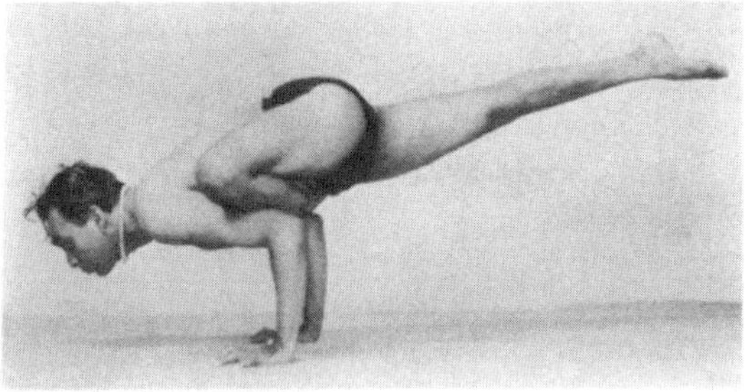

433

158. *Dwi Pāda Kouṇḍinyāsana* Twenty-two* (Plate 458)

Dwi Pāda (dwi = two or both; pāda = leg or foot) means both feet.

Kouṇḍinya was a sage belonging to the family of Vasiṣṭha and founded the Kouṇḍinya Gotra (sect). This āsana is dedicated to him.

Technique

1. Perform Sālamba Śīrṣāsana II. (Plate 192)

2. Exhale and lower the legs straight together until they are parallel to the floor. (Plate 434.) Pause here and take a few breaths.

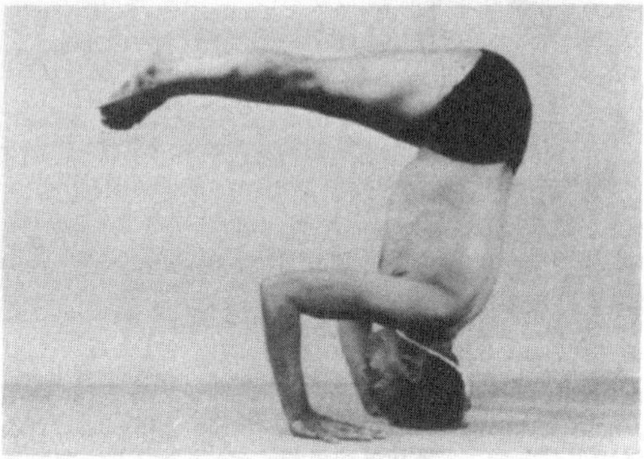

434

3. Exhale, turn the trunk slightly to the right and move both legs sideways to the right. (Plate 435.) Lower both legs together over the right arm so that the outer side of the left thigh above the knee rests on the back of the upper right arm as near the armpit as possible. (Plate 436)

Figure 11 Reproduction of pages 330–1 from B. K. S. Iyengar's *Light on Yoga*. Reprinted by permission of HarperCollins Publishers Ltd. © B.K.S. Iyengar 1966

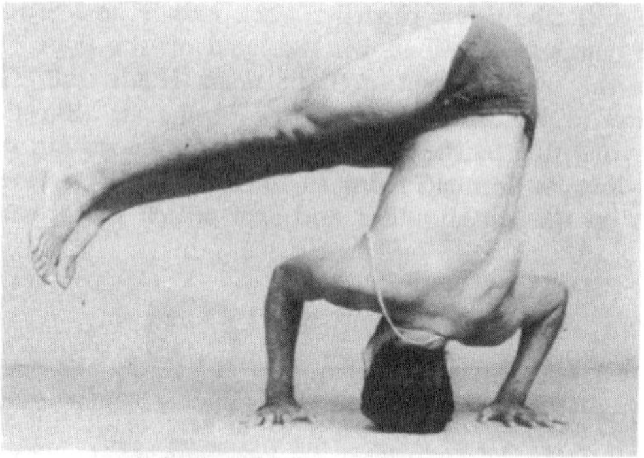

435

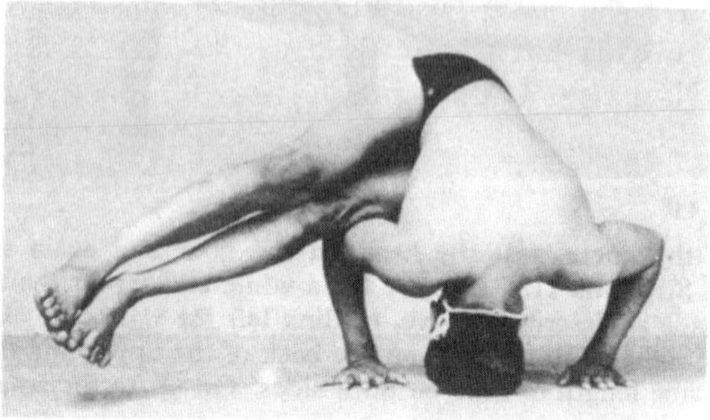

436

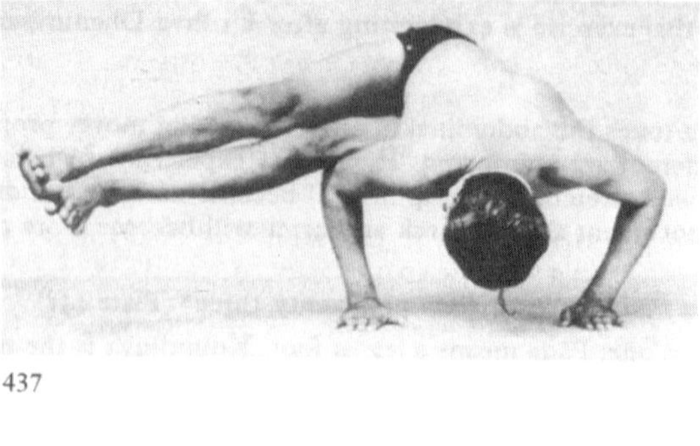

437

332 *Light on Yoga*

4. Balance and take a few breaths. Then exhale and firmly pressing down both palms to the floor, lift the head off the floor. (Plate 437.) Then raise the trunk and stretch the neck. (Plate 438.) This is the final position in which the legs will be in the air almost parallel to the floor, while due to the twist of the trunk, breathing will be fast. Balance as long as you can from 10 to 20 seconds. Greater pressure will be felt on the left shoulder and arm which are apparently free.

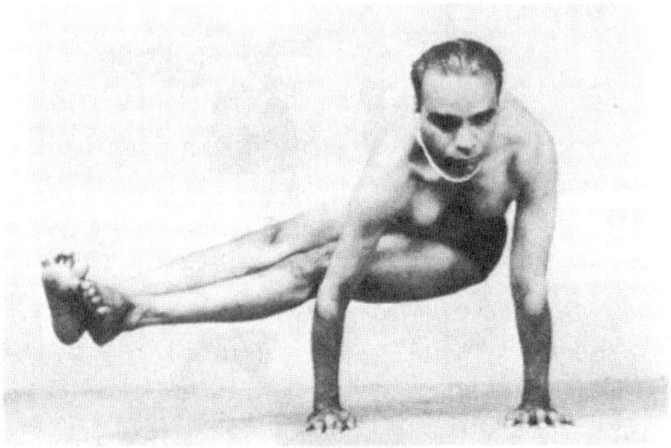

438

5. Bend the knees, rest the head on the floor and again go up to Sālamba Śīrṣāsana II. Rest here for a while and repeat the āsana on the left side as described above, reading left for right and vice versa. Here the right thigh will rest on the back of the upper left arm. Stay for the same length of time on both sides. Go up to Śīrṣāsana again.

6. To complete the pose, either lower the legs to the floor and relax or do Ūrdhva Dhanurāsana (Plate 486) and stand up in Tāḍāsana. (Plate 1.) When one has mastered Viparīta Chakrāsana (Plates 488 to 499), this exercise is exhilarating after Ūrdhva Dhanurāsana.

Effects

The pose tones the abdominal organs. The colon moves properly and toxins therein are eliminated. It requires experience to balance with the legs well stretched. The spine will become more elastic due to the lateral movement and the neck and arms will become more powerful.

159. *Eka Pāda Kouṇḍinyāsana I* Twenty-three* (Plate 441)

Eka means one. Pāda means a leg or foot. Kouṇḍinya is the name of a sage.

Figure 12 Reproduction of pages 332–3 from B. K. S. Iyengar's *Light on Yoga*. Reprinted by permission of HarperCollins Publishers Ltd. © B.K.S. Iyengar 1966

Yogāsanas, Bandha and Kriyā 333

Technique

1. Perform Sālamba Śīrṣāsana II. (Plate 192)

2. Exhale, lower the legs straight together until they are parallel to the floor. (Plate 434.) Pause here and take a few breaths.

3. Exhale, bend the legs and move the left leg sideways to the right. Place the left leg over the back of the upper right arm so that the outer side of the left thigh above the knee rests as near the right armpit as possible. (Plate 439.) Take a few breaths and balance.

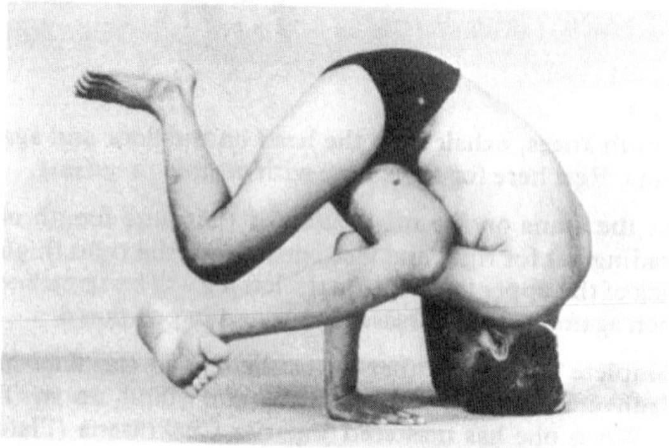

439

4. Stretch the left leg straight sideways and the right leg straight back. (Plate 440.) Take two breaths.

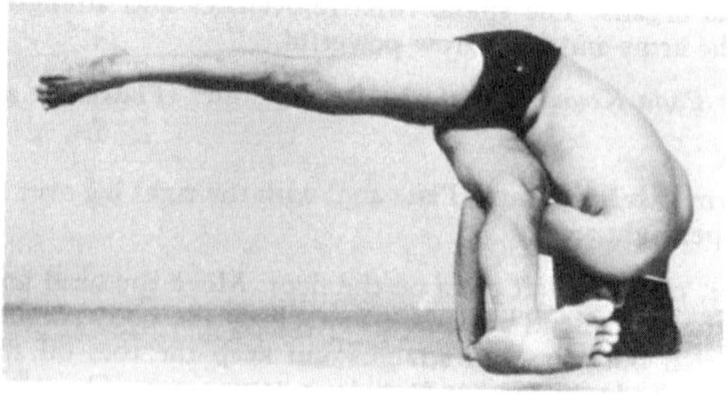

440

5. Exhale, raise the head above the floor, extend the arms and balance on the hands. Keep both legs straight and taut at the knees. (Plate 441.)

74), another "is beneficial ... for horsemen" (*ibid.*: 89), yet another "can be tried conveniently by the elderly" (*ibid.*: 88); and more wide-ranging human wishes are also catered for: practice of some postures will "enable us to grow old gracefully and comfortably" (*ibid.*: 114), others will help "to keep one ... fresh and alert in mind" (*ibid.*: 403). Concerns over physical appearance are not forgotten: *āsanas* can be used "to reduce body weight" (*ibid.*: 85), "to reduce the size of the abdomen" (*ibid.*: 257), to make "the leg muscles more shapely and sturdy" (*ibid.*: 74). And all this in the comfort of one's own home and at no expense since yoga practice "requires no special apparatus or gymnasiums. The various parts of the body supply the weights and counterweights" (*ibid.*: 282).

But one of the great attractions of the Iyengar system to the modern mind rests on the fact that it develops these medical and fitness themes along even more detailed and comprehensive self-help lines. Instructions are given on how to use *āsanas* to combat stress,[3] to recover more promptly after illness (*ibid.*: 216), to relieve as varied a range of conditions as depression and over-excitement (*ibid.*: 93) or constipation (*ibid.*: 170). The effects of *āsana* practice are indeed remarkable and, it would seem, almost miraculous: "Continuous practice will change the outlook of the practiser. He will discipline himself in food, sex, cleanliness and character and will become a new man" (*ibid.*: 60).[4]

Western practitioners could feel comfortable with following the book's instructions. The tone of Part II on *āsana* is, in the main, down-to-earth, and the anatomico-physiological and medical language and descriptions are reassuring due to the familiar, 'scientific' terminology. References to haṭhayogic practices and models of the human being are sparse and 'impersonal' enough so that they can be conveniently ignored if one so chooses. Besides, the rather basic *haṭhayoga* tenets and terminology employed in *LOY* were already fairly commonplace by 1966, thus they added spice to the text and could be linked up with more in-depth knowledge or teachings if the reader wished to. But in *LOY* Iyengar seems to be more reporting on them than recommending or describing these practices from

3. "The stresses of modern civilisation are a strain on the nerves for which Śavāsana is the best antidote" (*ibid.*: 424. *Śavāsana* or 'corpse pose' entails lying on one's back and stilling all sense and mental activity, but without falling asleep; see also section on "The incorporation phase" in Chapter 8).
4. Iyengar consistently employs the masculine gender to indicate both men and women.

experience. The postural, medical and anatomico-physiological teachings, on the other hand, are presented in strong first-hand experiential tones. The visual impact of *LOY* is also remarkable, as the book contains over 600 photographs of the author demonstrating the over 200 postures and practices described.

As the above suggests, *LOY* follows on, from a certain point of view, in the footsteps of earlier *haṭhayoga* texts: only the claims concerning the effects of the practices are expressed in contemporary language and address contemporary needs and preoccupations. And, of course, as we saw in the preceding chapters, the social, religious and institutional dimensions of MPY are very different from earlier, classical forms of yoga.

MPY theory in Light on Yoga

While *LOY* is replete with detailed practical explanations, the related MPY theory is only expressed in embryonic terms over relatively few pages.[5] Most of Iyengar's formative influences and the three MPY theoretical elements discussed at the beginning of the present chapter are, however, well in evidence.

Formative influences are seen in the range of texts quoted: Iyengar repeatedly refers (whether directly or indirectly) to classical texts such as the *Upaniṣads*, the *Bhagavad Gītā* and the *Yoga Sūtras*. Haṭhayogic lore is also well represented, with numerous borrowings from the *Gheraṇḍa Saṃhitā*, the *Śiva Saṃhitā* and the *Haṭha Yoga Pradīpikā*. Purāṇic contributions are also found.[6] Strong Neo-Vedāntic influences are seen in quotations from Mahadev Desai (*LOY*: 19), Mohandas Karamchand Gandhi (*ibid.*: 33), Vinoba Bhave (*ibid.*: 39, 50), Sarvepalli Radhakrishnan (*ibid.*: 117–18), and in echoes of Vivekananda's writings,[7] in the use of Christian formulas

5. About 40 pages out of 544.
6. While classical texts are mainly used to expound yoga philosophy throughout Part I (*LOY*: 17–53), haṭhayogic references are found both in Part I and in the much lengthier Part II, treating the actual practice of *āsana*. Purāṇic stories are mainly drawn upon in Part II to explain the name of *āsanas* dedicated to ancient Indian sages.
7. For example, when Iyengar mentions four main yoga *mārgas* ("yoga paths") as *karma, bhakti, jñāna* and *rāja* (*ibid.*: 22).

and imagery,[8] and of scientific similes inspired by Western applied sciences.[9] Iyengar's own devotionalism and Viśiṣṭādvaita-inspired theology are also relatively prominent in *LOY*, where 'God', the 'Lord' or 'Creator' is often mentioned,[10] while the *Bhagavad Gītā* is considered "the most important authority in Yoga philosophy" (*ibid.*: 19). A budding Harmonialism is also seen in Iyengar's individualistically oriented elaborations of the concept of 'self' (*ātman*).[11] When this happens, the focus shifts from an external God to the inner realm of the practitioner. "The yogi," in fact, "does not look heavenward to find God. He knows that HE [*sic*] is within, being known as the Antarātmā (the Inner Self)" (*ibid.*: 21). In this case the wider framework of yoga is also reinterpreted: rather than as a process of surrender (*prapatti*), yoga is now seen as the "the conquest of the Self" (*ibid.*: 24).

Two specific aspects of Modern Yoga theory

Two theoretical teachings of *LOY* are worth commenting upon because they are central to almost all Modern Yoga elaborations: (a) that the practice of yoga should go hand in hand with the performance of voluntaristic 'good works', and (b) that 'self-improvement' is at the heart of yoga practice. These recommendations have no matching counterparts in classical yoga and can therefore be singled out as distinctive characteristics of modern forms of yoga. The first teaching may be seen to derive from Neo-Vedāntic elaborations of the Puritan ethic, the second from a Metaphysically oriented psychologization of yoga.

8. As when Iyengar uses the Commandments while discussing yoga philosophy ("Thou shalt not steal"; *ibid.*: 34; "Thou shalt not covet"; *ibid.*: 47), or when he describes *samādhi* as a state in which there is "peace that passeth all understanding" (*ibid.*: 52, 436), or again when he recommends the *sādhaka* to pray with the words "Thy will be done" (*ibid.*: 40).
9. "Brahmacharya is the battery that sparks the torch of wisdom" (*ibid.*: 35). For other instances see *ibid.*: 20, 51, 130, 141, 379, 425, 436, 439.
10. See, for example, *ibid.*: 19, 23, 25, 28, 31, 32, 33, 37, 38, 44.
11. Iyengar uses various translations for this key term: self (*ibid.*: 22, 38), Self (*ibid.*: 30, 33, 36, 117), inmost Self (*ibid.*: 49), human soul (*ibid.*: 30), individual soul (*ibid.*: 28) Supreme Soul (*ibid.*: 117, 440, and in Glossary: 515), spirit (*ibid.*: 44), Brahman (*ibid.*, in Glossary: 515). Not all occurrences of every term are listed. Cross-referencing between the text, the Glossary and the Index shows that this and other key terms are translated in varied and not always consistent ways.

Neo-Vedāntic ethics

About 'good works', *LOY* states:

> Yoga is a method by which the restless mind is calmed and the energy directed into constructive channels. As a mighty river which when properly harnessed by dams and canals, creates a vast reservoir of water, prevents famine and provides abundant power for industry; so also the mind, when controlled, provides a reservoir of peace and generates abundant energy for human uplift. (*Ibid.*: 20)

What we find here is a pragmatic and humanitarian interpretation of yoga, ultimately inspired by a Brahmo type of ethic and exemplified in Vivekananda's conceptualizations of yoga as "Practical Religion".[12] A few pages on, two choices – traditional and modern, theistic and voluntaristic – are presented as equally valid alternatives: the reader is told that the yogi "cuts the bonds that tie himself [*sic*] to his actions by dedicating their fruits *either to the Lord or to humanity*" (*LOY*: 31, emphasis added). Similarly, while discussing the term *karuṇā* ("pity, compassion"), found in *YS* I. 33,[13] Iyengar states that

> [The yogi's] compassion [is] coupled with devoted action to relieve the misery of the afflicted. [He] uses all his resources – physical, economic, mental or moral – to alleviate the pain and suffering of others. He shares his strength with the weak until they become strong. He shares his courage with those that are timid until they become brave by his example ... He becomes a shelter to one and all. (*LOY*: 26)

This is far more proactive and voluntaristic than the *Yoga Sūtras* or any of the classical commentaries on it enjoin and, like the previous quotations, shows the influence of a Vivekananda-style humanistic interpretation of yoga.

12. See, for example, "Practical Religion: Breathing and Meditation" (*CW* 1: 513–21); and, of course, his famous concept of "Practical Vedanta" (*CW* 2: 289–358). As is almost always the case in this kind of text, the technological simile is a sign of Neo-Hindu ideological derivation.
13. The *sūtra* reads: *maitrī-karuṇā-muditopekṣāṇāṃ sukha-duḥkha-puṇyāpuṇya-viṣayāṇāṃ bhāvanātaś citta-prasādanam* ||. In Yardi's translation (1979): "Through cultivation of friendship, compassion, joy and forbearance respectively towards the happy, the miserable, the virtuous and the wicked, the mind becomes purified."

The concept of 'self-improvement'

More specifically linked to actual Modern Yoga theory and practice is the second teaching. The 'self-improvement' theme can be exemplarily illustrated by analysing Iyengar's treatment of the concept of *svādhyāya*. This Sanskrit term signifies the "reciting or repeating or rehearsing to oneself, repetition or recitation of the Veda" (Monier-Williams 1994 [1899]: 1277) and can be literally translated as "one's own study", usually of Hindu sacred texts. In the ideal framework of classical India, such study was undertaken by all twice-born males during the *brahmacarya* (student) stage of life, and was enjoined on the Brahmins as a lifelong task because of this group's traditional role as preservers and transmitters of revealed texts.[14] Iyengar, however, interprets the word in typically modern fashion along individualistic and eclectically pluralistic lines:

> Sva means self and adhyāya means study or education.[15] Education is the drawing out of the best that is within a person. Svādhyāya, therefore, is the education of the self ... The person practising svādhyāya reads his own book of life, at the same time that he writes and revises it...
>
> ...it is essential to study regularly divine literature ... The sacred books of the world are for all to read. They are not meant for the members of one particular faith alone. As bees savour the nectar in various flowers, so the sādhaka absorbs things in other faiths which will enable him to appreciate his own faith better. (*LOY*: 38–9)

A couple of pages before he had rendered *svādhyāya* as "study of the Self" (*ibid.*: 36). Not surprisingly, these psychological universalistic interpretations of yoga have found favour with esoterically and occultistically inclined practitioners already accustomed to the language of Jungian and Transpersonal psychology. As we saw in Chapter 5, rapprochements between yoga and the psychological sciences are already to be found in *Rāja Yoga*, and have been constantly explored ever since.[16] Today, adaptations of yoga inspired by

14. For a general discussion of this question and for related bibliographical sources see Klostermaier (1989: 342ff.).
15. Translating *sva* as 'self' is correct, but turning 'self' into a noun is not. *Sva* in this case means 'self' in the sense of 'own'.
16. C. G. Jung's interest in oriental religions and more specifically in yoga is well known. Other examples of rapprochement are Coster (1935) and Mishra (1973).

psychotherapy are encouraged in some British schools,[17] and grass-roots elaborations along these lines are pervasive (own field data). Indeed, Iyengar himself must have been mirroring the speculations of existing literature and the elaborations of his students when formulating these concepts.[18]

Another example, bringing together both of the themes discussed here, is found in Iyengar's treatment of the Sanskrit term *upekṣa*, "overlooking, disregard, negligence, contempt, ... endurance, patience" (Monier-Williams 1994 [1899]: 215). *Upekṣa* is one of four means recommended by Patañjali in *YS* I. 33 to attain "a calming of the mind" (*cittaprasādana*) by reacting in appropriate fashion to a number of standard relational situations.[19] As is usual in the *sūtra* style, the passage is open to a number of interpretations. However, the main classical commentators show a rather unsentimental approach to the question. Vyāsa points out that these means are recommended in order to achieve an aim, which in turn will make the practitioner progress on the yogic path.[20] Vācaspati Miśra echoes the same argument by elaborating along the same utilitarian lines. King Bhoja is even more explicit: "All these conscientiously cultivated attitudes have only one common purpose, viz. to prepare the ground for effective concentration" (Ghosh 1980: 213). Iyengar's attitude is quite different, and brings to mind Christian soul-searching and modern guilt complexes rather than yogic cool-headed expediency:

> Upekṣa ... is not merely a feeling of disdain or contempt for the person who has fallen into vice (apuṇya) or one of indifference or superiority towards him. It is a searching self-examination to find out how one

17. Viniyoga Britain, for example, structures teacher/pupil interaction along one-to-one sessions explicitly inspired, at least to some degree, by psychotherapeutic models.
18. The well-stocked library of the Iyengar Yoga Institute in Pune, containing in excess of 6,000 volumes in 1992 (Ramamani Iyengar Memorial Yoga Institute 1992: 19) has a section dedicated to psychology. The ongoing stream of Iyengar Yoga pupils visiting the Institute from all over the world keep the library up to date with whatever is fashionable in Modern Yoga circles, as books are often presented to the library or left behind once read. Iyengar himself spends time at his desk in the library most afternoons when not otherwise engaged. Impromptu discussions on yoga and other topics may also take place at this time with visitors and/or with whoever is present in the library (own field data, 1997).
19. See this *sūtra*'s text in note 13 above.
20. *evamasya bhāvayataḥ śuklo dharma upajāyate, tataśca cittaṃ prasīdati prasannam-ekāgraṃ sthitipadaṃ labhate* ||. In Yardi's translation (1979): "As he cultivates these sentiments, white [i.e. pure] deeds proceed from him and his mind, becoming serene and one-pointed, attains a state of steadiness."

> would have behaved when faced with the same temptations. It is also an examination to see how far one is responsible for the state into which the unfortunate has fallen and the attempt thereafter to put him on the right path. The yogi understands the faults of others by seeing and by studying them first in himself. This self-study teaches him to be charitable to all. (*LOY*: 27)

Iyengar's concept of 'self-study', then, is intended to be part of a multifaceted effort towards self-improvement and is also meant to inform the 'good works' that the practitioner should perform. In *LOY*, Iyengar also uses other locutions to refer to such endeavour: "character building" (*ibid.*: 38), "study ... of [one]self" (*ibid.*: 47), "self-examination" (*ibid.*: 48). But all represent propaedeutic strategies aimed at the attainment of Neo-Vedānta style "spiritual evolution" (*ibid.*: 37), culminating in "Self-realization". We do not actually find the latter expression in *LOY*, but Iyengar goes close enough to it when he writes about the yogi who "realises his self (ātman)" (*ibid.*: 22), or when he quotes a *Kaṭha Upaniṣad* passage as: "The Self is not to be realised by study ..."[21]

"Self-realization": a chameleonic concept

The concept of "Self-realization" will increasingly gain in importance in Iyengar's thought (a clear indication of this is its growing prominence in indexes),[22] but its beginnings can already be seen in *LOY*. It is mainly by holding on to this concept that our author will be able to adapt his own synthesis of classical and Neo-Vedāntic tenets to the general ideological temper of the Counterculture[23] and of the New Age. The marvellous ambiguities of this concept, whether used by Iyengar or by other MPY representatives, allow it to become all things to all people. Iyengar uses the term "self" to translate the Sanskrit *ātman* (for example, *LOY*: 51), but he also uses "soul" and "spirit", at times with added qualifiers (see note 11 here). This multiplicity of translations can be somewhat confusing. However, if one overlooks the rather loose terminology a certain synthetic overview of his use of the word can be brought to light: the "Self" (often

21. *Kaṭha Upaniṣad* 2.23, where "not to be realised" is translated from "*na ... labhyaḥ*".
22. "Self-realization" is not listed in *LOY*, appears as a sub-entry of 'self' in *LOP* and as a full entry in *LOYSP*.
23. This term is used with reference to Roszak's standard work on the subject (1995 [1969]).

capitalized) is either a part of (*ibid.*: 21, 22, 41, 50) or identical with (*ibid.*: 30, 49) God, even though in some cases instead of God we find a less obviously theistic entity such as "Supreme Soul" (*ibid.*: 22, 438, 440) or "divine spirit" (*ibid.*: 50). Essentially, the aim of yoga – and indeed the aim of human life in general – is to *realize* the union between the two (*ibid.*: 22, 28, 30, 48, 51, 438). This formulation, in all its vagueness – or rather due to it – is very consonant with Neo-Vedāntic formulations of the same tenets.

This brief terminological discussion also provides us with a demonstration of why the term "Self-realization" has become so successful in Neo-Vedāntic (and related) discourses: its ambiguity as descriptive of both material and intellectual operations works perfectly well in whichever way the relationship between the two terms 'self' and 'God' is defined. And if such relation is *not* defined, or defined in contradictory ways within the same text (as is often enough the case in Modern Yoga sources), the readers will be free to interpret it according to their inclination: whether the two entities are identical, or whether one is part of the other, or whether the two are completely distinct, the term 'realization' works. Indeed, it can even be made to accommodate non-theistic, materialistic, sceptical or agnostic convictions if instead of 'self' and 'God' one uses terms such as "living spirit" and "divine spirit" (*ibid.*: 50) or "individual soul" and "Divine Universal Soul" (*ibid.*: 28). Still, as far as *LOY* is concerned and in line with its overarching theistic and devotional interpretation of yoga, Iyengar keeps to terms clearly indicative of strong theistic beliefs.

Light on Prāṇāyāma (1981): the Consolidation period

It is really only in the last two developmental phases that Iyengar Yoga comes into its own. During the Popularization period Iyengar was still, so to speak, in the position of the apprentice. During the Consolidation period this changes: the practices and connected ideology become distinctive, Iyengar is fully established as a widely reputed yoga master, and the school's institutional profile is heightened by the worldwide diffusion of its teachers, many of whom run their own yoga centres by this time.

The evidence we find in Iyengar's texts shows that he continues to explore the previously mentioned main MPY themes: Neo-Vedāntic ethics, *haṭhayoga* teachings, Western occultistic motifs and personal religious allegiance. None of these elaborations, however, lead to significant changes in his practice or thinking, the one exception being Western occultistic motifs. It is in the area of practice, in other words, and in the theoretical interpretations directly connected with it, that innovations and transformations take place. This does not mean that Iyengar's protracted study and reflection on other topics does not help him to deepen his personal practice or understanding of yoga or, more generally, of life. But it does mean that the main recorded evidence of developments is to be found in the practical and theoretical elaborations of *aṣṭāṅgayoga* and more specifically of *āsana* and *prāṇāyāma*.

*Fully-fledged Neo-*Haṭhayoga

As we saw in the previous chapter, the institutional developments of Iyengar Yoga during the Consolidation period were essentially positive in the sense that the school gained in overall influence and strength. We also noticed that, at least to start with, Iyengar Yoga was more successful in the West than in India. Maybe inevitably, therefore, Iyengar's conceptual constructs started to be substantially influenced by the Countercultural and New Age milieus in which his teachings flourished. Iyengar himself does not seem to have been aware of the shift: indeed, such a gradual change of position would have hardly been noticeable under the circumstances. As has been shown, much overlap and dialogue between Indian and Western forms of esotericism and occultism had taken place in Modern Yoga circles from the start. We also saw how Vivekananda brought yoga within the scope of alternative medicine and hence of unchurched and cultic religiosity. This was already an accomplished fact before Iyengar's birth. By the time he became professionally active, Modern Yoga had developed specific forms and discourses in this sense, a trend that was only to grow and develop further from the 1960s and beyond, by this time with Iyengar's full participation. Also, because Iyengar lacked any formal training in the classical Indian intellectual tradition, and furthermore subscribed to the generally anti-intellectual Modern Yoga ethos, he is unlikely to have been too concerned about the role and value of theoretical contents and backgrounds.

From the vantage viewpoint of the analytical observer, however, we can detect a series of momentous, if subtle, shifts. For example, the failings of the human condition are no longer to be righted by addressing what was described in *LOY* (in typical Neo-Vedāntic fashion) as our congenital metaphysical ignorance and ensnaring sensuality. *LOP*'s stress is, instead, on neutralizing our shortcomings through the implementation of a yogic regime aimed at redressing imbalances and eliminating impurities from our psychosomatic being. Whereas according to *LOY* individuals resort to yoga in order to go "beyond the realms of illusion and misery with which our world is saturated" (*LOY*: 36) and to eradicate desires without doing which "there [could] be no peace" (*ibid.*: 24), according to *LOP* our most important commitment is to keeping "the human body in a balanced state of *health* and *perfection*" (*ibid.*: xix, emphasis added; it will be noted how the two terms are conceptually brought together). *LOY*'s unwieldy attempt to blend a strongly practical and utilitarian physiotherapeutic emphasis with a markedly theological religio-philosophical framework has been abandoned. In *LOP* Iyengar develops what in the early days was only an embryonic discourse: yoga as a form of holistic healing based on the uniqueness of individual experience. By the time *LOP* was published it is clear that Iyengar's position had undergone a substantial evolution. His *personal* commitment to Vaiṣṇava devotionalism remained intact, but it contributed more sporadically to his elaborations of theory and practice. By and large, it was the cultivation of human potential within a haṭhayogic framework that now engaged him.

The enthusiastic, self-assured theoretical and theological certainties of *LOY* are also gone (albeit not as personal convictions): Iyengar is now aware that his religious, cosmological and metaphysical assumptions are not going to be accepted unquestioningly, and he aligns his speculative approach to the more flexible and polyvalent (read secular) models found in cultic circles. Introducing in the very first page of *LOP* the fundamental categories of "God (Puruṣa) … nature (prakṛti), religion (dharma) and Yoga", he states: "Since it is so difficult to define these concepts, each man has to interpret them according to his understanding" (*ibid.*: 3.1–2). From the relative safety of his original Śrīvaiṣṇava/Neo-Vedāntic background; from the lofty, old-fashioned rhetoric of God and of 'nation building', our author is catapulted to the fast globalizing, pluralistic, deconstructionist and much more ideologically and socially unsteady late modern world. The main priority in this context, at least as far as the Modern Yoga practitioners are concerned, is to satisfy their longing for healing and personal growth: to restore, most importantly, a sense of integrity to fragmented individualities.

We now find that the 'self-improvement' of the Brahmo ethic has become the 'personal development' of the New Age.[24] Thus in the brief cosmological introduction to *LOP* Iyengar states that after man appeared on the earth he "began to realise his own potential" (*LOP*: 3), and "realised that he should keep his body healthy, strong and clean in order to follow Dharma and to experience the divinity within himself" (*ibid.*). *Dhyāna*, on the other hand, is described as "the expansion of consciousness", having attained which "the soul of man permeates his whole body" (*ibid.*: 225). This latter theme prefigures the way in which the *Samādhi* Model will eventually be integrated within the Iyengar system during the Acculturation phase: through practices of 'culturing' or 'diffusing awareness'. As we shall see, such modes will come to replace Vivekananda's cruder, more exclusively physical instructions for proprioception. The ideological roots of such speculations, however, are the same: *haṭhayoga* on the one hand and occultistic mesmerism on the other. The never-quite-successful assimilation of the two is based on attempts to combine the magico-transcendental assumptions of the former with the mechanistic and evolutionary principles of the latter.

Thus the occultistic mix of Harmonial tenets and *haṭhayoga* started by Vivekananda comes to full fruition in the latter half of the twentieth century. Here Iyengar emerges as one of the most innovative and successful representatives of Neo-*Haṭhayoga*, the modernistic and secularized version of classical *haṭhayoga* lying at the heart of MPY.

In *LOP* Iyengar establishes the foundations of his own interpretation of yoga, which he will then go on to refine throughout the rest of the Consolidation and Acculturation periods. Despite being a text on *prāṇāyāma*, this book is much concerned with *āsana* theory and practice, thus retaining Iyengar's specialist focus (see Figure 13). In its rather substantial theoretical parts (about half of the book) it keeps returning to and expanding on the subject of *āsana* in general,

24. I.e. the 'personal development' that brings us to 'Self-realization', as for example in the title of Waters' 1996 New Age book: *Dictionary of Personal Development: An A–Z of the Most Widely-used Terms, Theories and Concepts.*

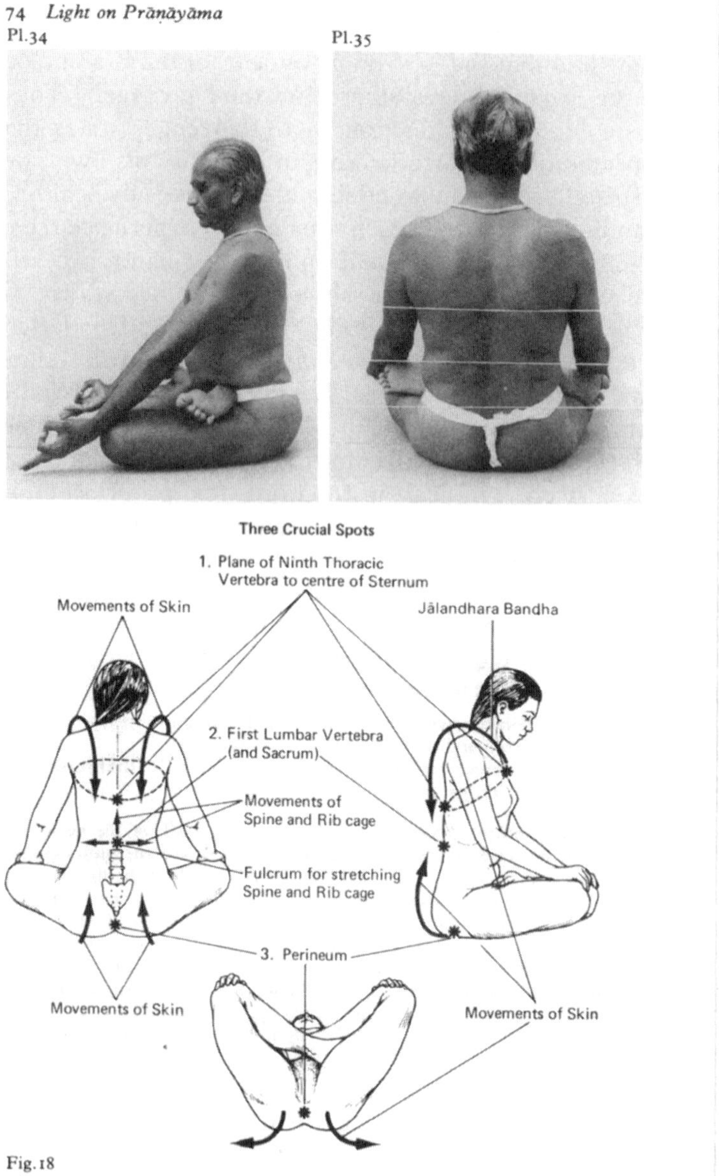

Figure 13 Reproduction of pages 74–5 from B. K. S. Iyengar's *Light on Prāṇāyāma*. Reprinted by permission of B.K.S. Iyengar and by agreement with HarperCollins Publishers Ltd and Crossroad Publishing (USA)

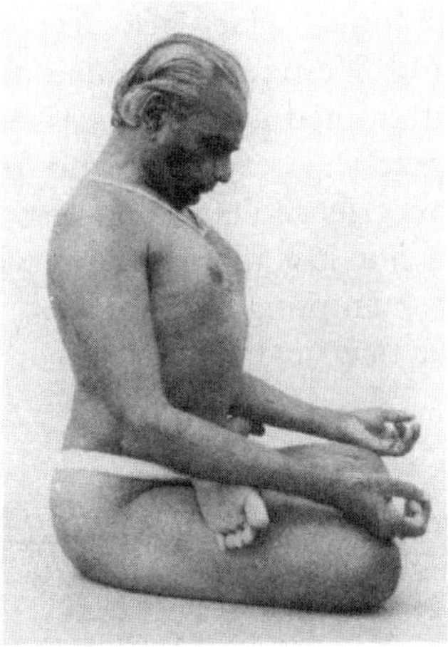

Pl.36

(corners of the torso) on either side. If the dorsal or the lumbar spine sags, the lungs do not expand properly. Only the correct movement and stretch of the skin at the back, the sides and the front of the torso enables the top lobes of the lungs to be filled.

Skin of the Torso
26. Like a bird spreading its wings in flight, keep the shoulder-blades down and open them away from the spine. Then the skin there moves down and the back of the armpits are slightly lower than the front ones. This prevents the back from drooping. The skin of the front is stretched sideways on each side as the breasts are lifted away from the armpits (Pl. 36).

27. The inner and the outer intercostal muscles inter-connect the whole rib cage and control diagonal cross-stretches. It is commonly understood that the action of the inner intercostal muscles is expiratory and the action of the outer intercostal muscles is inspiratory. Normal deep breathing techniques differ from that of prāṇāyāma techniques. In prāṇāyāma, the inner-intercostal muscles at the back initiate inspiration and the outer intercostal muscles at the front initiate expiration. In internal retention (see Ch. 15) the sādhaka has to balance evenly and fully the muscles of the chest wall throughout to release tension in the brain. The muscles and skin at the back must act in unison, as if interwoven, both in prāṇāyāma as well as in meditation (dhyāna).

and of the more physical aspects of *prāṇāyāma* in particular.[25] The importance and effects of postural practice are often highlighted.[26] Iyengar's interpretation of yoga in *LOP* veers more and more towards *haṭha* themes and terminology.[27] He also repeatedly attempts to homologize haṭhayogic and Western anatomico-physiological models,[28] which he had not attempted in *LOY*.[29] Also, contrary to what happened in *LOY*, practical teachings and related interpretations are now expressed as experienced facts and personally recommended instructions. Iyengar is not just reporting on what is found in *haṭhayoga* texts, but actively attempting to build such tenets into his system of psychosomatic practice on the basis of his own experience.

MPY theory and practice in Light on Prāṇāyāma*: the consolidation of the* Prāṇa *Model*

In the previous chapter we introduced the standard anthropological distinction between biomedical and alternative types of medicine. When Iyengar started his career as a yoga teacher, forms of Modern Yoga had already been more or less successfully applied to both types of medicine. In the case of biomedicine, the recognized applications of yoga had been mainly in the field of prevention and the maintenance of general health and fitness. Throughout the Popularization

25. For example, Chapter 2 in *LOP*, "Stages of Yoga", discussing the eight limbs, dedicates twelve sections out of twenty-two to *āsana* and Chapter 10, "Hints and Cautions", dedicates nineteen sections out of sixty-three to "Posture". Other instances are found throughout the book.
26. See, for example, the following passages in *LOP*: paragraph 14 (pp. 9–10; quoted in full below), and paragraphs 11(p. 14), 1–3 (p. 48), 38–40 (p. 61). That Chapter 11, "The Art of Sitting in Prāṇāyāma" (pp. 64–85), should expand on *āsana* is probably understandable. The same cannot be said of Chapter 12, supposedly on "The Art of Preparing the Mind for Prāṇāyāma", which is full of postural details. And while giving guidelines for meditative practice, Iyengar reiterates that mastering "[t]he art of sitting correctly . . . is essential" (p. 227). At length, one gets the impression that physical posture is more important than anything else.
27. See *ibid.*, Chapters 3–5, and Sections II and III (*passim*).
28. For example, the definition of *prāṇāyāma* as a system "to keep the involuntary or autonomous controlling systems of the human body in a balanced state of health and perfection", combining physical (implicit reference to the nervous system), 'subtle' (*prāṇāyāma* itself) and 'spiritual' ("perfection") levels (*ibid.*: xix). Also see the first paragraph of Chapter 5, where *nāḍīs* and *cakras* are said to be all "tubes, ducts or channels" whether in the physical, "subtle" or "spiritual" bodies (*ibid.*: 32); further details are given in paragraph 17 (p. 36). Finally, the effects of *prāṇāyāma* are described in *LOP* (pp. 48–9.1–10) in altogether modern anatomico-physiological terms.
29. One finds only hints in this direction (*LOY*: 273, 348, 439).

period Iyengar mainly kept his teaching within the bounds of biomedicine thus understood. But as he was making more substantial imports from *haṭhayoga*, and interacting with pupils and institutions that took for granted that Modern Yoga was a branch of alternative and complementary medicine, so this theme came to the fore in his system.

In *LOP*, both of these types of medicine are brought to bear. The biomedical model is mainly resorted to in order to provide anatomical and physiological explanations,[30] or when describing the therapeutic effects of practices.[31] It is, however, the alternative medical model, applied especially in its Harmonial and mesmeric aspects, that stands at the centre of Iyengar's somato-energetic theory of *āsana* and *prāṇāyāma*.

The theoretical core of Iyengar Yoga practice, i.e. the rules on which Iyengar Yoga orthoperformance is based, is relatively straightforward. The problem is that it is never explicitly set out as such.[32] In the absence of a single straightforward statement from Iyengar we shall try to collate one by extracting key concepts from selected quotations. In the second chapter of *LOP*, Iyengar states:

> āsanas purify the body and mind and have preventive and curative effects ... They cause changes at all levels from the physical to the spiritual. Health is a delicate balance of body, mind and spirit. By practising āsanas the sādhaka's physical disabilities and mental distractions vanish and the gates of the spirit are opened.
>
> Āsanas bring health, beauty, strength, firmness, lightness, clarity of speech and expression, calmness of the nerves and a happy disposition ... the essence distilled from practising āsanas is the spiritual awakening of the sādhaka. (pp. 9–10)

We note first of all that the concepts of "health" and of "spiritual awakening" are conflated within an altogether alternative medicine/

30. See, for example, *LOP*, Chapter 4.
31. As in the description of the effects of *ujjāyī prāṇāyāma* (stage III): "This preliminary practice is good for those suffering from low blood pressure, asthma and depression ..." (*ibid.*: 132).
32. This is partly due to Iyengar's style of address, whether oral or written: he is very precise in his action-oriented, meticulously detailed and well-ordered *practical* yoga instructions, but his language becomes rather inspirational/literary (and thus more impressionistic than instructional) when elaborating on the more theoretical or abstract aspects of his teachings.

Harmonial definition of health as "a delicate balance of body, mind and spirit". Secondly, *āsana* performance is said to "purify", "cure", and "change" the individual "at all levels"; it dissolves "mental distractions", it "calms", "beautifies" and results, eventually, in "spiritual awakening". Further,

> Through the abundant intake of oxygen by [*prāṇāyāma*'s] disciplined techniques, subtle chemical changes take place in the sādhaka's body. The practice of āsanas removes the obstructions which impede the flow of prāṇa, and the practice of prāṇāyāma regulates that flow of prāṇa throughout the body. It also regulates all the sādhaka's thoughts, desires and actions, gives poise and the tremendous will-power needed to become a master of oneself. (*Ibid.*: 14.12)

How this transformation is achieved, the second quotation explains, is by diffusion of *prāṇa* "throughout the body". As *prāṇāyāma* is said to increase the "intake of oxygen", thus bringing about "subtle chemical changes", and to "regulate the flow of prāṇa" and "all the sādhaka's thoughts, desires and actions", biomedical and alternative medicine frameworks are powerfully (if not explicitly) brought together. The causal relations between biomedical and alternative models said to regulate access to spiritual gnosis are further explained in the following extract, implicitly equating the anatomical nervous system and prāṇic channels:

> The body is trained by practice of āsanas, which keep the channels free from obstruction for the flow of the prāṇa. Energy does not radiate through the body if the nāḍīs are choked with impurities. If the nerves are entangled [*sic*], it is impossible to remain steady, and if steadiness cannot be achieved the practice of prāṇāyāma is not possible. If the nāḍīs are disturbed, one's true nature and the essence of things cannot be discovered. (*Ibid.*: 86)

This is not all, however. The diffusion of fluidic *prāṇa* must be altogether 'even' (i.e. equally and symmetrically distributed) in order to produce the desired effects. This is achieved by seeking perfection in musculo-skeletal alignment and even in the 'positioning' of air flow during *prāṇāyāma*. *Padmāsana* provides us with a perfect example of how, according to Iyengar, body posture influences prāṇic distribution and the psychosoma in general. In this position

> all the four areas of the body[33] ... are evenly balanced ... and the brain rests correctly and evenly on the spinal column, giving psychosomatic equilibrium. The spinal cord passes through the spinal column. In padmāsana, the adjustment and alignment of the spinal column and the ridges on either side move uniformly, rhythmically and simultaneously [*sic*]. The prāṇic energy flows evenly, with proper distribution of energy through the body. (*Ibid.*: 66.13–14)[34]

As for the effect of 'evenly-inspired air', Iyengar states that:

> Precise and sensitive adjustments with the thumb and the ring and little fingers of the right hand on the nose [while performing *nāḍī śodhana prāṇāyāma* or alternate nostril breathing] will make the breath flow simultaneously over the same location in both nostrils creating clarity in the brain and stability in the mind. (*Ibid.*: 158)[35]

We then see that, in its mature form, Iyengar Yoga propagates a system of practice in which a perfect harmonization of the somato-energetic being (*annamayakośa* plus *prāṇāmayakośa*) brings about all manner of healing: physical, psychological and 'spiritual', effectively culminating in "Self-realization", or in the attainment of the ultimate religio-spiritual goal, however described. Harmonization is brought about by (progressively more accurate)[36] orthopractical performance of *āsana* and *prāṇāyāma* according to principles of musculo-skeletal alignment and even prāṇic diffusion. An analysis of these principles, as offered above, clearly reveals the kind of materialistic and mechanistic presuppositions of causality that characterize occultistic teachings. In a nutshell: 'perfect' physical alignment allows 'perfect' diffusion of *prāṇa*, which automatically results in the perfected condition of "Self-realization".

Most further elaborations of Iyengar Yoga revolve around this

33. That is (a) the lower limbs, (b) the torso, (c) the arms and hands, and (d) the neck and head (*ibid.*: 66.11)
34. For other examples of how alignment is causally linked to extensive psychosomatic effects, see *ibid.*: 15, 75, 77.
35. *Ibid.* (p. 167.18) provides numerous further details, including the (causally significant) statement that "The correct adjustment of nasal passages will control the flow of breath from the external, measurable area of the nostrils to the immeasurable depth within."
36. Later in life, Iyengar will write: "In the beginning, effort is required to master the *āsanas*. Effort involves hours, days, months, years and even several lifetimes of work ..." (*LOYSP*: 28), thus justifying lifelong engagement (or engagement over multiple lives) in yoga practice.

central somato-energetic core: the proliferation of anatomical detail and of 'adjustments' in its practical teachings;[37] the ingenious and pervasive use of props to improve postural performance and alignment;[38] the imaginative anatomico-dynamic teaching vocabulary devised by Iyengar and propagated by his teachers;[39] the clever subdivision of postures by type of movement and corresponding psychosomatic effect;[40] the training and fitness principles used to devise postural sequencing[41] – all may be suitable and effective for a

37. Anatomical and proprioceptive 'adjustments' are gross to start with, and become subtler as the pupil progresses. The following teaching instructions presuppose a fair amount of experience of the Iyengar method:

    > Sit on the base of the pelvis after doing padmāsana. Rest both buttocks evenly on the floor. If you sit more on one than the other, the spine will be uneven. Press the thighs down to the floor, bringing the thigh bones deeper into the hip sockets. Stretch the skin of the quadriceps towards the knees. This creates freedom round the knees to move diagonally and circularly from the top of the outer to the bottom of the inner knees. Bring the hamstring muscles closer in order to lessen the distance between the thighs... (*LOP*: 67)

    This trend of minute description has been actively cultivated in the school, and plays a crucial role in its teachings past the beginner's stage.
38. The use of props was scanty during the Popularization phase, but has become pervasive in the mature system. The aim of props is to help practitioners to improve their postural performance while also becoming more aware of the role played by various body parts (Mehta, S. *et al.* 1990: 13). Props are also used to adapt postures for people with medical conditions or with limited mobility (*LOP*: 123). Virtually anything can be used as a prop: blankets, pillows and bolsters, belts, pieces of furniture, structural parts of a building such as walls, stairs, window sills, etc. However, a whole range of specialized props has been developed for specific Iyengar Yoga use, and these are the ones that characterize the Iyengar Yoga studio: ropes hanging from walls and ceilings, special benches of various shapes and sizes, non-slip mats, foam blocks, wooden bricks and so on. Photos of props and their use may be seen in *LOP* (pp. 123–7, 252–3). Since the publication of *LOP*, props have become much more prominent and varied in Iyengar Yoga. A pamphlet produced by cabinet maker François Lozier (1994) lists over 50 designs of, and (when applicable) building specifications for, benches, boxes, stools, tables, trestles, bricks, blocks, planks, sticks, cylinders, ropes, hooks, pillows, belts, weights, etc.
39. See Clennell (1994), from which some examples include: "Suck the outer calf muscle into the bone" (*ibid.*: 2); "Rotate from the pit of the abdomen" (*ibid.*: 6); "The *moon* between the inner heel and the inner ankle has to grow from a half moon to a full moon", where "*Moons* are used to describe different areas of the body that need to become illuminated ... 'The consciousness should be felt there' " (*ibid.*: 7).
40. "[T]he standing poses give vitality, the sitting poses are calming, twists are cleansing, supine poses are restful, prone poses are energising, the inverted poses develop mental strength, balancings bring a feeling of lightness, backbends are exhilarating and the jumpings develop agility" (Mehta, S. *et al.* 1990: 12).
41. Beginners' classes, for example, are structured to reinforce the pupils' frames and to make them flexible in preparation for more advanced practice. An advanced class may typically build up through preparatory, more localized stretches to a few demanding poses, then slow down with calming *āsanas* to end in relaxation. Specific rules for class structuring and management are given in teacher training courses (own field data).

number of utilitarian applications, but are ideally and ultimately oriented towards the perfect harmonization of all levels of being.

What this amounts to, however, when looked at from the perspective of intellectual history, is a continuation of Vivekananda's *Prāṇa* Model – though with the further specification that Iyengar's elaborations are worked out in much more detail and are more firmly rooted in the body, or rather in what goes under the name of 'bodywork' in contemporary alternative medicine circles. We must bear in mind that over three-quarters of a century elapsed between the publication of *Rāja Yoga* and *LOP*: many theoretical speculations and healing methods were experimented with, all of which are part of the culture of in-body healing absorbed by Iyengar during his yogic career. Out of this connecting chain of relevant links, which would well deserve a separate study, we will only mention two.

Firstly, the now almost paramedical disciplines of chiropractic and osteopathy, healing systems originally based on a Harmonial and mesmeric "belief in the power of physical manipulation to realign the body with a higher spiritual power" (Fuller 1989: 65).[42] Secondly, the orgone and 'muscular armour' theories of the psychiatrist Wilhelm Reich (1897–1957), who may be regarded as a seminal figure for all types of modern 'bodywork' systems of healing. The orgone energy, "supposed to permeate the cosmos and possess healing powers" (Honderich 1995: 753), is clearly linked to mesmeric speculations, but also calls to mind MPY's understandings of *prāṇa*. The muscular armour theory postulates the existence of a set of somatically engrained defensive attitudes that a person would adopt to protect herself against physical or emotional hurt.[43] The attempt to 'dissolve' such an armour, often conceptualized in terms of mis-*alignments* or wrong postural habits, is at the root of most 'bodywork' approaches to healing. As the Iyengar Yoga system reaches its maturity in the Consolidation phase, the assimilation of MPY among the New Age styles of 'bodywork' therapy (ultimately aimed at the cultivation of personal growth) is completed.[44]

42. For this author's extensive treatment of these two disciplines see Fuller (1989, Chapter 4).
43. Honderich (1995: 753). For an excellent study on Reich see Rycroft (1971).
44. Etic evidence of this assimilation is provided by the sociologist of (contemporary) religion J.G. Melton, who dedicates a whole chapter (out of eight) of his *New Age Almanac* to yoga, i.e. Modern Yoga (1991: 147–65).

Light on the Yoga Sūtras of Patañjali (1993): the Acculturation period

By the end of the 1980s Iyengar had established all the practice-related foundations necessary for the ongoing development of his system. Always willing to take up new challenges, he is now ready to review his system of practice in the light of Patañjali's seminal yoga text, the *Yoga Sūtras*. The result of this will be *LOYSP*, published in 1993.

In the meantime Modern Psychosomatic Yoga (MPsY) is becoming, generally speaking, more and more secularized. Taught now mainly by Westerners in the West, at least at grassroots level, and adopted by substantial Expressivist minorities[45] and even more widely by individuals seeking various standards of health and fitness, it naturally undergoes a process of acculturation. As it becomes further assimilated into secularized milieus, it is itself further secularized. Iyengar, however, now in his full maturity, his school safely established, does not quite go along with this. While maintaining (and indeed always refining) his system of *practice*, at the level of *theory* (i.e. of belief and philosophical speculation) he turns back, as will soon become apparent, to his Śrīvaiṣṇava roots. In his new synthesis Iyengar will also, importantly, attempt to assimilate the *Samādhi* Model more fully into his Neo-*Haṭhayoga* system. Let us see how.

The Samādhi *Model in Iyengar's Neo-*Haṭhayoga

It is not easy to find one's way through Iyengar's *LOYSP*. The *Yoga Sūtras* are a difficult text at the best of times, and Iyengar's somewhat over-elaborated commentatorial style may be inspiring and enriching with regard to detail but, overall, feels rather unstructured.[46] If one reduces this text to its foundational themes, however, its contribution to Iyengar Yoga theory and practice appears quite straightforward.

45. 'Humanistic Expressivism' is a useful category employed by sociologists of religion to indicate a substantial minority group, estimated at 10 per cent of British and USA populations (Heelas 1996: 115). The same author describes this category as being composed of "those who have faith in what the inner psychological realm has to offer" and value "'awareness', 'insight', 'empathy', 'creativity', ... and seeking 'fulfilment'" (*ibid.*: 115). They are further "intent on discovering and cultivating their 'true' nature, delving within to experience the wealth of life itself ... What matters is ... personal 'growth', 'meaningful' relationships, being in tune with oneself" (*ibid.*: 156).
46. The reader may get an overall impression of the scope and eclecticism of Iyengar's text by looking at the form and content of its Glossary (*LOYSP*: 301–32).

Essentially, its practical teachings expand the *Prāṇa* Model to include the *Samādhi* one, while its more theoretical contributions hark back to Iyengar's Vaiṣṇava roots by creatively reconfiguring them in patterns suited to contemporary use and to integration with the other elements of the school's teachings.

Let us first look at what *LOYSP* has to say about practice. The key dynamis here is one in which, in Iyengar's own words, the movements of consciousness are "at once centripetal and centrifugal" (*LOYSP*: 66). Or, more technically, "we reach a state when skin-consciousness moves toward the centre of being, and the centre radiates toward the periphery" (*ibid.*). This, according to our author, reflects the central teaching of "Eastern thought", which

> takes one through the layers of being, outwards from the core, the soul, towards the periphery, the body; and inwards from the periphery towards the core. The purpose of this exploration is to discover, experience and taste the nectar of the soul. The process begins with external awareness: what we experience through the organs of action ... and proceeds through the senses of perception ... That awareness begins to penetrate the mind, the intelligence, the ego, the consciousness, and the individual self (*asmitā*) until it reaches the soul (*ātma*). These sheaths may also be penetrated in the reverse order. (*Ibid.*: 9)

At a more microcosmic level the above theorizations give rise to explanations of practice such as what we may call Iyengar's theory of 'cellular enlightenment': "While performing the *āsanas*, one has to relax the cells of the brain, and activate the cells of the vital organs and of the structural and skeletal body. Then intelligence and consciousness may spread to each and every cell" (*ibid.*: 28). Thus employed, "*Āsanas* act as bridges to unite the body with the mind, and the mind with the soul ... Through *āsana*, the *sādhaka* comes to know and fully realize the finite body, and merge it with the infinite – the soul ... This is the essence of a perfect *āsana*" (*ibid.*: 29).

A further example of such theorizations provides us with a more heavily anatomized explanation of practice:

> The seat of logic is in the front brain, the seat of reasoning in the back brain, the imprinting of pleasure and pain takes place in the base and the seat of individuality, the 'I' or 'Me' is in the top. When all four lobes of the brain are cultured and blended together, the brain becomes superconscious. (*Ibid.*: 105, note*; reproduced in Figure 14)

Here we find an obvious anchoring of practice in the body, but it should be noted that the use of 'culturing' and similar terms, which is very prominent in *LOYSP*, points to the main way in which Iyengar proceeds to psychologize the *Prāṇa* Model into the *Samādhi* Model. These inward and outward movements are in fact described in terms of "study" and of "culture of consciousness" (*ibid.*: 13), and Iyengar explicitly states that "The culture of consciousness entails cultivation, observation, and progressive refinement of consciousness by means of yogic disciplines" (*ibid.*: 13). What is consciousness then? This term is Iyengar's translation for the *Yoga Sūtras'* keyword *citta*, which he defines as "a composite word for mind, intellect and ego" (*LOYSP*: 308). In this context the yogic training of "mind" (and hence meditative practice, however interpreted) lies at the root of all yogic endeavour:

> Patañjali begins the treatise on yoga by explaining the functioning of the mind so that we may learn to discipline it, and intelligence, ego and consciousness may be restrained, subdued and diffused, then drawn towards the core of our being and absorbed in the soul. This is yoga. (*Ibid.*: 13)

At yet another level, the integration of the two models is operated by way of an homologization of *citta* and *prāṇa*. After two long paragraphs explaining that the whole cosmos is pervaded by *prāṇa*, for example, Iyengar goes on to state: "This self-energizing force is the principle of life and consciousness [*citta*]" (*ibid.*: 153). And further: "*Prāṇa* (energy) and *citta* (consciousness) are in constant contact with each other. They are like twins. *Prāṇa* becomes focussed where *citta* is, and *citta* where *prāṇa* is" (*ibid.*). There is, in other words, a shift from a more quantitative-spacial theory of even diffusion (as predominantly found in *LOP*) to a more qualitative one: in Iyengar's *Samādhi* Model the quality of the 'culturing of consciousness' is postulated to be just as important (if not more so) than the quality of somato-energetic alignment.

While in *LOP* the emphasis was on diffusing the *prāṇa* as evenly as possible, in *LOYSP*, more oriented towards the mental aspects of yoga, the emphasis is on even 'diffusion' of "intelligence", "consciousness" or "awareness". When this is achieved, *āsana* itself becomes meditation:

> In *āsana*, there is a centrifugal movement of consciousness to the frontiers of the body, whether extended vertically, horizontally or circumferentially, and a centripetal movement as the whole body is brought into a single focus. If the attention is steadily maintained in this manner, meditation takes place... (*ibid.*: 169)

Thus in the advanced practice of *āsana*,

> the rhythmic flow of energy and awareness is experienced evenly and without interruption both centripetally and centrifugally throughout the channels of the body [, and eventually a] pure state of joy is felt in the cells and the mind. The body, mind and soul are one. This is the manifestation of *dhāraṇā* and *dhyāna* in the practice of *āsana*. (*Ibid.*: 150)

Similar principles – but this time going back all the way to the *puruṣa* – are employed to explain the state of *samādhi* in a full and more explicit translation into the *Samādhi* Model:

> *Samādhi* is the tracing of the source of consciousness – the seer [i.e. *puruṣa*] – and then diffusing its essence, impartially and evenly, throughout every particle of the intelligence, mind, senses and body.
>
> ...the enticing prospect of *samādhi*, revealed so early in [Patañjali's] work, serves as a lamp to draw us into yogic discipline, which will refine us to the point where our own soul becomes manifest. (*Ibid.*: 4)

Of course the 'diffusion' theory also supports the Iyengar method's strong emphasis on *āsana* practice. Indeed, in his more extreme theorizations, Iyengar has been known to interpret the process of meditative *saṃyama* in rather unorthodox ways – at least from the point of view of strictly dualistic Classical Yoga. Most prominently, such 'radical' elaborations are found in *Yoga Vṛkṣa: The Tree of Yoga* (or *YV*; 1988), an edited collection of Iyengar's discourses published at the end of the Consolidation period. In some passages of this book *dhāraṇā, dhyāna* and *samādhi* are stated to follow altogether mechanically from the practice of the other five limbs of yoga (which in turn are said to hinge on *āsana* practice). Here is how Iyengar expresses this view:

> Yoga can ... be seen as having three tiers: external, internal and innermost, or physical, mental and spiritual. Thus the eight limbs of

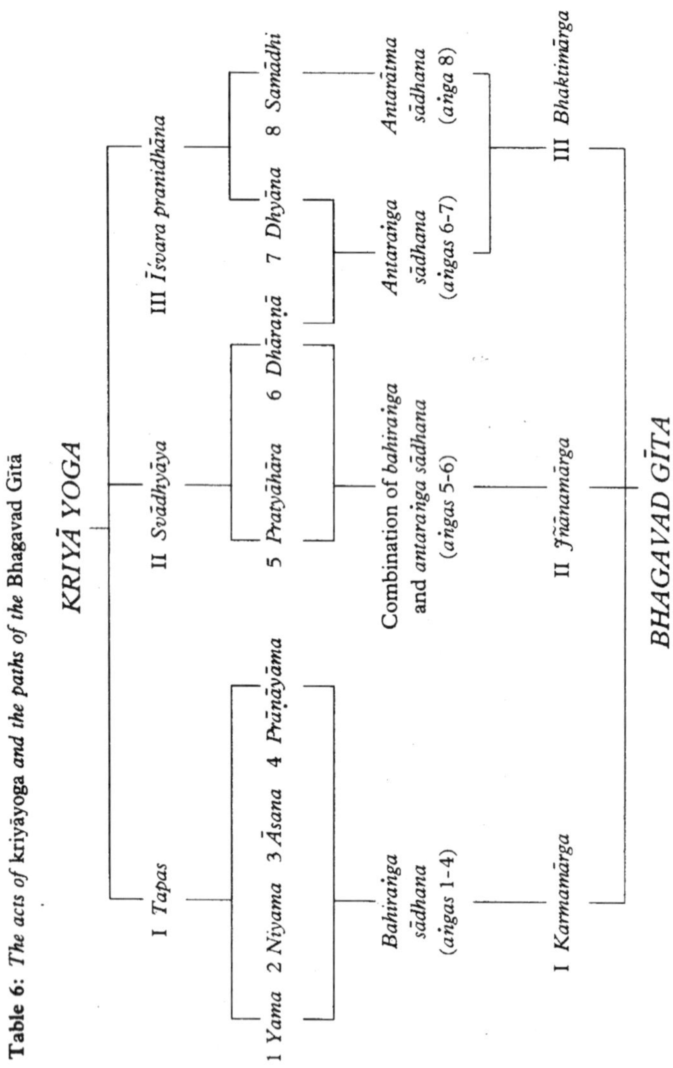

Figure 14 Reproduction of pages 104–5 from B. K. S. Iyengar's *Light on the Yoga Sūtras of Patañjali*. Reprinted by permission of HarperCollins Publishers Ltd. © B.K.S. Iyengar 1993

अविद्याऽस्मितारागद्वेषाभिनिवेशाः क्लेशाः ।३।

II.3 *avidyā asmitā rāga dveṣa abhiniveśaḥ kleśāḥ*

avidyā	lack of spiritual knowledge, spiritual ignorance
asmitā	ego, pride, 'I' or 'me'
rāga	desire, attachment, love, passion, affection, joy, pleasure, musical mode, order of sound
dveṣa	hate, dislike, abhorrence, enmity
abhiniveśaḥ	love of life, fear of death, clinging to life, application, leaning towards attachment, intent, affection, devotion, determination, adherence, tenacity
kleśaḥ	affliction, pain, distress, sorrow, trouble

The five afflictions which disturb the equilibrium of consciousness are: ignorance or lack of wisdom, ego, pride of the ego or the sense of 'I', attachment to pleasure, aversion to pain, fear of death and clinging to life.

Afflictions are of three levels, intellectual, emotional and instinctive. *Avidyā* and *asmitā* belong to the field of intelligence; here lack of spiritual knowledge combined with pride or arrogance inflates the ego, causing conceit and the loss of one's sense of balance. *Rāga* and *dveṣa* belong to emotions and feelings. *Rāga* is desire and attachment, *dveṣa* is hatred and aversion. Succumbing to excessive desires and attachments or allowing oneself to be carried away by expressions of hatred, creates disharmony between body and mind, which may lead to psychosomatic disorders. *Abhiniveśa* is instinctive: the desire to prolong one's life, and concern for one's own survival. Clinging to life makes one suspicious in dealings with others, and causes one to become selfish and self-centred.

The root causes of these five afflictions are the behavioural functions and thoughts of the various spheres of the brain. *Avidyā* and *asmitā* are connected with the conscious front brain, and the top brain is considered the seat of the 'I' consciousness. *Rāga* and *dveṣa* are connected with the base of the brain, the hypothalamus. *Abhiniveśa* is connected with the 'old' brain or back brain which is also known as the unconscious brain, as it retains past subliminal impressions, *saṁskāras**.

* According to Patañjali the five fluctuations (*vṛttis*), the five afflictions (*kleśas*) as well as the maturity of intelligence through *savitarka*, *nirvitarka*, *savicāra*, *nirvicāra*, *ānanda* and *asmitā* are all functions of the four lobes of the brain. The seat of logic is in the front brain, the seat of reasoning in the back brain, the imprinting of pleasure and pain takes place in the base and the seat of individuality, the 'I' or 'Me' is in the top. When all four lobes of the brain are cultured and blended together, the brain becomes superconscious (see I.17).

> yoga can be divided into three groups: yama and niyama are the social and individual ethical disciplines; āsana, prāṇāyāma and pratyāhāra lead to the evolution of the individual, to the understanding of the self; dhāraṇā, dhyāna and samādhi are the effects of yoga which bring the experience of the sight of the soul, but they are not as such part of its practice. (*YV*: 5)

Soon after this, and after having explained the simile of *aṣṭāṅgayoga* as a tree,[47] Iyengar states that when a tree is well cared for it "gives its natural culmination which is the fruit"; thus *saṃyama* "is the effect or the fruit of sādhana" (*ibid.*: 6). He further postulates that "The mastery of āsanas and prāṇāyāma leads *automatically* towards concentration and meditation" (*ibid.*: 8, emphasis added), an idea that he elaborates more fully later in the book (*ibid.*: 138–9), eventually concluding that "dhāraṇā, dhyāna and samādhi ... are the effects of the practice of āsana, prāṇāyāma and pratyāhāra, but in themselves do not involve practice" (*ibid.*: 138).

At first sight, and especially if the reader relies on the more radically dualistic interpretations of meditative practice, such a reading of *saṃyama* may well appear unorthodox, even shockingly so. By proposing it, Iyengar seems to overlook (or disregard) centuries, even millennia of speculations and theorizations about meditative practice as found in countless Hindu, Buddhist and Jain texts; he seems to bypass innumerable testimonials, beliefs, folk tales and statements scattered throughout the lore of these traditions, all of which insist on the efficacy, worthiness and power of the meditative enterprise.

The dispassionate analyst should, however, carefully take into consideration Iyengar's hermeneutical situation and the impact that his personal and cultural motivations may have had on the shaping of his system. It will then become possible to argue that his 'automatization' of *saṃyama*, apart from answering the needs of a practice strongly oriented towards *āsana* and *prāṇāyāma* orthoperformance[48] also, and more importantly, defines the orthodoxy of what finally emerges as Iyengar's Neo-Viśiṣṭādvaita synthesis.

47. "The root of the tree is yama ... Then comes the trunk, which is compared to the principles of niyama ... From the trunk of the tree several branches emerge ... These branches are the āsanas ... From the branches grow the leaves ... They correspond to prāṇāyāma ... The bark ... corresponds to pratyāhāra ... The sap of the tree is dhāraṇā ... [D]hyāna, meditation, is the flower of the tree of yoga. Finally, when the flower is transformed into a fruit, this is known as samādhi" (*YV*: 7–8).
48. For which the Iyengar School continues, on and off, to be criticized (own field data).

The Neo-Viśiṣṭādvaita synthesis

Within such a synthesis, and at its more mundane level, this interpretative strategy could have been adopted not on the basis of conscious speculation, but simply as an intuitive solution to a perceived practical problem. The problem, as Iyengar himself put it in 1985, is that "[a]sanas bring the mind closer to the self without losing the contact with the external world, whereas *in meditation, people get completely lost*" (*ILW*: 228, emphasis added). A passage in *LOYSP* clarifies his thought further:

> There are many examples ... of people ... experiencing *saṃyama* even if they have been following no fixed path of yogic discipline ... This is undoubtedly a moment of grace, but it is not the same thing as enlightenment...
>
> The modern fancy of '*kuṇḍalini* [*sic*] awakening' has probably arisen through these freakish experiences of 'integration' [viz. *saṃyama*] ... It is, however, clear that many who undergo an overwhelming experience of fusion with the universal consciousness reap, through their unpreparedness, more pain than benefit ... The eightfold path [*aṣṭāṅgayoga*] ... is ultimately a path of spiritual evolution whose [*sic*] motto might well be 'safety first'. The foundation must be secure, as Patañjali emphasizes when he places *yama* and *niyama* first, and when he marks a definite step up between *āsana* and *prāṇāyāma*. (*Ibid.*: 173)

These perceived dangers, along with Iyengar's keenness to cultivate postural orthoperformance, could easily have resulted in the elaboration of a Neo-Viśiṣṭādvaita position which is rather conservative towards 'enlightenment' and altered states of consciousness, especially when compared with overall New Age attitudes towards such phenomena. Iyengar's reliance on postural orthoperformance may thus be explained as a buttress used to 'steady' the general (and often ambiguous) Neo-Vedāntic and New Age reliance on "Self-realization". We should not forget that many of his first generation students were sons and daughters of the 'tune in, turn on, drop out' culture of the 1960s: a culture which, differently from other modern *gurus*, Iyengar has never wished to patronize, let alone adopt. Such a position could then be construed, quite tenably, as Iyengar's attempt to keep his followers 'out of trouble'.

From the more crucial point of view of religious allegiance, however, Iyengar's position can be explained by reminding ourselves about the standard Viśiṣṭādvaita diffidence towards meditative practice. In the section on yogic experience in classical Vedānta at the end of Chapter 5 we reviewed Rāmānuja's basic position with regard to the Yoga *darśana*: meditative practice is to be interpreted exclusively as a devotional exercise based on progressively more sustained remembrance of the Supreme Person (*paramapuruṣa*), while *samādhi* is not even taken into consideration. It may be argued that, along with his other Neo-*Haṭhayoga* interpretations, Iyengar elaborates a parallel, or rather intertwining, Neo-Viśiṣṭādvaita one in which devotional dedication and concentration (*dhyāna*) on one's orthoperformative practice substitutes the classical, *samādhi*-oriented sitting meditation. As in Rāmānuja's case, the ultimate aim would be an enhancement of devotion rather than the attainment of a transcendent state. Whatever samādhic or other state such practice may or may not result in, one could imagine Iyengar affirming, will be the will of God, and there should be no expectation or striving for results on the part of the practitioner.

A number of passages in *LOYSP* substantiate this thesis; we will discuss three representative ones. The first two are found at key junctures in the text, the first at the beginning of Iyengar's actual translation and commentary of the *Yoga Sūtras*,[49] the second at its very end. In the first passage Iyengar echoes Vyāsa's well-known gloss on *YS* I. 1[50] but also adds a strong devotional element to it by stating: "*Samādhi* means yoga and yoga means *samādhi*: both mean profound meditation and *supreme devotion*" (*LOYSP*: 43, emphasis added). In the second passage Iyengar summarizes his teachings, this time echoing the *Gītā*, by affirming that the yoga adept should "seek refuge by surrendering all actions as well as himself to the Supreme Spirit or God", so that he may journey "from Self-Realization to God-Realization" (*ibid.*: 269). These two programmatic affirmations hold, as it were, the whole text within explicitly theistic brackets.

Such 'devotionalization' of yoga and particularly of *saṃyama* is further expressed in one of *LOYSP*'s numerous tables (*ibid.*: 104, Table 6; reproduced in Figure 14), where correspondences are given for the various components of three central types of yoga: *kriyāyoga* (*YS* II. 1), *aṣṭāṅgayoga* (middle section of the table), and the yoga of the *Bhagavad Gītā*. Iyengar homologizes devotion and the meditative

49. I.e. after a lengthy Prologue.
50. The relevant part of which reads: "*yogaḥ samādhiḥ*".

aspects of *aṣṭāṅgayoga* (*dhāraṇā*, *dhyāna* and *samādhi*, i.e. *saṃyama*) by matching the latter with the more theistic aspect of *kriyāyoga* (*īśvarapraṇidhāna*, or "placing [all] in the Lord"; *YS* II. 1) on the one hand and to the *Gītā*'s *bhaktimārga* (way of devotion) on the other.

We also know from Iyengar's writings and speeches that throughout his career he has consistently relied on the *Bhagavad Gītā*, along with the *Yoga Sūtras* and key haṭhayogic texts, as his main authority on yoga.[51] In *LOYSP* the *Gītā* is often referred to and occasionally quoted at length.[52] Such an intellectual position provides Iyengar with strong theistic and devotional themes, which he willingly cultivates. Not surprisingly, this is very obvious in Iyengar's translation of, and commentary on *YS* I. 23–9 on *Īśvara* ("the Lord"), which he treats in full theistic fashion. What is more revealing in the context of the present discussion is that his treatment of this passage is at variance with many of those found in New Age or New Age-oriented publications.[53] One example of Iyengar's Neo-Viśiṣṭādvaita rendition, as found in his treatment of *sūtra* I.23, will suffice here:

> "Or, the *citta* may be restrained by profound meditation upon God and total surrender to Him".[54]
>
> To contemplate God, to surrender one's self to Him, is to bring everything face to face with God. *Praṇidhāna* is the surrender of everything: one's ego, all good and virtuous actions, pains and pleasures, joys and sorrows, elations and miseries to the Universal Soul. Through surrender the aspirant's ego is effaced, and the grace of the Lord pours down upon him like torrential rain. (*LOYSP*: 73)

Such devotionalism is very strong in certain passages of the text, but it is in no way pervasive. Indeed, quantitatively speaking, the Neo-*Haṭhayoga* element is the prevailing one. By now it will be easy to guess why: our author, as most MPY teachers, is keen to preserve the polyvalence of his teachings and practices so that all may be able to access them. He knows very well that he is talking to globalized, multifaith, multicultural audiences. This is part and parcel of the

51. As stated at the beginning of this chapter, according to Iyengar "the *Bhagavad Gītā* ... is the most important authority on Yoga philosophy" (*LOY*: 19).
52. See for example *LOYSP*: 251, 266, 228–9.
53. The latter may be exemplified by Feuerstein's influential (as it is widely used in Modern Yoga circles) *Yoga Sūtras* translation, which explains the concept of *Īśvara* in terms of a Neo-Jungian archetypal function (1989: 42–5).
54. The Sanskrit *sūtra* reads: *īśvarapraṇidhānādvā*.

Modern Yoga ethos, at least insofar as most of its international MPsY ramifications are concerned. But such an observation does not detract from the evidence suggesting that, ultimately, the Iyengar method rests upon a foundation of Neo-Viśiṣṭādvaita devotionalism.

To sum up: in order to understand Iyengar's position in the fullness of the Acculturation phase we should combine (a) Iyengar's Neo-Viśiṣṭādvaita interpretation of *saṃyama* as resulting 'automatically' from the practice of the other limbs of yoga, (b) a related insistence on the power of devotion, (c) his Neo-Vedāntic understanding of ethics, and (d) his Neo-Haṭhayogic reading of orthoperformance and of "Self-realization". Thus when Iyengar describes the aims of the *Yoga Sūtras* he states that Patañjali's text

> guide[s] the aspirant ... towards full knowledge of his own real nature. This knowledge leads to the experience of perfect freedom, beyond common understanding. Through ardent study of the sūtras, and through devotion, the *sādhaka* is finally illumined by the lamp of exalted knowledge. Through practice, he radiates goodwill, friendliness and compassion. This knowledge ... gives him boundless joy, harmony and peace. (*LOYSP*: 3)

Here what must be known is one's "own real nature" (part of New Age "Self-realization") and this happens by studying and practising the teachings of the *Sūtras* in a devotional spirit (Neo-Haṭhayogic and Neo-Viśiṣṭādvaita elements). This "exalted knowledge" leads to "perfect freedom", impeccable ethical behaviour and "boundless joy, harmony and peace" (mixture of New Age and Neo-Vedāntic aims).

All of the strands found in most MPY speculations are present, though as far as Iyengar is concerned the central ones, ultimately, will have to be (*āsana*-based) "practice" and "devotion":

> Some say that it is possible to acquire mastery of *āsana* by surrendering to God. How can this be so? In yoga we are on a razor's edge and in *āsana* perfection must be attained through perseverance, alertness and insight. Without these we remain dull and make no progress. Surrender to God alone does not make us perfect, although it helps us to forget the stresses of life and of our efforts, and guides us towards humility even when perfection in *āsana* has been attained. (*LOYSP*: 151)

After a basic understanding of Iyengar's Neo-Viśiṣṭādvaita synthesis has been achieved, what remains to be asked is whether his and other MPY masters' vision and projects reflect what actually goes on at the grassroots level of everyday practice: are their theorizations really widespread among MPY practitioners? Why is MPY successful, and what exactly do practitioners find in it? In the next chapter we shall attempt to sketch some possible answers to these questions. This will be done by interpreting field data and a selection of primary sources in the light of some well-known anthropological models of ritual.

8. Conclusion: Modern Postural Yoga as healing ritual of secular religion

> Ultimately, yoga practice is the process of discovering who we are, and how and why we continue to exist. Through yoga practice our consciousness can be raised to a new vantage point from which to view life. Yoga theory conveys to us that we must look within our own physical bodies and our own minds to find truth. The process of uplifting our consciousness begins by uplifting the energy level in our body. Our natural heritage is one of cosmic consciousness, but this can be realized only as we remove the dust of the body and illusions of the mind, say the yoga masters.
>
> (Smith and Boudreau 1986: 10)

MPY in everyday life

Modern Postural Yoga (MPY) has become a widespread and popular activity. Most people will have heard about 'yoga', and may even have tried it themselves. Indeed, in colloquial English, 'yoga' has come to mean a session of MPY.

The way MPY has been practised throughout the twentieth century is of course worlds apart from all forms of classical yoga. The schools which first started, in the 1920s, to elaborate MPY practice in India used it to construct a sort of indigenized (and 'spiritualized') version of British education. Yoga-inspired routines of physical exercise would train the body, and a yoga-inspired self-control and morality would further 'character building'. This was still principally (but not exclusively) a Neo-Hindu development.[1] But, as MPY became more

1. For further details on the history and teaching of these schools see Alter (2000, Part II; and forthcoming) and De Michelis (1995; 2002).

deeply rooted and assimilated in Western (and progressively also Indian) esoteric and occultistic milieus, Harmonial developments came to the fore.

By the middle of the twentieth century what would become the standard international MPY classroom format was taking shape. This went hand in hand with drastic changes in *mores*, which in turn brought about changes in popular ideals of body image and identity. As journalist Veronica Horwell reports (1998: 12), in the postwar period

> The Americans ... brought [to Europe] a new concept of pleasure: they were young and their idea of bliss was to be even younger ... In just over a decade, in two locations, the Med[iterranean] and Los Angeles, the ultimate sexy dream place changed from a perfumed boudoir in a sophisticated city to a beach under the sun with a dazzle on the ocean. Erotic fantasies of hook-and-eye underwear removed privately were replaced by the proto-bikini...

Such developments resulted in increasing attention and importance being given to physical grooming, including fitness and the cultivation of youthful looks. These predilections were not new in themselves, the most obvious precedent being Ancient Greece. What was unprecedented, however, was (and is) the attention, value and energy given to their cultivation in the latter part of the twentieth century and beyond. Quite naturally, the more exoteric aspects of MPY came to play a part in these phenomena, and this discipline thus established itself at the margins of the 'sports' category.[2]

The other great boost to MPY was provided by the recognition of 'stress' as a specific (if not univocally defined) psychosomatic syndrome.[3] Speculations on links between the fast pace of modern urban living and "nervousness" were already in evidence by the last quarter of the nineteenth century,[4] but the beginnings of the formulation of the concept of 'stress' as we now know it are found in research published by the scientist Hans Selye from the 1930s onwards.[5] Like

2. It is significant that, as already pointed out, MPY practice in Britain is regulated by the Sports Council.
3. Both Cox (1978, Chapter 1) and King *et al.* (1987, Chapter 1) provide interesting overviews of the various ways in which stress has been defined.
4. See George Beard, *American Nervousness* (New York: G. P. Putnam, 1881), as discussed in Fuller (1989: 63–4).
5. Selye (1957) is considered the seminal text. Selye's definition of stress is spelt out over twelve pages (*ibid.*: 53–64).

earlier medical researchers, Selye speculated that it was "the individual frustration arising out of constricted urban living, rather than life's major causes of worry, which [made] people illness-prone" (Inglis 1980: 114). The constellation 'urban living – stress – MPY' is not random. Modern conditions of urban living are notoriously frustrating, and this type of lifestyle is also highly conducive to sedentariness. Hence the need for fitness and de-stressing, both of which can be supplied by MPY. But there are deeper sources of frustration, insecurity and anxiety, linked to the gradual secularization of developed societies.

As Fuller reminds us, the term 'secularization' refers, in a general sense, "to the gradual decline of [institutionalized] religion as a consequence of the growth of scientific knowledge and [to] the continued diversification of social and ethnic groups in the Occident" (1989: 118). All of these elements would be especially prominent in conditions of 'urban living', and it is in such environments that MPY grows and thrives. Adopted and cultivated in conditions of marked privatization and relativization of religion, MPY is successful, like other Harmonial belief systems, because it provides "experiential access to the sacred" (*ibid.*: 119).

Such experiential access to the sacred, epitomized by the 'secular ritual' of the MPY practice session, represents the third key to understanding the current success of MPY, along with its fitness and de-stressing applications. These three elements constitute, *guṇa*-like, the 'root contents' and main facets of MPY's polymorphism: the flexibility and adaptability of this discipline depends on their presence and on the multiplicity of their possible combinations.

Analysed in their religio-philosophical underpinnings, these three elements also reveal the ambiguous polyvalence characteristic of occultistic teachings. The 'fitness' discourse relates to mainstream anatomical and physiological assumptions, but also, at a more esoteric level, to MPY's "*mechanical* power to revolutionize our whole being" (*LOYSP*: 139, emphasis added). The 'de-stressing' discourse, relating to psychosomatic medicine on the one hand and to Neo-Haṭhayogic understandings of healing on the other, is hybrid by definition. It tries to bridge the gap not only between body, mind and spirit, but also between orthodox and alternative styles of medicine, and between mechanistic and holistic models of the human being. The religio-philosophical discourses that shape and validate the ritual dimension of the MPY session, finally, bring to bear both traditional religious concepts (God, transcendence, devotion, etc.) and modern understandings of 'spirituality' as awareness of and participation in/attunement to a holistic and evolutionary universe. Throughout its history, MPY displays varied modulations of these basic themes, but the key agenda remains the eminently occultistic attempt to harmonize and connect tradition and modernity, revelation and rationality, the sacred and the profane.

Thus the MPY session becomes a ritual which affords various levels of access to the sacred, starting from a 'safe', mundane, tangible foundation of body-based practice. In such DIY forms of spiritual practice, there is room for the practitioner to decide whether to experience her practice as 'spiritual' or as altogether secular. Except in cases of thoroughly utilitarian (fitness or recreational) performance, however, some notion of healing and personal growth is likely to provide the deepest rationale for practice.

One may begin to map such shifting patterns of ritual semantics by relating them to standard anthropological interpretative models. Because of the necessary limits of this study, this will only be done in a circumscribed manner, the aim being to disclose the 'everyday appeal' of MPY practice.

The MPY practice session

Without special reference to any one school, we shall describe a typical MPY class as might be experienced by any beginner. Once the structure, pace and at least a few basic assumptions of MPY theory and practice have been transmitted to the practitioner, the ritual value of the session will become operative.

The one to one-and-a-half hours of the standard MPY session is usually divided into three parts: (i) introductory quietening time: arrival and settling in (about ten minutes); (ii) MPY practice proper: instruction in postural and breathing practice given by the instructor through example, correction and explanation; (iii) final relaxation: pupils lie down in *śavāsana* ("corpse pose")[6] for guided relaxation, possibly with elements of visualization or meditation (ten to twenty minutes). This period includes a short 'coming back' time at the end of the relaxation session.

6. I.e. lying on one's back doing 'nothing' (see also note 3, Chapter 7).

Within this overall framework there may be many variations: the actual classroom may be a gym, or community centre hall, or the more soothing atmosphere of a yoga centre or a teacher's living room. There may be introductory and/or final short readings or theoretical 'instructions'; different styles of yoga will be characterized by a slower or faster pace, or different paces will be found across various sessions of the same style of yoga; some styles of yoga or sessions will be run with a greater sense of 'social' or 'communal' event, others will emphasize inwardness and quiet individual work, etc. – but the overall structure remains.

MPY as healing ritual of secular religion

The emergence of the threefold pattern in the practice session is not by chance, and may be explained with reference to Arnold van Gennep's classic work on rites of passage (1965 [1908]). His well-known discussion defines the fundamental structure of ritual as consisting of three phases: (i) separation or preliminal state; (ii) transition or liminal state; and (iii) incorporation or postliminal state (*ibid.*: 11). This basic structure, as we discuss below, is obviously correlated to the three phases of the standard MPY practice session.

(i) The separation phase (introductory quietening time in MPY)

Elaborating on van Gennep's model, Turner (1982 [1969]: 94) comments that this first phase "comprises symbolic behaviour signifying the detachment of the individual or group either from an earlier fixed point in the social structure, from a set of cultural conditions ... or from both". Detachment from both social and cultural points of reference is well in evidence in the MPY session.

Spatially, practitioners remove themselves from the hustle and bustle of everyday life to attend the yoga class in a designated 'neutral' (and ideally somewhat secluded) place. As the teacher and the relevant literature recommend, they should leave their social persona, responsibilities, commitments, plans and worries behind for the time being. As Iyengar says, these should be left outside the practice room along with one's 'ego' and one's shoes (own field data).

Some amount of deference towards the teacher is usually expected, especially in forms of Modern Yoga established by Indians. Indeed, some of the more "intense" teachers will expect pupils to act like the liminal *personae* ("threshold people") described by Turner (*ibid.*: 95):

> Their behaviour is usually passive or humble; they must obey their instructors implicitly, and accept arbitrary punishment without complaint. It is as though they are being reduced or ground down to a uniform condition to be fashioned anew and endowed with additional powers to enable them to cope with their new … life.

Such 'intensity', as Iyengar explains, may just be part of a wider strategy to draw the practitioner into a different, sacralized time and space, the time of the 'here and now':

> One of the reasons why, as a teacher of *āsana*, I am so intense … is that I want to give the students one and a half hours of present life in a lesson. As I shout at them to straighten their legs in *Śīrṣāsana* (headstand), they cannot be wondering what is for dinner or whether they will be promoted or demoted at work. For those who habitually flee the present, one hour's experience of 'now' can be daunting, even exhausting, and I wonder if the fatigue felt by some students after lessons is due more to that than to the work of performing *āsanas*. Our perpetual mental absences are like tranquillizing drugs, and the habit dies hard. (*LOYSP*: 221)

Turner (1982 [1969]: 95) also points out that persons in a liminal state will often "be represented as possessing nothing": they are divested of outside markers to show that "they have no status, property, insignia, [or] secular clothing indicating rank or role". Similarly, practitioners attending an MPY session are expected to dress in standardized and simple fashion and not to wear jewellery or other accessories. When the weather is hot the reduced amount of clothing and the sheer physicality of the practice may call to mind ritual nakedness symbolizing, as in more complex traditional rituals, the womb and the grave, death and rebirth (*ibid.*: 28).

Even when one is practising on one's own, there is a sense in which time and the space used are 'other'. One tries to practise at a time and place where there will be no disturbance or interruption. One's 'yoga gear' – a cushion or other seat, props, dedicated clothing, but especially the blanket or mat used for practice – will represent the minimum expanse of this 'cordoned off' space. As in the case of the Islamic prayer mat (the parallel is structurally closer than may appear at first sight), the yoga mat becomes a special object, not to be trodden on, not to be soiled, and not to be used for other purposes. Opening it up on the floor instantly creates a 'special' time and space in which certain practices, ritual-like, are repeated at regular intervals.

Vivekananda already recommended in *Rāja Yoga* that the practitioner should, if at all possible, "have a room for this practice alone" (*CW* 1: 145). Such a room, he continued, should be "kept holy" by adorning it with flowers and pleasing pictures, by "burning incense morning and evening" and by being used only when the person is in a pure state: "bathed", "clean in body and mind", without "anger" or "unholy thought", as this would eventually create "an atmosphere of holiness" (*ibid.*).

This initial phase of quiet and resting is more about turning away from the external world and settling into the different dimension of the MPY session than about active practice. After a short while, another ritual marker signifies the passage to the next phase: a brief sitting meditation, the chanting of 'OM',[7] or a few words of address by the teacher indicating the actual start of the session. At the Iyengar Institute in Pune, a Sanskrit invocation to Patañjali is always chanted at this point.[8] Here the practitioners ready themselves to enter, to use Iyengar's expression, "the temple of [their] own body" (*LOP*: 55.20).

(ii) The transition phase (MPY practice proper)

It is at this point that the dynamics of the *Prāṇa* and *Samādhi* Models discussed in the previous chapters come into play. As the teacher

7. "All words are said to be but various forms of the one sound – *om* – according to the Upaniṣads. It represents the Divine and the power of God. It is the sound symbol of the ultimate Reality" (Grimes 1996: 216).

8. The invocation is as follows:

> *yogena cittasya padena vācāṃ/malaṃ śarīrasya ca vaidyakena /*
> *yopākarottaṃ pravaraṃ munīnāṃ / patañjaliṃ prāñjalirānato'smi //*
> *ābāhu puruṣākāraṃ / śaṇkha cakrāsi dhāriṇam /*
> *sahasra śirasaṃ śvetaṃ / praṇamāmi patañjalim //*

and the (fairly free) translation used within the Iyengar school reads:

> Let us bow before the noblest of sages, Patañjali, who gave yoga for serenity and sanctity of mind, grammar for clarity and purity of speech, and medicine for perfection of health.
>
> Let us prostrate before Patañjali, an incarnation of Ādiśeṣa, whose upper body has a human form, whose arms hold a conch and a disc, and who is crowned by a thousand-headed cobra. (*LOYSP*: ix)

This Sanskrit invocation is a traditional one, probably dating back at least to the eighteenth century (see Woods 1992 [1914]: xiv).

instructs the pupils, theoretical tenets are passed on, more or less explicitly, along with practical instructions. In this strongly psychosomatic universe, the practitioner learns experientially to feel and to perceive in novel ways; most of all inwardly, though in ways that are also likely to affect external awareness and behaviour.

MPY orthoperformance may in fact be understood, to use Mary Douglas' concept, as a 'framing' ritual, as a focusing mechanism and method of mnemonics which helps us, through practice and repetition, not only to control, but to create experience:

> ritual focusses attention by framing: it enlivens the memory and links the present with the relevant past. In all this it aids perception. Or rather, it changes perception because it changes the selective principles. So it is not enough to say that ritual helps us to experience more vividly what we would have experienced anyway. It is not merely like the visual aid which illustrates the verbal instructions for opening cans and cases. If it were just a kind of dramatic map or diagram of what is known it would always follow experience. But in fact ritual does not play this secondary role. It can come first in formulating experience. It can permit knowledge of what otherwise would not be known at all. It does not merely externalise experience, bringing it out into the light of day, but it modifies experience in so expressing it. (Douglas 1988 [1966]: 63–4).

Much in MPY practice, as we saw in the preceding chapters, is about assimilating new modes of feeling and perception. This may lead us, ultimately, to look at the world in a different way, so that we may "discover ... who we are" (Smith and Boudreau 1986: 10).

One is encouraged to "become silent and receptive" in order to cultivate "inward dispositions that help destructure the ego-dominated rationality of modern Western life" (Fuller 1989: 123). The temporary suspension of these secular interpretative habits, along with the altered sense of body awareness created by postural and breathing practice, further contribute to 'reframe' one's identity and sense of being. In this ritual space, the body and the mind are strengthened and trained, time after time, by cycle upon cycle of repetitive practice.

These actions are transformative: correct practice "brings lightness and an exhilarating feeling in the body as well as in the mind and a feeling of oneness of body, mind and soul" (*LOY*: 60). So there may be curing as in relieving or resolving a backache. But also, and more momentously, there is a 'making whole' or healing of the self, of one's own being and history:

> This actuality, or being in the present, has both a strengthening and a cleansing effect: physically in the rejection of disease, mentally by ridding our mind of stagnated thoughts or prejudices; and, on a very high level where perception and action become one, by teaching us instantaneous correct action; that is to say, action which does not produce reaction. On that level we may also expunge the residual effects of past actions. (*LOYSP*: 28–9)

At this "very high level", a connection may also be made with the metaphysical: by looking within "our own physical bodies and our own minds [we] find truth" (Smith and Boudreau 1986: 10).

In this hieratic context all is charged with meanings that go well beyond the individual person and the present situation. In Iyengar's case, devotional and theological aspects also come in at this stage:

> While performing āsanas, the student's body assumes numerous forms of life found in creation – from the lowliest insect to the most perfected sage – and he learns that in all these there breathes the same Universal Spirit – the Spirit of God. He looks within himself while practising and feels the presence of God. (*LOY*: 60)

Ultimately, the MPY practitioner embodies, and is trained to perceive, the identity of microcosm and macrocosm:

> At this subtlest level, when we are able to observe the workings of *rajas*, *tamas* and *sattva* in one toe, and to adjust the flow of energy in *iḍā*, *piṅgalā* and *suṣumnā* (the three principal *nādis* [*sic*], or energy channels) the macrocosmic order of nature is perceived in even the smallest aspects. And when the student then learns how the minutest modifications of a toe can modify the whole *āsana*, he is observing how the microcosm relates to the whole, and the organic completeness of the universal structure is grasped. (*LOYSP*: 29)

In this context the teacher, especially if charismatic and/or knowledgeable, experienced and perceived as wise, may also (as in Iyengar's case) take on the role of the healer,[9] the individual "who is

9. Apart from running numerous 'Remedial Classes', Iyengar is widely recognized as having both curing and healing capabilities (own field data; see also *ILW*: 357–418).

understood to be in special rapport with higher cosmic powers" (Fuller 1989: 123).

Strong psychosomatic practice, finally, with suitably planned postural content and progression, and enhanced by implicit or explicit theoretical 'framing', can bring about noticeable mood changes, and even more or less pronounced hypnotic trance states. Depending on which of two overall practice patterns is used, one can obtain a relaxed and focused calm (good against tension and stress), or a fairly durable state of mild euphoria (useful in cases of depression or apathy). This, along with relief from physical ailments, is one of the main reasons why people carry on practising Postural Yoga to start with. Indeed, from a psychosomatic point of view the health-related advantages of yoga are undeniable. But relevant studies on addiction have also shown that physical exercise is a double-edged sword: voluntarily induced psychosomatic highs can become addictive and can take, under certain circumstances, pathological overtones. While this is not likely to happen in the case of gentler forms of yoga, such a scenario is theoretically possible in the case of more strenuous forms of the discipline, especially if reinforced by extreme claims concerning their effects as 'religious' or 'revelatory' events.[10] Maybe this gives us some clue as to one of the reasons why secrecy warnings were so often reiterated in classical yoga texts.

(iii) The incorporation phase (final relaxation in MPY)

Śavāsana is recommended in classical *haṭhayoga* as a posture to be used for rest and recovery (*Haṭha Yoga Pradīpikā* I. 32). It is true that at a purely physiological level, the quality and depth of relaxation will be greater after well-coordinated and suitably demanding physical practice. The practice of *śavāsana* at the end of an MPY session obviously takes advantage of this.

In MPY, however, this practice is given a much wider range and depth of meaning: it is interpreted as an exercise in sense withdrawal and mental quietening, and thus as a first step towards meditative practice. It is also seen as a cleansing/revivifying process and,

10. Committed practitioners remark often enough how after missing one or two days of practice they feel deflated. This is a normal reaction in people who exercise regularly. In rare cases, however, situations may develop in which the intensity of the practice and the practitioner's apparent psychological dependence on it may seem to border on the obsessive.

ultimately, as a symbolic death and renewal of self. Here the appellation "corpse pose" takes on its full range of meanings. In this sense, this practice may be interpreted as the key step in a secular (hence implicit) ritual of initiation into our "heritage ... of cosmic consciousness" (Smith and Boudreau 1986: 10).

Fuller (1989: 121) has observed how Eliade's speculations on the death and rebirth symbolism found in initiatory rites of primitive religions may also be applied to the healing rituals of alternative medicine. Such rituals "help structure a process through which individuals are induced to discard a no longer functional identity and discover a new, 'higher' self" (*ibid.*). The same may be said for the MPY session, and especially for *śavāsana* practice, described by Iyengar as "the experience of remaining in a state as in death and of ending the heart-aches and the shocks that the flesh is heir to", but also as "recuperation" and as "the most refreshing and rewarding" of postural practices (*LOP*: 232.1).

At a deeper or subtler level, Iyengar states, *śavāsana* means accessing "that precise state [in which] the body, the breath, the mind and the brain move towards the real self (Ātma)" (*ibid.*: 232.3). Making a direct connection with the higher stages of yoga (and of being), he adds that the famous Upaniṣadic *turīya*, the "fourth" state of ultimate metaphysical awakening,[11] may be accessed "in perfect śavāsana" (*LOP*: 233.8). This may seem a rather outsized claim for what appears as a rather undemanding practice. But when Iyengar explains that in *śavāsana* the practitioner should "surrender ... his all – his breath, life and soul – to his Creator" (*ibid.*: 249.22) in order to "merge ... in the Infinite (Paramātmā)" (*ibid.*: 251.29), we understand that he is explaining the standard MPY ritual of healing and renewal in Neo-Viśiṣṭādvaita terms. Other teachers will use different imagery and religio-philosophical constructs to explain the same practices. What remains unchanged is the structure and purpose of the ritual.

It is this element of sacralized personal transformation and healing, ultimately, which motivates the practice: "That such changes are regarded as real and important is demonstrated by the recurrence of rites, in important ceremonies among widely differing peoples,

11. Out of the Upaniṣadic terminological variants *turīya* (*Bṛhadāraṇyaka Upaniṣad* 5.14.3, 4, 6, 7), *caturtha* (*Māṇḍūkya Upaniṣad* 7), and *turya* (*Maitri Upaniṣad* 6.19; 7.11.7), *turīya* came to be the accepted technical term in all later philosophical treatises (Hume 1991 [1877]: 392).

enacting death in one condition and resurrection in another" (van Gennep 1965 [1908]: 13).

To sum up, the *śavāsana* practice which concludes the standard MPY session represents the final, assimilative phase of the healing ritual which is, through it, integrated and consolidated. At this point practitioners are ready, after a brief but important 're-emergence' phase (another ritual marker), to return to the 'normal' world of everyday concerns and commitments, their lives regenerated by contact with the sacred (Fuller 1989: 123). As the initiates discussed by van Gennep (1965 [1908]: 82), MPY practitioners "retain ... a special magico-religious quality" as a result of this passage through the domain of the sacred.

The ritual progression, rhythm and meaning of the MPY session as analysed above finds perfect emic expression and confirmation in the following description (from a Canadian Modern Yoga magazine) of what it means for the practitioner to attend an MPY class:

> When I enter the familiar centre where I take my Hatha classes, I already feel as though I have separated myself from the hectic outside world. I deposit my street shoes, my daytimer and my cell phone along with my stress and deadlines in a cubbyhole. All of my worries aside, I enter the sanctuary of my yoga classroom.
>
> The room has a wall of windows and a skylight illuminating the wooden floors and soft, cream-coloured walls with natural light. The calming sounds playing from a nature tape, and a few hanging plants help to create the illusion that I have just entered a secret garden.
>
> I find a place for my mat among twenty or so other students, mostly women, who seem also to have left their stress at the door. Our instructor, Beth, is sitting in lotus position at the front of the room, greeting us with a welcoming smile as we settle into our own versions of the lotus position.
>
> She begins the class with a prayer. Her voice emanates calm, helping me to let my eyes rest and my body relax so that my mind can focus. From there, we go through a series of stretches. With each pose, I find a new muscle to bend and loosen into with the help of my breath. Despite the slow motion, my body is working hard to hold each pose and I can feel sweat on my back as my body heats up.
>
> I welcome the final relaxation pose and meditation. As I lie still, Beth's calm, soothing voice guides me through a prayer, which reminds

> me that my efforts were in devotion to something beyond myself. (Dalton 2001: 37)

Thus historical, textual and field findings all concur in showing that MPY has been adopted and acculturated in developed societies as a healing ritual of secular religion. Flexible in its suitability to varied applications secular and sacred, MPY propagates polyvalent teachings which may similarly be 'read' and adopted at various levels. The lack of pressure to commit to any one teaching or practice, the cultivation of "Self" and of privatized forms of religiosity make MPY highly suitable to the demands of contemporary developed societies. The enhancement of physical fitness and psychosomatic relaxation granted by MPY practice are similarly much in demand.

If actual "Self-realization" is likely to be perceived as an achievable goal only by enthusiastic young novices or by those who truly partake of the forceful spirit of *haṭhayoga*, it will still remain as a respected far-off goal in a distant (maybe reincarnational) future for some practitioners. The ultimate teleology of "God-" and "Self-realization" may or may not be adopted by followers, but it will nevertheless remain as a possible background option. Even if practitioners' commitments and beliefs are differently structured, it is likely that MPY will be able to offer some solace, physical, psychological or spiritual, in a world where solace and reassurance are sometimes elusive. As such, MPY has obviously found a place in our society.

Bibliography

Abhishiktananda, S. (1984 [1974 first English edn]) *Saccidananda: A Christian Approach to Advaitic Experience*. ISPCK, Delhi.

Almond, P. C. (1988) *The British Discovery of Buddhism*. Cambridge University Press, Cambridge.

Alter, J. S. (1997) "A Therapy to Live By: Public Health, the Self and Nationalism in the Practice of a North Indian Yoga Society", *Medical Anthropology*, 17: 309–35.

—— (2000) *Gandhi's Body: Sex, Diet, and the Politics of Nationalism*. University of Pennsylvania Press, Philadelphia.

—— (forthcoming) *Yoga in Modern India: The Body Between Philosophy and Science*. Princeton University Press, Princeton, NJ.

Apte, V. S. (1991 [1890?]) *The Student's Sanskrit-English Dictionary*. Linguasia, London.

Aranya, S. H. (1983 [1977]) *Yoga Philosophy of Patañjali* (revised edn). State University of New York Press, Albany, NY.

Arnold, D. and Sarkar, S. (2002) "In Search of Rational Remedies: Homoeopathy in Nineteenth-century Bengal", in W. Ernst (ed.), *Plural Medicine, Tradition and Modernity, 1800–2000*. Routledge, London and New York, pp. 40–57.

B. K. S. Iyengar 60th Birthday Celebration Committee (1987) *Iyengar: His Life and Work*. Timeless Books, Porthill, ID.

Banerji, G. C. (1931) *Keshab Chandra and Ramkrishna*. (No publisher), Allahabad.

Basu, S. P. and Ghosh, S. B. (1969) *Vivekananda in Indian Newspapers*. D. B. B. Bhattacharya & Co. (PVT) Ltd, Calcutta.

Bayly, C. A. (1996) "Colonial Rule and the 'Informational Order' in South Asia", in N. Crook (ed.), *The Transmission of Knowledge in South Asia*. Oxford University Press, Delhi, pp. 280–315.

Bernard, T. (1982 [1944]) *Hatha Yoga*. Rider & Company, London.

Bevir, M. (1994) "The West Turns Eastwards: Madame Blavatsky and the Transformation of the Occult Tradition", *Journal of the American Academy of Religion*, LXII, 3: 747–67.

Bharati, A. (1970) "The Hindu Renaissance and Its Apologetic Patterns", *Journal of Asian Studies*, 29, 2: 267–88.

—— (1976) *The Light at the Center: Context and Pretext of Modern Mysticism*. Ross-Erikson, Santa Barbara, CA.

—— (1992 [1965]) *The Tantric Tradition*. Rider, London.

BKSIYTA (1992) *Members' Handbook*. BKSIYTA, UK.

Blavatsky, H. P. (1967 [?]) *Collected Writings* (2nd edn). Theosophical Publishing House, Wheaton, L.

Brockington, J. L. (1989 [1981]) *The Sacred Thread: Hinduism in its Continuity and Diversity*. Edinburgh University Press, Edinburgh.

Brooks, D. R. (1992) "Encountering the Hindu 'Other' ", *Journal of the American Academy of Religion*, LX, 3: 405–36.

Burke, M. L. (1983–87) *Swami Vivekananda in the West: New Discoveries* (3rd edn). Advaita Ashrama, Calcutta.

Campbell, C. (1972) "The Cult, the Cultic Milieu and Secularization", *A Sociological Yearbook of Religion in Britain*, 5: 119–36.

—— (1978) "The Secret Religion of the Educated Classes", *Sociological Analysis*, 39, 2: 146–56.

Ceccomori, S. (2001) *Cent Ans de Yoga en France*. Edidit, Paris.

Chadwick, O. (1990 [1975]) *The Secularisation of the European Mind in the Nineteenth Century*. Cambridge University Press, Cambridge.

Chaudhuri, N. (1973) *Maharshi Devendranath Tagore*. Sahitya Akademi, New Delhi.

Chetananda, S. (1995) *Vivekananda: East Meets West: A Pictorial Biography*. Vedanta Society of St Louis, Missouri.

Chowdhury-Sengupta, I. (1996) "Reconstructing Spiritual Heroism: The Evolution of the Swadeshi Sannyasi in Bengal", in J. Leslie (ed.), *Myth and Mythmaking*. Curzon Press, Richmond, Surrey: 124–43.

—— (1998) "Reconstructing Hinduism on a World Platform: The World's First Parliament of Religions, Chicago 1892", in: W.

Radice (ed.), *Swami Vivekananda and the Modernization of Hinduism*. Oxford University Press, Callcutta: 17–35.

Christy, A. (1932) *The Orient in American Transcendentalism: A Study of Emerson, Thoreau and Alcott*. Columbia University Press, New York.

Clennell, B. (1994) *Iyengar Yoga Glossary*. Privately published pamphlet.

Collett, S. D. (ed.) (1871) *K. C. Sen English Visit*. Strahan & Co, London.

Coster, G. (1935 [1934]) *Yoga and Western Psychology: A Comparison*. Oxford University Press, London.

Cox, T. (1978) *Stress*. Macmillan, London.

Cox, H. (1979 [1977]) *Turning East: The Promise and Peril of the New Orientalism*. Allen Lane, London.

Criswell, E. (1989 [1987]) *How Yoga Works: An Introduction to Somatic Yoga*. Freeperson Press, Novato, CA.

Cushman, A. (1997) "Iyengar Looks Back", *Yoga Journal*, 137: 85–91, 156–65.

Cushman, A. and Jones, J. (1999 [1998]) *From Here to Nirvana*. Rider Books, London.

Dalton, T. (2001) "Yoga in the City", *Ascent*, 11 (Fall): 37.

Damen, F. L. (1983) *Crisis and Religious Renewal in the Brahmo Samaj (1860–1884): A Documentary Study of the Emergence of the "New Dispensation" under Keshub Chandra Sen*, Orientalia Lovaniensia Analecta 9. Katholieke Universiteit, Leuven.

Dars, S. (1989) "Au pied de la montagne", *Viniyoga*, 24: 4–13.

Dechanet, J.-M. (1993 [?]) *Yoga per i Cristiani*. S. Paolo, Cinisello Balsamo, Milan.

De Mello, A. (1984 [1978]) *Sadhana: A Way to God*. Doubleday, New York.

De Michelis, E. (1995) "Some Comments on the Contemporary Practice of Yoga in the UK, with Particular Reference to British Haṭha Yoga Schools", *Journal of Contemporary Religion*, 10, 3: 243–55.

—— (2002) "Notes on the historical development of Modern Yoga, including comments on the problem of knowledge transmission and on Modern Yoga's relation to Western scientific thought", paper presented at the Sanskrit Tradition in the Modern World (STIMW) conference, University of Newcastle upon Tyne, UK.

Devdutt (1997) "Yoga a tool not a belief", *Yoga and Total Health*, XLII, 6: 20–1.

Douglas, M. (1988 [1966]) *Purity and Danger*. Ark Paperbacks, London.

Dvivedi, M. N. (1890 [1885]) *Rāja-Yoga: Being a Translation of the Vākyasudha or Dṛgdṛśyaviveka of Bhāratitirtha* [Part I] *and the Aparokṣānubhuti of Śri Śankarāchārya* [Part II] (*sic*), *with Introduction and Notes*. (No publisher), Ahmedabad.

ElFeki, S. (1999) "Dr. Nature's Surgery", in *The World in 2000*. The Economist Publications, London, pp. 142–3.

Eliade, M. (1973 [1954 in French]) *Yoga: Immortality and Freedom*. Princeton University Press, Princeton, NJ.

Faivre, A. (1992) "Ancient and Medieval Sources of Modern Esoteric Movements", in A. Faivre and J. Needleman (eds), *Modern Esoteric Spirituality*. Crossroad, New York, pp. 1–70.

—— (1994 [1986 in French]) *Access to Western Esotericism*. State University of New York Press, Albany, NY.

—— (1997) "Renaissance Hermeticism and the Concept of Western Esotericism", in R. Van Den Broek and W. Hanegraaff (eds), *Gnosis and Hermeticism from Antiquity to Modern Times*. State University of New York Press, Albany, NY, pp. 109–23.

Falk, M. (1986) *Il Mito Psicologico nell' India Antica*. Adelphi, Milan.

Farquhar, J. N. (1977 [1914]) *Modern Religious Movements in India*. Munshiram Manoharlal, New Delhi.

Feuerstein, G. (1989 [1979]) *The Yoga-Sūtra of Patañjali: A New Translation and Commentary*. Inner Traditions International, Rochester, VT.

Fields, R. (1992 [1981]) *How the Swans Came to the Lake: A Narrative History of Buddhism in America* (3rd revised and updated edn). Shambala, Boston, MA.

Freedman, F. Barbira and Hall, D. (2000 [1998]) *Yoga for Pregnancy*. Cassell, London.

Friedberger, J. (1991) *Office Yoga*. HarperCollins, London.

Fuchs, C. (1990) *Yoga im Deutschland: Rezeption-Organisation-Typologie*. Kohlhammer Verlag, Stuttgart.

Fuller, R. C. (1989) *Alternative Medicine and American Religious Life*. Oxford University Press, New York and Oxford.

Gellner, E. (1993 [1985]) *The Psychoanalytic Movement: The Cunning of Unreason*. Fontana Press, London.

Ghosh, S. (1980) *The Original Yoga*. Munshiram Manoharlal, New Delhi.

Ghurye, G. S. (1995 [1953]) *Indian Sadhus*. Popular Prakashan, Bombay.

Godwin, J. (1994) *The Theosophical Enlightenment*. State University of New York Press, Albany, NY.

Godwin, J., Cash, P. and Smith, T. (eds) (1990) *Paul Bruton: Essential Readings*. Crucible (Thorsons Publishing Group), Wellingborough.

Gombrich, R. and Obeyesekere, G. (1988) *Buddhism Transformed: Religious Change in Sri Lanka*. Princeton University Press, Princeton, NJ.

Goring, R. (1995 [1992 as *The Chambers Dictionary of Beliefs and Religions*]) *The Wordsworth Dictionary of Beliefs and Religions*. Wordsworth Reference, Ware, Hertfordshire.

Gould, R. F. (1920 [1882–87, 2 vols]) *A Concise History of Freemasonry* (Abridged, revised, rewritten and updated edn). Gala & Polder, London.

Gregory, R. L. (ed.) (1987) *The Oxford Companion to the Mind*. Oxford University Press, Oxford.

Grimes, J. (1996 [1989]) *A Concise Dictionary of Indian Philosophy: Sanskrit Terms Defined in English* (new and revised edn). State University of New York Press, Albany, NY.

Gupta, M. (1978 [1907]) *Condensed Gospel of Sri Ramakrishna* (translated by M. Gupta). Sri Ramakrishna Math, Mylapore, Madras.

—— (1984 [1942]) *The Gospel of Sri Ramakrishna* (translated by Swami Nikhilananda). Ramakrishna-Vivekananda Center, NY.

Halbfass, W. (1988 [1981 in German]) *India and Europe: An Essay in Understanding*. State University of New York Press, Albany, NY.

Hanegraaff, W. J. (1995) "Empirical Method in the Study of Esotericism", *Method & Theory In the Study of Religion*, 7, 2: 99–129.

—— (1996) *New Age Religion and Western Culture: Esotericism in the Mirror of Secular Thought*. Brill, Leiden.

Hardy, F. (1984) "How 'Indian' are the New Indian Religions in the West?", *Religion Today*, 1, 2–3: 15–18.

—— (ed.) (1990 [1988]) *The Religions of Asia*. Routledge, London.

Harthan, B. (1977) "London Branch, The BKS Iyengar Yoga Insti-

tute", *B. K. S. Iyengar Yoga Teachers' Association & Associates Newsletter*, 1: 9.
—— (1985) "The First Anniversary of the Institute", *Dīpikā, London Iyengar Yoga Institute*, 13, Autumn: 14–16.
—— (1987) "In Defence of Iyengar", *Yoga Today*, 12, 6: 37.
Hasselle-Newcombe, S. (2002) "Yoga in Contemporary Britain: A Preliminary Sociological Exploration", unpublished MSc dissertation, London School of Economics and Political Science.
Hastings, W. (1785) "To Nathaniel Smith, Esq.", in *The Bhagavat-Geeta* (translated by C. Wilkins). C. Nourse, London.
Hay, S. (ed.) (1988) *Sources of Indian Tradition. Volume Two: Modern India and Pakistan* (2nd edn). Columbia University Press, New York.
Health Education Authority (1990) *Exercise, Why Bother?* Health Education Authority, London.
—— (1995) *Becoming More Active*. Health Education Authority, London.
Heelas, P. (1996) *The New Age Movement: The Celebration of the Self and the Sacralization of Modernity*. Blackwell, Oxford.
Helman, C. G. (1994 [1984]) *Culture, Health and Illness* (3rd edn). Butterworth-Heinemann, Oxford.
His Eastern and Western Disciples (2000 [1912]) *The Life of Swami Vivekananda*. 2 Vols (6th edn, 4th reprint). Advaita Ashrama, Calcutta.
Honderich, T. (ed.) (1995) *The Oxford Companion to Philosophy*. Oxford University Press, Oxford.
Horwell, V. (1998) "First time here?", *The Guardian Travel, The Guardian*, London, 29 August: 12.
Hume, R. E. (1991 [1877]) *The Thirteen Principal Upanishads* (2nd edn). Oxford University Press, Delhi.
Indrananada, S. (2000) "Yoga, a Perennial Science", *The Hindu Today: Newsletter of the National Council of Hindu Temples (UK)*, 7: 2.
Inglis, B. (1980 [1979]) *Natural Medicine*. Book Club Associates, London.
Iyangar, S. (1994 [1972 reprint of 2nd edn, thoroughly revised; 1893 first edn]) *The Haṭayogapradīpikā of Svātmārāma, with the Commentary Jyotsnā of Brahmānanda and English Translation*. The Adyar Library and Research Centre, Madras.

Iyengar, B.K.S. (1983 [1981]) *Light on Prāṇāyāma: Prāṇāyāma Dīpikā*. Unwin Paperbacks, London.
—— (1984 [1966]) *Light on Yoga: Yoga Dipika*. Unwin Paperbacks, London.
—— (1988) *Yoga Vṛkṣa: The Tree of Yoga*. Fine Line Books, Oxford.
—— (1993) *Light on the Yoga Sūtras of Patañjali: Patañjala Yoga Pradīpikā*. The Aquarian Press, London.
—— (1993 [1985]) *The Art of Yoga*. Indus, New Delhi.
—— (2001) *Yoga, the Path to Holistic Health*. Dorling Kindersley, London.
Iyengar Yoga Institute (1988) "Institute Teaching Policy", *Dīpikā*, 17, Summer: 16–17.
Iyengar Yoga News, The Joint Magazine of LOYA (UK) and BKSIYTA (2002) "Guruji Honoured by the Indian Government", (UK) 1, Spring.
Jackson, C. T. (1975) "The New Thought Movement and the Nineteenth Century Discovery of Oriental Philosophy", *Journal of Popular Culture*, 9: 523–48.
—— (1994) *Vedanta for the West: The Ramakrishna Movement in the United States*. Indiana University Press, Bloomington, IN.
Judge, W. Q. (1889) *The Yoga Aphorisms of Patanjali*. The Path, New York.
—— (1980) *Echoes of the Orient: The Writings of William Quan Judge* (compiled by D. Eklund). Point Loma Publications, Inc., San Diego, CA.
Karambelkar, P. V. (n.d.) *Patanjala Yoga Sutras*. Kaivalyadhama, Lonavla, Maharashtra.
Kent, H. (1993) "Yogis of the World Unite!", *Yoga Life*, 24, 9: 14–17.
Killingley, D. H. (1977) "Rammohun Roy's Interpretation of the Vedānta", unpublished PhD thesis, SOAS, University of London.
—— (1993) *Rammohun Roy in Hindu and Christian Tradition: The Teape Lectures 1990*. Grevatt & Grevatt, Newcastle upon Tyne.
King, U. (1978) "Indian Spirituality, Western Materialism: An Image and its Function in the Reinterpretation of Modern Hinduism", *Social Action*, 28, 1: 62–86.
—— (1980) "Who is the Ideal Karmayogin: the Meaning of a Hindu Religious Symbol", *Religion*, 10, Spring: 41–59.

King, M., Stanley, G. and Burrows, G. (1987) *Stress: Theory and Practice*. Grune & Stratton, Inc., Sydney.

King, R. (1999) *Orientalism and Religion: Postcolonial Theory, India and "the Mystic East"*. Routledge, London.

Klostermaier, K. K. (1989) *A Survey of Hinduism*. State University of New York Press, Albany, NY.

Kopf, D. (1969) *British Orientalism and the Bengal Renaissance*. University of California Press, Berkeley, CA.

—— (1979) *The Brahmo Samaj and the Shaping of the Modern Indian Mind*. Princeton University Press, Princeton, NJ.

Kripal, J. J. (1995) *Kali's Child: The Mystical and the Erotic in the Life and Teachings of Ramakrishna*. University of Chicago Press, Chicago, IL.

Lasater, J. (1995) *Relax and Renew*. Rodmell Press, Berkeley, CA.

Lavan, S. (1984 [1977]) *Unitarians and India: A Study in Encounter and Response* (2nd edn). Skinner House, Boston, MA.

—— (1995 [1981]) "The Brahmo Samaj: India's First Modern Movement for Religious Reform", in R. D. Baird (ed.), *Religion in Modern India*. Manohar, New Delhi, pp. 1–25.

Lester, R. C. (1976) *Rāmānuja on the Yoga*. The Adyar Library and Research Centre, Madras.

Lipner, J. J. (1998) "A Meeting of Ends? Swami Vivekananda and Brahmabandhab Upadhyay", in W. Radice (ed.), *Swami Vivekananda and the Modernization of Hinduism*. Oxford University Press, Delhi, pp. 61–76.

Lozier, F. (1994) *Working Plans of Iyengar Yoga Props Used at the Ramamani Iyengar Memorial Yoga Institute, Pune, India*. Privately published pamphlet, Toronto.

Manor, J. (1977) *Political Change in an Indian State: Mysore 1917–1955*. Manohar, New Delhi.

Marshall, P. J. (1970) *The British Discovery of Hinduism in the Eighteenth Century*. Cambridge University Press, Cambridge.

Masson, J. (1994 [1993]) *My Father's Guru: A Journey through Spirituality and Disillusion*. HarperCollins, London.

McGuire, M. B. (1985) "Religion and Healing", in P. E. Hammond (ed.), *The Sacred in a Secular Age: Towards Revision in the Scientific Study of Religion*. University of California Press, Berkeley, CA, pp. 268–84.

Mehta, S., Mehta, M. and Mehta, S. (1990) *Yoga: The Iyengar Way*. Dorling Kindersley, London.

Mehta, G. (1993 [1979]) *Karma Cola: Marketing the Mystic East.* Penguin Books India, New Delhi.

Melton, J. G. (1991) *New Age Almanac.* Visible Ink Press, Detroit, MI.

Michaël, T. (1980 [1975 as *Clefs pour le Yoga*]) *Introduction aux Voies de Yoga.* Editions du Rocher, Monte Carlo.

Mill, J. (1997 [1817, 3 vols]) *The History of British India, With Notes and Continuation by Horace Hayman Wilson* (Facsimile of 1858 edn. London, Madden). Routledge/Thoemmes, London.

Miller, B. Stoler (1996) *Yoga, Discipline of Freedom: The* Yoga Sutra *Attributed to Patanjali.* University of California Press, Berkeley, CA.

Mishra, R. S. (1973 [1963]) *Yoga Sutras: The Textbook of Yoga Psychology.* Anchor Press, Garden City, NY.

Monier-Williams, M. (1994 [1899]) *Sanskrit English Dictionary* (new enlarged and improved edn). Munshiram Manoharlal, New Delhi.

Mukherjee, S. N. (1968) *Sir William Jones: A Study in Eighteenth-Century British Attitudes to India.* Cambridge University Press, Cambridge.

Naidu, G. R. (1895) *A Short History of the Brahmo Samaj.* Chengalroya Naicker's Orphanage Press, Madras.

Neevel, W. G. (1976) "The Transformation of Śrī Rāmakrishna", in B. L. Smith (ed.), *Hinduism: New Essays in the History of Religion.* Brill, Leiden, pp. 51–97.

Nikhilananda, S. (1984 [1942]) "Introduction", in M. Gupta, *The Gospel of Sri Ramakrishna* (translated by Swami Nikhilananda). Ramakrishna-Vivekananda Center, New York, pp. 3–73.

O'Malley, L. S. S. (ed.) (1968 [1941]) *Modern India and the West.* Oxford University Press, London.

Olivelle, P. (1998) *The Early Upaniṣads: Annotated Text and Translation.* Oxford University Press, New York.

Osborne, A. (1994 [1954]) *Ramana Maharshi and the Path of Self-Knowledge.* Jaico, Bombay.

Patañjali (1904) *Pātañjalayogasūtrāṇi.* Ānandāśrama, Puṇyākhya-pattana.

Paul, N. C. (1888 [1850]) *A Treatise on the Yoga Philosophy.* Tukaram Tatya, Bombay.

Perez-Christiaens, N. (1976) *B. K. S. Iyengar: Un mystique hindou ivre de Dieu.* Institut de yoga B. K. S. Iyengar, Paris.

Philosophico Literary Research Dept. of Kaivalyadhama SMYM

Samiti (1991 [1972]) *Yoga Kośa: Yoga Terms Explained with Reference to Context* (new enlarged edn). Kaivalyadhama SMYM Samiti, Lonavla, Pune.

Pillai, B. P. (1986 [1979]) *Yoga: A Way of Life*. P. Indirabai, Kerala.

Prabhavananda, S. and Isherwood, C. (1953) *How to Know God: The Yoga Aphorisms of Patanjali*. Allen & Unwin, London.

Ramamani Iyengar Memorial Yoga Institute (1992) *Know Your Institute*. Ramamani Iyengar Memorial Yoga Institute, Pune.

Rambachan, A. (1994) *The Limits of Scripture: Vivekananda's Reinterpretation of the Vedas*. University of Hawaii Press, Honolulu.

Reese, W. L. (1996) *Dictionary of Philosophy and Religion: Eastern and Western Thought* (2nd enlarged edn). Humanities Press, Atlantic Highlands, NJ.

Robertson, B. C. (1995) *Raja Rammohan Roy: The Father of Modern India*. Oxford University Press, Delhi.

Rocher, R. (1983) *Orientalism, Poetry and the Millennium: The Checkered Life of Nathaniel Brassey Halhed, 1751–1830*. Motilal Banarsidass, Delhi.

Rolland, R. (1966 [1930]) *La vie de Vivekānanda et l'évangile universel*. Stock, Paris. Translated from the French as: *The Life of Vivekananda and the Universal Gospel* (1984), Advaita Ashrama, Calcutta.

Roszak, T. (1995 [1969]) *The Making of a Counter Culture: Reflections on the Technocratic Society and its Youthful Opposition*. University of California Press, Berkeley, CA.

Rycroft, C. (1971) *Reich*. Fontana/Collins, London.

Said, E. (1978) *Orientalism*. Pantheon, New York.

Sastri, S. N. (1911) *History of the Brahmo Samaj*. R. Chatterji, Calcutta.

Schatz, M. P. (1992) *Back Care Basics: A Doctor's Gentle Yoga Program for Back and Neck Pain Relief*. Rodmell Press, Berkeley, CA.

Schwab, R. (1984 [1950 in French]) *The Oriental Renaissance: Europe's Rediscovery of India and the East, 1680–1880*. Columbia University Press, New York.

Selye, H. (1957 [1956]) *The Stress of Life*. Longmans, Green & Co., London.

Sen, K. C. (1885) *Yoga or Communion with God*. The Brahmo Tract Society, Calcutta.

—— (1901) *Lectures in India I.* Cassell, London.
—— (1904) *Lectures in India II.* Cassell, London.
Sen, P. K. (1938) *Keshub Chunder Sen.* Keshub's Birth Centenary Committee, Calcutta.
Sharf, R. H. (1995) "Buddhist Modernism and the Rhetoric of Meditative Experience", *Numen*, 42: 228–83.
Siegel, L. (1991) *Net of Magic: Wonders and Deceptions in India.* University of Chicago Press, Chicago, IL.
Sil, N. P. (1993) "Vivekānanda's Rāmakṛṣṇa: An untold Story of Mythmaking and Propaganda", *Numen.* 40: 38–62.
—— (1997) *Swami Vivekananda: A Reassessment.* Susquehanna University Press, Selinsgrove, PA.
Sinclair, J. M., general consultant (1999) *Collins English Dictionary.* BCA–HarperCollins–Market House Books Ltd, Aylesbury.
Sivananda Yoga Centre (1993 [1983]) *The Book of Yoga: The Complete Step-by-Step Guide.* Ebury Press, London.
Sjoman, N. E. (1996) *The Yoga Tradition of the Mysore Palace.* Abhinav Publications, New Delhi.
Slade, H. E. W. (1973) *Meeting Schools of Oriental Meditation.* Lutterworth Educational, Guildford and London.
Slater, T. E. (1884) *Keshab Chandra Sen and the Brahma Samaj.* Society for Promoting Christian Knowledge, Madras.
Smart, N. (1982) "Asian Cultures and the Impact of the West: India and China", in E. Barker (ed.), *New Religious Movements: A Perspective for Understanding Society.* Edwin Mellen Press, New York, pp. 140–54.
—— (1992 [1989]) *The World's Religions.* Cambridge University Press, Cambridge.
Smith, B. and Boudreau, L. (1986 [1981]) *Yoga for a New Age: A Modern Approach to Hatha Yoga.* Smith Productions, Seattle.
Stewart, M. (1995) *Yoga Over 50.* Little, Brown & Co., Boston, MA.
Stewart, M. and Phillips, K. (1992) *Yoga for Children.* Vermillion, London.
Stirk, J. (1988) *Structural Fitness.* Elm Tree Books, London.
Strauss, S. (1997) "Re-Orienting Yoga: Transnational Flows from an Indian Center", PhD thesis, University of Pennsylvania.
—— (2000) "Locating Yoga: Ethnography and Transnational Practice", in V. Amit (ed.), *Constructing the Field.* Routledge, New York, pp. 162–94.
—— (2002a) "Swamiji: A Life in Yoga", in L. Walbridge and A.

Sievert (eds) *Personal Encounters in Anthropology: An Introductory Reader*. McGraw-Hill Publishing Co., New York, pp. 180–4.

—— (2002b) "The Master's Narrative: Swami Sivananda and the Transnational Production of Yoga", *Journal of Folklore Research*, 39, 2/3: 217–41.

—— (2003) "'Adapt, Adjust, Accommodate:' The Production of Yoga in a Transnational World", *History and Anthropology*, 13, 3: 231–51.

Sweetman, W. (forthcoming) *Mapping Hinduism: 'Hinduism' and the Study of Indian Religions 1600–1776*. Verlag der Franckesche Stiftungen zu Halle, Halle.

Sykes, M. (1997) *An Indian Tapestry* (revised edn). William Sessions Ltd, York.

Tagore, D. (1909) *The Autobiography of Maharshi Devendranath Tagore*. S. K. Lahiri & Co., Calcutta.

Tagore, S. (1909) "Introduction", in D. Tagore (ed.), *The Autobiography of Maharshi Devendranath Tagore*. S. K. Lahiri & Co., Calcutta, pp. i–xxiv.

Taylor, K. (1996) "Arthur Avalon: The Creation of a Legendary Orientalist", in J. Leslie (ed.), *Myth and Myth Making*. Curzon, Richmond, Surrey, pp. 144–64.

Teich, M. and Porter, R. (eds) (1990) *Fin de Siecle and Its Legacy*. Cambridge University Press, Cambridge.

Thomas, T. (1988) "East Comes West", in T. Thomas (ed.), *The British: Their Religious Beliefs and Practices, 1800–1986*. London, Routledge, pp. 72–100.

Tilak, B. G. (1935 [1915]) *The Hindu Philosophy of Life, Ethics and Religion:* Om-tat-sat Śrīmad Bhagavadgītā Rahasya *or* Karma-yoga-śāstra. *Including an external examination of the* Gītā, *the Original Sanskrit Stanzas, their English Translation, Commentaries on the Stanzas, and a Comparison of Eastern and Western Doctrines, etc.* Translated from the Marathi by Bhalchandra Sitaram Sukthankar. R. B. Tilak, Poona.

Troeltsch, E. (1931) *The Social Teachings of the Christian Churches*. Macmillian, New York.

Turner, V. W. (1982 [1969]) *The Ritual Process: Structure and Anti-Structure*. Cornell University Press, Ithaca, NY.

van Gennep, A. (1965 [1908 in French]) *The Rites of Passage*. Routledge & Kegan Paul, London.

Versluis, A. (1993) *American Transcendentalism and Asian Religions*. Oxford University Press, New York.

Viniyoga Editors (1989) "Principaux ouvrages de Shri T. Krishnamacharya". *Viniyoga*, 24: 94.

Vishnudevananda, S. (1988 [1960]) *The Complete Illustrated Book of Yoga*. Harmony Books, New York.

Vivekananda, S. (1896) *Rāja Yoga: Conquering the Internal Nature*. Longmans, Green, and Co., London.

—— (1907–97) *The Complete Works*. [Years of publication consulted: Vol. 1, 1907, Vol. 2, 1995, Vol. 3, 1984, Vol. 4, 1995, Vol. 5, 1995, Vol. 6, 1995, Vol. 7, 1996, Vol. 8, 1985, Vol. 9, 1997.] Advaita Ashrama, Calcutta.

—— (1994 [1896]) *Rāja Yoga: Conquering the Internal Nature*. Advaita Ashrama, Calcutta.

—— (1995 [1896]) "Rāja Yoga", in S. Vivekananda (ed.), *The Complete Works of Swami Vivekananda*, Vol. 1. Advaita Ashrama, Calcutta, pp. 119–314.

Walker, P. M. B. (ed.) (1997 [1995]) *Larousse Dictionary of Science and Technology*. Larousse, Edinburgh.

Ward, R. (1994) "LOYA (UK) and the BKSIYTA – Time for an Arranged Marriage?" *LOYA News, The Magazine of the Light on Yoga Association (UK)*, 17: 8–10.

Warrier, M. (2000) "Hindu Conceptions of Self: Reconciling the Real and the Ideal in the Mata Amritanandamayi Mission", unpublished paper based on PhD thesis submitted at the University of Cambridge, 2000, under the title *The Appeal of Modern God-persons in Contemporary India: The Case of Mata Amritanandamayi and her Mission*.

Waters, M. (1996) *Dictionary of Personal Development: An A–Z of the Most Widely-used Terms, Theories and Concepts*. Element, Shaftesbury, Dorset.

White, D. G. (1996) *The Alchemical Body: Siddha Traditions in Medieval India*. University of Chicago Press, Chicago, IL.

Whitmarsh, K. (1989) *Concordance to the Gospel of Sri Ramakrishna: Based on the Translation of the Gospel by Swami Nikhilananda* (revised edn). Vedanta Press, Los Angeles, CA.

Williams, G. M. (1974) *Quest for Meaning of Svāmi Vivekananda*. New Horizons Press, Chico, CA.

—— (1995a [1981]) "The Ramakrishna Movement: A Study in

Religious Change", in R. D. Baird (ed.), *Religion in Modern India*. Manohar, New Delhi, pp. 55–85.
—— (1995b [1981]) "Svami Vivekananda", in R. D. Baird (ed.), *Religion in Modern India*. Manohar, New Delhi, pp. 372–401.
Wilson, B. (1979 [1976]) *Contemporary Transformations of Religion*. Clarendon Press, Oxford.
—— (1988) "'Secularisation': Religion in the Modern World", in S. Sutherland, L. Houlden, P. Clarke and F. Hardy (eds), *The World's Religions*. Routledge, London, pp. 953–66.
Wood, E. (1982 [1959]) *Yoga* (revised edn). Penguin, Harmondsworth.
Woods, J. H. (1992 [1914]) *The Yoga-System of Patañjali*. Motilal Banarsidass, Delhi.
Yardi, M. R. (1979) *The Yoga of Patañjali*. Bhandarkar, Pune.
Yogacharya B. K. S. Iyengar's 70th Birthday Celebrations (1990) *70 Glorious Years of Yogacharya B. K. S. Iyengar: Commemoration Volume*. Light on Yoga Research Trust, Bombay.
Yoga Journal Editors (1994) "Guess Who's Coming to Yoga?", *Yoga Journal*, 118: 47–8.
Yogananda, P. (1950 [1946]) *Autobiography of a Yogi*. Rider, London.
Young, A. (1982) "The Anthropologies of Illness and Sickness", *Annual Review of Anthropology*, 11: 257–85.

Index